Interviewing Children and Adolescents

Interviewing Children and Adolescents

*Skills and Strategies
for Effective DSM-IV Diagnosis*

James Morrison
and
Thomas F. Anders

The Guilford Press
New York / London

© 1999 The Guilford Press; revisions © 2001
A Division of Guilford Publications, Inc.
72 Spring Street, New York, NY 10012
www.guilford.com

Printed in the United States of America

This book is printed on acid-free paper.

Last digit is print number: 9 8 7 6 5 4

Library of Congress Cataloging-in-Publication Data

Morrison, James R., 1940–
    Interviewing children and adolescents : skills and strategies for
effective DSM–IV diagnosis / James Morrison, Thomas F. Anders.
        p. cm.
    Includes bibliographical references and index.
    ISBN 1-57230-501-0 (hard. : alk. Paper) ISBN 1-57230-717-X (pbk.)
    1. Interviewing in child psychiatry. 2. Interviewing in
adolescent psychiatry. 3. Mental illness—Diagnosis. I. Anders,
T. F. (Thomas F.) II. Title.
    [DNLM: 1. Mental Disorders—diagnosis—Adolescence. 2. Mental
Disorders—diagnosis—Child. 3. Interview, Psychological—
Adolescence. 4. Interview, Psychological—Child. 5. Interviews—
methods. WS 350 M879i 1999]
RJ503.6.M67 1999
618.92′89075—dc21
DNLM/DLC   99-43058
for Library of Congress   CIP

DSM-IV is a trademark of the American Psychiatric Association.

For Eric, a chip off the old step-block.

—J. M.

To my family, Connie, Michael, Geoff, and Max, for their loving support; to Judith Williams, PhD, and Susan McDonough, PhD, who helped in teaching "Talking with Children" and inspired me; and to the children and their families who really taught me.

—T. F. A.

About the Authors

James Morrison, MD, received his medical and psychiatric training at Washington University in St. Louis, Missouri. He has spent his career providing psychiatric care and writing on mental health issues and is the author of *The First Interview, DSM-IV Made Easy,* and *When Psychological Problems Mask Medical Disorders.* Dr. Morrison is currently Chief of Staff at the Department of Veterans Affairs Medical Center in Coatesville, Pennsylvania, and Clinical Professor of Psychiatry at Temple University, Philadelphia.

Thomas F. Anders, MD, received his medical training at Stanford University, Stanford, California, and his psychiatric and psychoanalytic training at Columbia University, New York, New York. He has chaired the divisions of child psychiatry at Stanford University and Brown University (Providence, Rhode Island) and the Department of Psychiatry at the University of California at Davis. Currently Associate Dean for Academic Affairs in the U.C. Davis School of Medicine, Dr. Anders has long pursued his research interests in pediatric sleep disorders and infant sleep–wake state development.

Acknowledgments

We express our appreciation to Emily Harris, MD, and Thomas Morrison, PhD, for their assistance with this material. Mary Morrison provided valuable criticism at various stages throughout the project. Our editor, Kitty Moore, and copyeditor, Marie Sprayberry, have given their usual all. We also acknowledge the assistance of Anna Brackett and Karen Stroker, as well as many others at The Guilford Press whose efforts made this book possible.

List of Abbreviations

ADHD	Attention-Deficit/Hyperactivity Disorder
ASD	Acute Stress Disorder
CDD	Childhood Disintegrative Disorder
CGAS	Children's Global Assessment Scale
CM	cytomegalovirus
CT	Computerized tomography ("cat scan")
DCD	Developmental Coordination Disorder
DSM	*Diagnostic and Statistical Manual of Mental Disorders*
EEG	Electroencephalogram
ELD	Expressive Language Disorder
EMG	electromyogram
GAD	Generalized Anxiety Disorder
GAF	Global Assessment of Functioning
GID	Gender Identity Disorder
GMC	general medical condition
HIV	human immunovirus
LSD	lysergic acid diethylamide
MDMA	methylenedioxymethamphetamine ("ecstasy")
MRELD	Mixed Receptive–Expressive Language Disorder
MRI	magnetic resonance imaging
MSE	mental status examination
NOS	not otherwise specified
OAD	Overanxious Disorder of Childhood
OCD	Obsessive–Compulsive Disorder

ODD	Oppositional Defiant Disorder
OSAS	Obstructive Sleep Apnea Syndrome
PCP	phencyclidine
PD	Perceptual Disturbance
PDD	Pervasive Developmental Disorder
PTSD	Posttraumatic Stress Disorder
RAD	Reactive Attachment Disorder
REM	rapid eye movement
SAD	Separation Anxiety Disorder
SMD	Stereotypic Movement Disorder
WISC	Wechsler Intelligence Scale for Children

Contents

Appendices

Introduction

By some estimates, just over 20% of all children and adolescents in the United States (more than 2 million) have a diagnosable mental disorder. Many of these are serious; that is, they cause significant distress or interfere with a child's or adolescent's ability to study or to relate to family or friends. Although some young people referred for mental health evaluation do not require treatment, hardly any referral we can imagine should be regarded as trivial. Nearly all referred children or adolescents will have worried someone, sometime. This thought underscores the importance of obtaining all the information relevant to the accurate diagnosis of each child or adolescent who comes to a mental health professional. At present there are far too few well-trained mental health professionals to evaluate more than a small fraction of all these potential patients.

Obtaining clinical information from young people, especially children under the age of 12, requires special technical skills and clinical experience in interviewing that are different from those necessary for interviewing adults.

1. In some cases, parents seek help for their child when the real problem is with them—marital conflicts, personal mental disorder, or the like. Diagnostically, parental and family disorders are beyond the scope of this book, but a mental health professional who treats children and adolescents must be alert to all of the possible causes of a patient's troubles.

2. Children's vocabularies are relatively limited, and their perspectives are somewhat more circumscribed than those of adults. Younger children have not yet begun to think in abstract terms; their thought processes tend to be concrete. It requires considerable interviewer sensitivity to use developmentally appropriate terms that are understandable to a young child without sounding condescending.

3. There is a danger that any patient may not reveal all the diagnostic information necessary, but a child patient especially may not realize the importance of forthright communication in a clinical evaluation.
4. Even a child who *can* be made to understand its importance may not realize what information is necessary to achieve full disclosure.
5. The stages of human development add complexity (and interest) to interviewing and the diagnostic process. A fundamental knowledge of development is essential for clinicians working with juveniles.
6. Flexibility and a sense of youthful playfulness are especially important capacities for mental health professionals who work with children and adolescents.

Talking *with* children and adolescents needs to be distinguished from talking *to* and *about* them. Parents[1] can talk to mental health professionals or teachers about their children. Parents and teachers also talk with young people. But most adults have goals that are different from those of the mental health professional who engages a child or adolescent in an evaluation. In this book, we focus on methods of talking with children and adolescents to elicit clinically relevant information. The methods necessarily vary according to the age and developmental stage of a young patient.

We view interview technique and mental diagnosis for children and adolescents as mutually interdependent. That is why we present them together in a single volume. To us, it seems hard to write about one without covering the other. In the first part of this book, we discuss the mental health interview as it applies to young people and their families; in the second, we describe the science (and art) of diagnosis.

PART I. INTERVIEWING CHILDREN AND ADOLESCENTS

Especially in the field of child and adolescent mental health, information should be gathered from multiple sources whenever possible, including the school. Because their broader experience and training provide them with a better opportunity to make comparisons, and because their self-esteem is usu-

---

[1]Throughout this book, we intend the term *parents* to include biological and adoptive parents, legal guardians, and "significant others"—in short, anyone who acts as a primary caregiver to a child or adolescent.

ally not at stake in the same way as that of parents, teachers may report certain childhood skills and behaviors more objectively than parents may. Bear in mind, however, that teachers also may be less involved personally with young people, are often overburdened by large class size and inadequate support, and may overgeneralize, using labels to facilitate the removal of boisterous children or obstreperous adolescents from the classroom. Some recommend medication to control behavior when a child's or adolescent's disruptiveness may actually be a response to stresses that originate *within* the classroom. A clinician must become adept at balancing all views and sources of information, using clinical and developmental judgment to establish a diagnosis that is in the best interest of a young person.

Certain general principles do seem universal to all successful approaches to interviewing techniques. They include listening carefully, directing conversation, establishing rapport, and following up on important clues. The most scholarly presentation of these principles has been that of Cox and colleagues, who in the 1980s published a series of studies based on interviews with parents whose children had been brought for evaluation. The principles they derived apply to nearly every patient, relative, friend or other informant encountered by a mental health professional. (See Appendix 1 for a reference to Cox et al.'s work.)

We hasten to point out that Part I is not intended as a textbook on interviewing. Rather, we present some of the methods commonly used to obtain information from patients and informants to make a diagnosis. Chapter 1 reviews material pertinent to any mental health interview. Chapter 2 discusses the steps needed to establish a relationship with a young mental health patient. Chapter 3 presents developmental information relevant to the initial interview, as well as a table of developmental milestones.

To demonstrate the principles of interviewing, the remainder of Part I comprises transcriptions of portions of actual interviews. In Chapter 4, we present something that has become much discussed and used in the past few years—an "infant/toddler interview," which is actually an interview with a mother while the clinician interacts with the infant or toddler. Chapters 5–7 contain interviews that demonstrate a variety of techniques useful for latency-age children: toys, drawing, and dolls. As you will note, clinicians often use all three modalities in a single interview. Chapter 8, containing an interview with a teenager, demonstrates many of the same interview techniques that apply to an adult patient. Chapter 9 presents an annotated initial interview with a mother and son that demonstrates the basics of conducting a family interview.

Because we believe that learning occurs best when it is illustrated by concrete examples, we rely throughout on verbatim transcriptions of actual patient interviews. These we have annotated with discussions of our impressions of the interviewers' goals, methods, and effectiveness, as well as with descriptions of other material that might be sought (or at least considered) in similar interviewing circumstances. We have not attempted to cover both sexes at every age. Although young patients of varying ages (and developmental stages) will inevitably require modifications and adaptations, the basic techniques remain much the same.

Finally, in Chapter 10, we discuss the written report. We cover formulation, in which we show how all the information gathered from records, informants, and the patient is brought together to create a clear statement of the problem; a list of most likely diagnoses (the differential diagnosis); and a working plan for further evaluation and treatment.

PART II. DSM-IV DIAGNOSES APPLICABLE TO CHILDREN AND ADOLESCENTS

In the second part of this volume, we present all of the mental diagnoses that are usually first made during childhood or adolescence, plus those from other sections of the American Psychiatric Association's *Diagnostic and Statistical Manual of Mental Disorders,* fourth edition (DSM-IV) that are often applied to young persons. We cover this material in several ways:

- At the beginning of each chapter, we include a Quick Guide that contains the necessary information for a rapid scan of the possible diagnoses, including those in other sections of DSM-IV.
- We present some of the basic information that mental health professionals need to know about the presentation, demographics, and possible causes of the disorders.
- We have rewritten the DSM-IV criteria for clarity and brevity, and we present these rewritten criteria in table form. In some cases (such as the substance-related disorders), we have condensed much diagnostic material about several disorders into a few tables that readers can consult at a glance, rather than flipping back and forth among many sections of the book. We have especially tried to do this when two or more criteria sets contain many items in common; we believe that this condensed format facilitates comparison and learning.

- For many diagnoses, we illustrate the symptoms with a clinical vignette.
- Following each vignette, a case discussion explains how the criteria are applied and presents the differential diagnosis.
- Each patient's diagnosis is written up in traditional DSM-IV five-axis format, complete with the appropriate code numbers and descriptive material.
- For each major diagnostic category, a special section addresses the problems and techniques of interviewing for the specific diagnoses. To help integrate the material from Parts I and II, age-specific interviewing skills and developmentally relevant diagnostic information are presented in these special sections. Whenever possible, we include material on differences in presentation that can be expected at various developmental stages. But note that the ages mentioned here are not set in stone; children can progress and mature at vastly different rates and still be normal.

Using the DSM-IV Multiaxial Classification

DSM-IV gets the most information into a compact space by using five coding areas (each is called an *axis*) on which to record information about the patient. The first three axes record the mental and physical diagnoses that apply to the patient; the clinician can use the others to note environmental or psychosocial problems and to assign a number that represents that patient's functioning during the previous year.

Axis I: Mental Disorders

On the line (or lines) for Axis I, record nearly every mental disorder that can be applied to a patient. Most children and adolescents referred for evaluation will have at least one Axis I diagnosis, and some will have two or more. Sometimes these diagnoses will be more or less independent; at other times they will interact with one another. When you are making multiple diagnoses, record one above the other; later, a number will be assigned to each Axis I disorder.

When a hospitalized patient has more than one diagnosis, the one that is felt to be mainly responsible for the admission is termed the *principal diagnosis*. This judgment is indicated by placing this diagnosis at the top of the list for Axis I. When an outpatient has multiple diagnoses, the one most responsible for occasioning that episode of care (and the one listed first) is termed the *reason for visit*.

Criteria. Once shorn of some excess verbiage, DSM-IV criteria are straight-forward and logical. The tables in this book presenting rewritten DSM-IV criteria sets include two types of individual criteria: mandatory and selective. Each mandatory criterion—in this text, marked with a bullet (•)—must be fulfilled for the patient to receive the diagnosis. The selective criteria—indicated by a check mark (✓)—are part of a list; only a certain number of these need be present. Besides the lists of symptoms, DSM-IV typically uses certain "boilerplate" criteria to help circumscribe the population addressed:

- Duration: for example, 6 months (as in Oppositional Defiant Disorder), 1 month (Pica).
- Age limits: for example, must begin prior to age 18 (as in Separation Anxiety Disorder or Mental Retardation), or after at least 2 years of normal development (as in Childhood Disintegrative Disorder).
- Statement of disability: for example, hinders educational or occupational achievement or social functioning (as in Stuttering, among many others) or causes distress (Enuresis). (Note, however, that stress or suffering by itself is never synonymous with mental disorder.)
- Exclusion of general medical conditions, as in Rumination Disorder and Chronic Motor or Vocal Tic Disorder.
- Exclusion of substance use disorders, as in Encopresis and Transient Tic Disorder.
- Exclusion of other mental disorders, as in Stereotypic Movement Disorder, where you must rule out the compulsions of Obsessive–Compulsive Disorder.

Severity. The criteria for some disorders automatically assign ratings of severity—Mental Retardation, Conduct Disorder, some mood disorders, and some substance-related disorders are examples. However, you may want to indicate the severity of the condition for other diagnoses. You can specify severity for *any* Axis I or Axis II disorder, using these generic guidelines:

Mild. The patient has few symptoms other than those necessary to fulfill the minimum criteria.

Moderate. This category is intermediate between Mild and Severe.

Severe. One or more of the following apply: The patient has many more symptoms than are needed to meet minimum criteria for diagnosis; or some of the symptoms (such as suicide attempts) are especially severe; or functioning at school or work, or in the family or with friends, is severely affected.

In Partial Remission. The patient has previously met full diagnostic criteria, some of which may remain but do not currently fulfill criteria.

In Full Remission. The patient has been free of symptoms for a period of time that seems clinically relevant to the diagnosis.

Prior History. Although the patient appears to have recovered from the disorder, you feel it is important to mention it.

Here is an example of an Axis I listing:

| Axis I | 312.8 | Conduct Disorder, Childhood-Onset Type, Severe |
| | 315.00 | Reading Disorder, Moderate |

Axis II: Mental Retardation and Personality Disorders

Its predecessors used Axis II to list a number of childhood disorders, but DSM-IV lists only Mental Retardation there. (The personality disorders are also listed on Axis II, but they are rarely applied to young people.) When an Axis II diagnosis is the main reason for the evaluation, but there is also an Axis I diagnosis, indicate the fact by including "(Principal Diagnosis)" after the Axis II diagnosis:

| Axis I | 315.31 | Expressive Language Disorder |
| Axis II | 317 | Mild Mental Retardation (Principal Diagnosis) |

Axis III: Physical Conditions and Disorders

On Axis III you can include any medical conditions that have a direct bearing on the Axis I or II diagnosis, or that may affect (or be affected by) the management of these mental disorders. In some cases, multiple Axis III diagnoses may be indicated.

Axis IV: Psychosocial and Environmental Problems

You should mention on Axis IV any environmental or psychosocial stresses or conditions that can affect diagnosis or management. Whether these are independent events or are caused by an Axis I or II disorder, they must have occurred within the year prior to the present evaluation. If they occurred earlier, they must have contributed to the development of the mental disorder or must be a focus of treatment. They should be listed on Axis IV as specifically as possible—you don't have to use the exact wording suggested. Here are some samples (many others are possible):

> **Economic Problems.** Poverty; inadequate public assistance or child support (these only affect children indirectly).
>
> **Housing Problems.** Homelessness; poor housing; dangerous neighborhood; move to a new house or school.
>
> **Problems with Primary Support Group.** Death of a relative; illness in a relative; family disruption through divorce or separation; remarriage of parent; physical or sexual abuse; disagreements with relatives; death or loss of pet; loss of best friend; change of teacher (from grammar school to junior high school).
>
> **Occupational Problems.** Some occupational problems only affect children indirectly through their effect on the parents; however, adolescents often feel financially disadvantaged compared to friends and have trouble finding gainful employment.
>
> **Educational Problems.** Academic problems; disagreements with classmates or teachers; illiteracy; poor school achievement, failure to make school team, poor grades.
>
> **Problems Related to the Social Environment.** Loss or death of friend; acculturation problems; racial or sexual discrimination; social isolation, loss of peer group.
>
> **Problems Related to Interaction with the Legal System/Crime.** Being arrested; being incarcerated; being a victim of crime.
>
> **Other Psychosocial Problems.** Disagreements with caregiving professionals (counselor, social workers, physician); exposure to war, natural disasters, or other catastrophes; unavailability of social service agencies; child abuse, neglect.
>
> **Problems with Access to Health Care Services.** Inadequate health care services; no or insufficient health insurance; unavailability of transportation to health care services.

Occasionally a psychosocial or environmental problem will be the focus for treatment or evaluation. Then it should be coded on Axis I and given the appropriate V-code number (see Chapter 27):

      Axis I   V62.3   Academic Problem (failing third grade)

Axis V: Assessments of Functioning

The Global Assessment of Functioning (GAF) is scored on a 100-point continuum. The steps from 1 to 90 represent progressively less severe degrees of psychopathology or inadequate functioning; the top 10 points are for functioning that is *better* than you would expect for the average individual. Despite the examples given in the GAF itself, it remains a subjective scale whose greatest utility may be in tracking across time changes in a given patient's level of functioning. The Children's Global Assessment Scale (CGAS) expresses the same concepts in terms relevant to the pediatric age group. Though it is not officially sanctioned by DSM-IV, the CGAS has been evaluated as reliable across time and between raters. We have reproduced the CGAS in Appendix 1. The GAF may be found in DSM-IV or in *DSM-IV Made Easy,* by James Morrison (see Appendix 1 for a reference). Because it is sanctioned by DSM-IV, we will report all Axis V coding in terms of the GAF.

Pointers for Making a Diagnosis

Here are some pointers to keep in mind when you are evaluating patients for a DSM-IV diagnosis.

1. Have you obtained all the data?

   - History of the present illness
   - Personal, familial, and social background
   - Sensitive subjects (substance use, suicide ideas/attempts, violence/ delinquency, physical/sexual abuse)
   - Medical history with review of systems
   - Physical exam (as relevant)
   - Family history (especially mental disorders)
   - Mental status examination
   - Testing

2. Select all possible areas of diagnosis:

More likely	*Less likely*
Mental Retardation	Psychotic disorders
Attention-Deficit/Hyperactivity Disorder	Pervasive developmental disorders
	Eating disorders
Learning disorders	Somatization Disorder

Mood disorders
Elimination disorders
Anxiety disorders
Conduct Disorder
Adjustment Disorder
Substance-related disorders

Tourette's Disorder
Stereotypic Movement Disorder
Separation Anxiety Disorder
Cognitive disorders
Gender Identity Disorder

3. Consult the introductory sections of DSM-IV, or the Quick Guides in the present book, for diagnostic possibilities (differential diagnosis).
4. Be sure to refer to the criteria; relying on memory breeds error. For each possible diagnosis, ask yourself:

   • Are inclusion criteria met?
   • Are exclusion criteria met?
   • Have you considered exclusion criteria?

5. What further information do you need—additional history or background material from informants, more interviews with the patient, time for observation?
6. Is a definitive diagnosis possible? Consider the possible ways of saying, "I'm not sure," expressed here for a patient with depressive symptoms and listed in more or less decreasing order of certainty:

   296.21   Major Depressive Disorder, Single Episode, Mild (Provisional)
   311   Depressive Disorder Not Otherwise Specified[2]
   296.90   Mood Disorder Not Otherwise Specified
   300.9   Unspecified Mental Disorder (nonpsychotic)
   799.9   Diagnosis or Condition Deferred on Axis I

7. Is it possible that a child or adolescent has *no* diagnosis? Consider these possibilities:

   V71.09   No Diagnosis or Condition on Axis I
   V71.09   No Diagnosis on Axis II

DSM-IV as It Applies to Children and Adolescents

Of course, much that we accept today about mental disorders in children and adolescents has been extrapolated from studies of adults. Furthermore, some DSM-IV criteria are based on research done on DSM-III-R diagnoses no longer

[2]But see the sidebar on page 175 for a caution about the use of Not Otherwise Specified diagnoses.

in use. As a result, the reliability of diagnosis in childhood and adolescence lags somewhat behind that in adulthood. This is not to say that we believe the criteria we have today are useless—only that some are based on information less solid than that used for the adult mental disorders. The mere fact of having well-defined (if not always proven) diagnoses provides a starting point for future studies that will eventually produce more reliable criteria.

Here are some additional thoughts about using DSM-IV with children and adolescents:

- DSM-IV is a snapshot in time. Hardly a child or adolescent diagnosis retains its criteria intact from the previous editions; 14% of such diagnoses are new in DSM-IV, suggesting that even now, new mental disorders of young people await description in DSM-V and beyond.

- In some cases, there have been few data-based studies. An example is Reactive Attachment Disorder, where clinical experience supports two subtypes, though the clinical studies are far from plentiful.

- Psychopathology in infants and toddlers, rarely fixed, is often dependent on context. Symptoms and prevalence rates change with age.

- Symptoms can cut across diagnostic boundaries. For example, inattentiveness can be found in Alcohol (and other Substance) Intoxication, Attention-Deficit/Hyperactivity Disorder, deliriums, Generalized Anxiety Disorder, Major Depressive Episode, and Manic Episode.

- Many children and adolescents turn out to have more than one diagnosis. Comorbidity is especially common in young people with Mental Retardation, anxiety disorders, learning disorders, and disorders of conduct and attentiveness. Mental Retardation also may be diagnosed in children or adolescents who have pervasive developmental disorders.

- When children develop diagnoses more commonly diagnosed in adults, the symptoms may be different. For example, a child with Posttraumatic Stress Disorder is likely to relive the event through repetitive play, rather than through flashbacks, dreams of specific content, or other adult manifestations. The Gender Identity Disorder criteria for children differ in almost every respect from those used for adults.

- Some diagnoses are not truly mental disorders, but are included in DSM-IV because they are useful in differential diagnosis or because they so often apply to young patients evaluated by mental health professionals. Examples include the communication disorders, learning disorders, and Developmental Coordination Disorder.

- There is a danger that unfamiliar diagnoses will be missed or made on incorrect or insufficient grounds. Of course, this caveat might be made for any patient; however, it is especially true for children and adolescents, in whom symptoms may be normal developmental variants whose symptomatic time course may not match DSM-IV criteria.
- DSM-IV facilitates multiple diagnoses, especially for Axis I. But there are many circumstances where a child clinician might doubt the utility of giving a variety of diagnoses to a single patient. For example, how valuable is it—regardless of how well the criteria may be met—to diagnose Attention-Deficit/Hyperactivity Disorder, Stereotypic Movement Disorder, or a mood disorder in a child with profound Mental Retardation?
- We acknowledge that not all diagnostic categories are useful for all clinicians (e.g., learning disorders, Phonological Disorder). But to promote wide differential diagnoses, as well as to encourage referrals, every clinician should be aware of each diagnosis.
- Although used the world over, DSM-IV is a distinctly American document that reflects U.S. experiences and tastes. European clinicians are much less likely to diagnose, for example, Attention-Deficit/Hyperactivity Disorder or Anorexia Nervosa. The prevalence of these conditions will be very different in series reported from abroad.
- Finally, we urge you again to refer repeatedly to the criteria when making a diagnosis. Even in those disorders most simply defined, reliance on memory breeds error.

APPENDIX 1

Appendix 1 presents general references for further reading, as well as citations of various structured and semistructured interviews that can be used to guide clinicians and researchers further in the quest for standardized assessments of children and adolescents.

APPENDIX 2

Appendix 2 lists all of the principal DSM-IV diagnoses with their appropriate code numbers, the approximate age at which each disorder begins, and the age range in which it is most commonly found.

PART I | Interviewing Children and Adolescents

A Background for Evaluating Children and Adolescents

CHAPTER 1 | Interviewing Informants: The Basics

To be sure, every part of the workup of a child or adolescent with mental or emotional problems is important. But if we had to assign some order of importance to the various steps in the process, obtaining reliable information from multiple informants would appear at the top of our list. With a young person, each observer may have a different viewpoint. Even a mother and father may differ in their description of how disruptive a problem may be. Certainly teachers and parents often differ in their view. Without multiple viewpoints from those who know your patient well, at best you will have a difficult time arriving at a correct diagnosis and appropriate treatment; at worst you might never get there.

A number of studies can guide us as we set about interviewing informants. For much of this discussion, we rely upon work that was done in Great Britain by Cox and colleagues. In a series of articles published in the early 1980s, these authors determined which interview techniques were most likely to succeed in obtaining different sorts of historical information. Their findings (see Appendix 1 for a reference) apply equally well to all types of informants—young patients themselves (especially older children and adolescents), parents, relatives and others.

TWO STYLES OF INTERVIEWING

Two fundamental styles of interviewing have been described: *directive* and *nondirective*. As a rule, young children usually respond better to more directed, structured, simple questions. Children who are preadolescent or younger don't usually respond well to nondirective, open-ended questioning, but usually do respond to play. Both techniques are useful in obtaining information from informants *about* children or adolescents.

Nondirective Interviewing

Nondirective interviewing allows the respondent maximum control over the course of the conversation. A nondirective style doesn't ask for "yes" or "no" answers; it doesn't present a multiple-choice format. It relies on open-ended questions, which allow the respondent to speak at length, perhaps to mention a variety of facts. It encourages people to think deeply, talk freely, and share feelings and intimate ideas about their families and themselves. When you use nondirective interviewing, you accomplish several important goals:

1. Because you haven't constrained the answer with requests for specific sorts of information, you increase the range of possible answers, some of which may surprise you.
2. You increase the accuracy of the answers. This is logical: When people respond at length and in their own words, they can express their ideas better than if they must limit their answers to a word or two.
3. Nondirective interviews promote rapport. A greater sense of relaxation and the opportunity to reveal something spontaneously about themselves helps informants feel that you are interested in them and in the young people being discussed.

Throughout this chapter, we illustrate some of the principles discussed here with examples—good and bad—from a session conducted by an inexperienced interviewer. The patient is 17-year-old Kevin, who has been brought to an adolescent inpatient unit.

Kevin's examiner begins well enough:

EXAMINER: Good morning. What brought you to the hospital?

KEVIN: I started thinking about killing myself. I tried to stab myself. My voices started to kick in.

Here are some other nondirective beginnings: "Why did you bring Sheila for counseling?" "What sort of difficulty has Jeremy had in school?"

Directive Interviewing

A directive style, which confines the patient to a narrow focus of the examiner's choosing, helps focus the respondent's attention on aspects of the problem that the interviewer finds especially important, and it increases the amount of information obtained. The minute or so of interview following the examiner's opening question (above) is given below in its entirety. Notice that each of the examiner's questions serves to direct Kevin's subsequent narrative.

EXAMINER: Tell me about those thoughts.

KEVIN: I don't remember, exactly. First I went over to my cousin's house and talked to him, and told him I wanted to see a therapist.

EXAMINER: What made you want to see a therapist?

KEVIN: I'm tired of thinking about killing myself.

EXAMINER: You've been thinking about killing yourself. How long has that been going on?

KEVIN: Four or five years. And then the voices.

Using directive requests, the examiner in this sequence follows up each of Kevin's key words or phrases: "killing" and "therapist." Typically for an adolescent, Kevin responds in short phrases that don't add much to the examiner's knowledge base.

Open- and Closed-Ended Questions

Many of the questions interviewers use to obtain information from patients and others are *open-ended;* that is, they allow informants maximum latitude to respond as they see fit. "Tell me more about that." "Tell me about your son's illness." "What happened next?" But *closed-ended* questions—those that can be answered in a word or two without elaboration—also have their place in mental health interviews. They are useful as probes of important areas already uncovered during an earlier, nondirective portion of the interview. And requests for yes–no (or sometimes multiple-choice) answers can help to rein in patients whose verbosity slows down an interview. The last question asked by the examiner in the excerpt above is a closed-ended one that yields a specific answer.

Conducting the Interview: Blending the Two Styles

From the discussion to this point, it should be clear that each of the two basic interviewing styles is important in an initial interview. In general, a nondirective, open-ended style of questioning is important during the early stages of an initial interview, when you want to give the respondent greatest leeway to volunteer important observations concerning the child's or adolescent's behavior and emotional life. Later on, as you come to understand the scope of your respondent's concerns, use questions that require short answers to increase the depth of your knowledge.

To elicit the informant's *chief complaint* (the reason the child or adolescent was brought for treatment), your first question should be directive yet open-ended. It will sound something like "Please tell me why you brought Jason for this evaluation." You'll probably hear something that is pretty specific, such as "He's seemed very depressed" or "He can't sit still in class." You can then respond with an open-ended encouragement, such as "Please tell me some more about that," and your interview will be off and running.

Occasionally your request for a chief complaint will be a response that tells you the informant doesn't really have much information about the circumstances of referral: "His mother made the appointment; he's only been staying with me for 4 days," or "His teacher said I should." Then you may have to direct the informant's thinking with specific questions about growth, development, emotions, scholastic achievement, moods, or social relationships. After you hit upon a fruitful topic, give the informant maximum leeway to discuss it fully. Remember that during the early part of the interview, you want to pick up the broadest range of information about the child or adolescent, as well as about family, friends, and the environment at home and at school. You also want to build a trusting relationship with the informant. Be respectful, listen carefully, and use body language (e.g., nodding assent, leaning toward the informant, smiling) that suggests acceptance and understanding. With children (and some adolescents), keep the questions simple, give examples, and use praise when indicated. "I know this is hard to talk about, but you're doing fine." Always be alert to hints of problems in the following major clinical areas:

- Difficulty thinking (cognitive disorders)
- Substance use
- Psychosis
- Mood disturbance (depression or mania)

- Anxiety, avoidance behavior, and arousal
- Physical complaints
- Developmental delay
- Socialization problems at school or at home
- Personality problems

Make a note about any of these areas that will require further investigation later in the interview. But for now, strive to keep out of the way and let the informant speak.

ENCOURAGEMENTS AND CLARIFICATIONS

Anything you say may distract your respondent. As long as you are obtaining material that is relevant to your patient's condition, you should just listen. But sooner or later your respondent will run out of steam, take a wrong turn, or simply look at you for guidance. Then a verbal or nonverbal encouragement can help shape the course of your interview for maximum efficiency and productivity.

The least intrusive encouragements you can make are nonverbal ones. A smile or nod of the head may be enough to indicate that the interview is going well and that you want to hear more. One clinician we know manages to do all this just by blinking his eyes! Maintaining eye contact can help establish a bond of sympathy and intimacy. By simply leaning forward, some clinicians subtly indicate support for someone who is recounting information that is particularly stressful. When it seems indicated, you can show sympathy and support without interrupting the flow of information by offering a box of tissues.

We now return to the interview with Kevin.

EXAMINER: The voices?

KEVIN: For about 3 years.

EXAMINER: Ah.

KEVIN: He [Kevin's cousin] was telling me the names of psychiatrists and everything, and he gave me the number, and I lost it. Then we went over to his homeboy's house and people started drinking. Then things got out of hand.

Notice from the sample above that a nearly nonverbal assent leads to more material. Here the examiner gets considerable good from a very few words. Sometimes a syllable or two—"I see" or "Uh-huh"—is all that's needed. At other points, especially when the interview seems to be stuck, you will need to be more articulate. Here are some suggestions:

1. Directly request information, as Kevin's examiner does next:

   EXAMINER: What got out of hand?
   KEVIN: My voices started telling me to kill myself. I got a knife and tried to stab myself.

   Another way of putting this question might be "Please tell me some more about what got out of hand." Similar questions in other cases might be "Please tell me more about Brad's drinking," or "Can you describe Tiffany's problems in school?"

2. If you don't understand an answer (or if your informant has mistakenly answered the wrong question), don't hesitate to ask your question again. You can make it seem less like an interrogation by saying something like this: "I still don't understand. [Ask your question again.]"

3. To ensure that you understand the broad outline of what your informant has been trying to say, you may occasionally want to offer a brief summary. This will be no more than a sentence or two, and will generally begin with "Do you mean that . . . " or "So you feel that . . . "

   EXAMINER: Do you mean that you tried to kill yourself?

TRANSITIONS

Your interview will work better if it flows naturally from one subject to the next, like a real conversation. To that end, you can provide *transitions,* or bridges from one topic to another. Wherever possible, try to follow the informant's lead. Such a process allows respondents to feel that they are full participants in the evaluation, allowed to convey all important facts.

As your interview moves out of the initial "free-form" phase, you will need to become more directive in the techniques you employ. Several of them can help you move comfortably from one topic to another. First, notice the *lack* of adequate transition in this exchange:

EXAMINER: Whom do you live with?

KEVIN: My mom and my grandma.

EXAMINER: Where's your dad?

KEVIN: Dead.

EXAMINER: So you were born in 1981. Did you start school when you were 6?

The abrupt shift of topic emphasizes the examiner's evident discomfort with Kevin's second response. You can reduce the abruptness of transitions by picking up on the last couple of words (or any recent thought) of your informant. In this fragment, notice how the interviewer uses Kevin's own words to encourage more detail:

EXAMINER: Earlier, you mentioned hearing voices . . .

To smooth out the flow of conversation, you can move from one topic to another by using any factor the topics may have in common, such as place, time, activities, or family relationships:

KEVIN: There are four voices. They're always telling me to do things. Right now they're just screaming, "Go to hell!"

EXAMINER: And what about the rest of your family—have they ever experienced anything like those screaming voices?

If you must make an abrupt change, say something that tells the informant that you realize you are changing gears. If your informant seems to have more to say on the first topic, you can offer to return to it later, when there's more time. Here is a possible way of doing this in Kevin's case:

EXAMINER: I think I understand about the problems with the voices. Now I'd like to hear about your problem with drinking alcohol.

PROBING FOR INFORMATION

After a few minutes of listening to the respondent's free-form reasons for the evaluation, you will reach a point of diminishing returns. To ensure that the main concerns have at least been touched upon, ask whether there are any other *major* problem areas (see the earlier list of such areas) that have not been covered. If not, you can begin to examine more closely the areas you have already identified.

Of course, any symptom has its own unique characteristics that require exploration. But common to all symptoms and behaviors are certain features you must probe to obtain more accurate detail. Consider, for example, how these questions would apply to a child's "aggressive behavior":

- Type—physical or verbal?
- Severity—scuffling or all-out fist fights?
- Frequency—daily, weekly, or only once or twice?
- Duration—how long ago did the behavior begin?
- Context—spontaneous or provoked, as by taunts or abuse of a parent?

Assess and record similar descriptors for virtually every problem area identified.

As you begin to seek specific details, you will need greater control over the responses you obtain. Here are some of the techniques you can use:

1. Begin to make your requests with closed-ended questions: "Did Matthew ever wet the bed?" "How old was he when he stopped?"
2. When you get a response that is brief, show your approval with smiles or nods.
3. Explicitly state what you need: "Now I'm going to ask you some questions that call for short answers."

However, when you want to assess feelings (concerning self, the patient, other family members, a situation), remember that open-ended questions provide the most accurate, complete information about emotions.

OTHER INTERVIEWING TIPS

Be careful not to let the way you phrase a question suggest the answer. For example, "Russell hasn't been using drugs, has he?" suggests a negative answer that may not be accurate.

Keep questions short. A complicated syntax that includes a lot of explanation is confusing and wastes time.

Don't try to save time by asking double questions; they will be confusing. If you ask, "Has Jessica ever run away from home or ditched school?", your respondent may focus on only half the question. Neither of you may realize that valuable material has been lost. Here's an unfortunate example from the interview with Kevin:

EXAMINER: How old were you when you and your mom moved in with Grandma?

KEVIN: Two or three.

EXAMINER: Does Grandma have any problems? And you've lived there ever since?

Encourage precision. If you are offered vague descriptions, ask for dates, time intervals, and numbers, as in this more productive line of questioning:

EXAMINER: Do you have any legal problems?

KEVIN: Not really.

EXAMINER: What do you mean?

KEVIN: I was never really arrested.

EXAMINER: Well, what kind of legal problems do you have?

KEVIN: Carjacking, robberies.

EXAMINER: So you've committed crimes that you've never been caught for?

KEVIN: Right.

EXAMINER: What sort were they?

KEVIN: Robbery.

EXAMINER: Like armed robbery?

KEVIN: Couple of times.

EXAMINER: Two armed robberies. Like a mugging?

KEVIN: No. Store robberies.

EXAMINER: Store robberies. For money?

KEVIN: Just to do it. To get the thrill of it.

EXAMINER: What else?

KEVIN: Shootings. Stabbings.

EXAMINER: How many people have you shot?

KEVIN: Maybe five or six.

EXAMINER: Have you ever killed anybody?

KEVIN: I'm not sure.

EXAMINER: So you don't know if any of these people died?

KEVIN: No.

EXAMINER: How is it that you've shot people, but never got arrested?

KEVIN: I throw the gun away or sell it.

EXAMINER: How many people have you stabbed?

KEVIN: About three people.

EXAMINER: Do you know any of the people that you shot or stabbed?

KEVIN: Some of them.

EXAMINER: Have you ever tortured animals?

KEVIN: I shot birds. I don't do it now, you know. When I was younger.

EXAMINER: Have you ever set fires?

KEVIN: Yes, when I was younger.

> *Despite the strongly positive history of antisocial and violent behavior obtained from this series of specific, quantitative questions, Kevin's veracity is difficult to determine. Potential exaggeration and grandiosity to impress the examiner are possible. For diagnostic purposes, this information needs corroboration from court records or statements from Kevin's mother or teachers.*

PARTS OF THE INITIAL INTERVIEW

The diagnostic mental health interview is traditionally divided into a number of discrete parts, the exact titles and content of which vary with the interviewer (and patient). However, the overall effect is always the same: to obtain the most complete account possible of the patient's life, problems, and potential. In the remainder of this chapter, we discuss these aspects under the following headings: "The Present Illness," "Personal, Familial, and Social Background," "Sensitive Subjects," "Medical History," "Family History," and "Mental Status Examination." We provide a more complete outline of the initial interview in Table 1.1.

The Present Illness

For each of the problem areas identified during the information-gathering process, the following lines of inquiry should be pursued:

What kind of stressors might have preceded the onset of symptoms? Try to understand what circumstances or precipitating events preceded the onset.

Changes in sleep and appetite ("vegetative symptoms") may be encountered even in young patients, especially those who have mood disorders.

For disorders that occur episodically (again, especially mood disorders), when did they start? Are the symptoms the same each time? Do they appear in a specific order? What is the first sign of disorder? What comes next? Do the symptoms resolve completely between episodes?

Almost regardless of the duration of symptoms, you will want to know about previous treatment. Was medication used? What effects did it have, wanted as well as unwanted (side effects)? How well did the patient and parents comply with the treatment regimen? If individual or family counseling was pursued, what was gained? What issues remained unresolved?

What have been the consequences of the illness for school attendance, relationships with siblings, and the patient's ability to make and maintain friendships? Have there been any legal consequences? Have interests changed (e.g., hobbies, reading, TV watching)?

In this excerpt, Kevin's examiner pursues details of the hallucinations:

EXAMINER: You said that about 3 years ago—you started to hear voices.

KEVIN: I think it was junior high. It was in the summer, I know.

EXAMINER: And how old were you then?

KEVIN: I don't . . . I can't even tell you. About 13 or 14.

EXAMINER: What were they like?

KEVIN: First I heard soft mumbling. Then as I started getting older, they started

TABLE 1.1. Outline of the Initial Mental Health Interview for a Child or Adolescent

Chief complaint

History of the present illness

Precipitating stressors? Onset? Symptoms?
Any previous episodes? If so, course and treatment (medication, hospitalization, counseling)?
Effects on patient, family, others?

Personal, familial, and social background

Patient's birthplace, number of siblings, sibship position?
Present family constellation? Patient's present residence?
Developmental history (milestones, possible traumatic events)?
Family ethnic background, religious preferences, cultural values?
Parents' relationship: Length/stability of marriage? Separation or divorce?
    Remarriages? Relationships within reconstituted families?
Physical/verbal violence or substance misuse in home?
Is patient adopted? If so, intra- or extrafamilially? At what age? Facts (if known) about natural parents? What does patient know?
Extended family involvement in caregiving? Foster care? Other alternative care?
Degree of family closeness?
Social supports for family?
Patient's age at puberty (if adolescent)? Dating and sexual history?
Education: Current or most recent grade? Scholastic problems? School refusal?
    Behavioral problems? Truancy? Suspensions/expulsions?
Hobbies/interests? Participation in sports/other activities? Any changes due to illness?
Friends? Strengths, positive qualities/outcomes? Sources of satisfaction? Self-esteem?

Sensitive subjects

Substance use by patient: Type of substance? Duration of use? Quantity? Effects?
    Consequences (medical, personal/interpersonal, school/job, legal, financial)?
Suicide ideas/attempts: Seriousness? Methods? Drug- or alcohol-associated?
    Consequences?
Violence/delinquency: Nature? History? Legal system involvement (arrests, incarcerations)? Illegal behaviors for which patient was not apprehended?
Physical or sexual abuse: Exact nature of events? Perpetrator? Legal system involvement? Effects on patient and family?

Medical history

Mother's health during pregnancy? Any problems at birth?
Physical health since birth: Major illnesses? Operations? Hospitalizations? Allergies (environmental, food, medication)? Medications (mental or nonmental) and their side effects? Physical impairments?
Review of relevant systems: Disorders of appetite? Head injury? Seizures? Chronic pain? Unconsciousness? Premenstrual syndrome (for adolescents)? Possible Somatization Disorder?

Family history

What are parents (and other close relatives) like?
Any history of mental disorder in relatives?

TABLE 1.1 (*continued*)

Mental status examination (make age-appropriate)

  Appearance: Apparent age? Race? Posture? Nutrition? Hygiene? Hairstyle? Body
    ornamentation? Clothing (style, cleanliness, neatness)?
  Behavior: Activity level? Tremors? Mannerisms? Smiles? Eye contact?
  Mood: Type? Lability? Appropriateness? Relation to examiner?
  Flow of thought: Word associations? Rate and rhythm of speech?
  Content of thought: Fantasies? Fears? Phobias? Anxiety? Worries? Obsessions,
    compulsions? Thoughts of suicide? Delusions? Hallucinations? Self-esteem?
  Language: Comprehension? Fluency? Naming? Repetitions? Reading? Writing?
  Orientation: Person? Place? Time?
  Memory: Immediate? Recent? Remote?
  Attention and concentration: Simple math? Count backward by 1's?
  Cultural information?
  Abstract thinking: Similarities, differences?
  Insight and judgment?

Personality characteristics

  Response to limit setting?
  Impulsiveness?
  Distractibility?
  Frustration tolerance?

getting stronger and stronger and became constant for longer periods of time.

EXAMINER: Where do they come from?

KEVIN: Just in the back of my mind.

EXAMINER: They don't call you from outside?

KEVIN: No, not at all.

EXAMINER: And they tell you to do what?

KEVIN: To rob people. To hurt other people, watch them suffer. Things like that.

EXAMINER: And what can you do to make them go away?

KEVIN: Sometimes I just try to go to sleep or smoke weed or drink.

EXAMINER: Can you describe the voices some more for me?

KEVIN: There are four voices, screaming.

EXAMINER: Do they talk about you among themselves?

KEVIN: Yeah, they think I'm a fag. And they're constantly telling me to do things.

EXAMINER: What kind of things?

KEVIN: Right now they're telling me to just grab you and start strangling you, because you want to lock me up.

A directive interviewing technique has revealed a great deal about these hallucinations—their type (auditory), location, intensity, number (of voices), content, when they occur, and Kevin's age when they first began. In this case, they are command hallucinations (they tell Kevin what to do). This requires further investigation.

EXAMINER: So they're screaming at you right now?

KEVIN: Yes.

EXAMINER: And they're telling you to grab me?

KEVIN: Grab you and try to get out of here.

EXAMINER: Are you able to control them right now?

KEVIN: I'm able to control them right now.

EXAMINER: Will you tell me if you're not?

KEVIN: Yes.

Although the nature of these voices seems exaggerated, as was Kevin's description of his antisocial behavior, the examiner is sensitive to the possibility that Kevin may be dangerous. Asking whether a patient intends to hurt an examiner is important. If the answer is "yes," then the examiner should seek help or terminate the interview. With a "no" answer, the examiner can proceed.

EXAMINER: Do you do what they say sometimes?

KEVIN: Sometimes.

EXAMINER: What kinds of things have they told you to do?

KEVIN: To rob people. Or when people come up and start saying something, start talking shit to them, or sometimes I'll black out.

EXAMINER: How many times have you blacked out?

KEVIN: Countless times.

EXAMINER: How long does it last?

KEVIN: Sometimes for hours, sometimes for a day.

EXAMINER: When did that start?

Blackouts may signal an organic or toxic etiology, so the interviewer veers off on a new tack to pursue possible causes. To Kevin, however, the change in course must seem barely perceptible.

KEVIN: Two or three years ago.

EXAMINER: Same time as the voices?

KEVIN: Probably before, or a little after.

EXAMINER: Ever lost consciousness for any reason?

KEVIN: No.

EXAMINER: Have you ever had a head injury?

KEVIN: No.

EXAMINER: Ever been in an accident?

KEVIN: No.

The examiner asks a number of closed-ended questions to pursue the specifics of Kevin's possible seizure disorder. Asking about head injuries and accidents may seem redundant, but the interviewer hopes that the repetition will jog Kevin's memory.

Personal, Familial, and Social Background

You will obtain much material about the patient's personal, familial, and social background as you pursue the details of the present illness. Many of these important details can be learned only from a parent or other close relative.

It is of course important to ask about the patient's birthplace, number of siblings, and position in the sibship (oldest, middle child, youngest).

Try to learn about the developmental history. Focus on developmental milestones and possible traumatic events, such as moves, deaths, and other losses. As an infant, at what age did the patient sit, walk, and speak words and sentences? If any of these were delayed, did the parents seek advice? Did they learn anything about the cause?

What can you learn about the ethnic background, religious preferences, and cultural values of the family?

Learn how well the parents get along. Have there been separations or a divorce? In the absence of a two-parent family, describe any remarriages, relationships with stepparents, and time spent with the noncustodial parent. Also, how is the patient disciplined? Is there violence at home, either physical or verbal? Are alcohol or drugs abused in the house?

If the patient was adopted, what were the circumstances? Was the adoption intra- or extrafamilial? At what age did the adoption take place? What, if anything, is known about the natural parents? What does the patient know of these matters? What has been the role of the extended family in the patient's rearing? Has the patient had any history of foster care or other alternative caregivers?

What does the family do for fun? What is dinnertime like? Who eats together? What is the routine at bedtime?

For an adolescent, determine the age at which puberty occurred (voice change, first menses). If dating has begun, at what age did it start? How sexually developed is the adolescent? If the patient is sexually active, is protection used regularly?

How far has the patient gone in school? Has there been any history of school refusal? Scholastic problems? Behavior problems in school? Truancy? Suspensions or expulsions? What collateral information is available from teachers and counselors at school? What kinds of friends does the patient have? Does the patient participate in sleepovers, in sports, in summer camps? Ask about strengths and positive outcomes as well. Is the patient popular? In what area is the patient successful? What gives the patient pleasure and a sense of satisfaction? How is the patient's self-esteem?

Sensitive Subjects

Several sensitive subjects must be broached even when you are inquiring about young children. Admittedly, parents and other adults may not know all that even latency-age children have been up to, but it is vital to avoid missing important information for want of asking. Even knowledgeable parents may feel reluctant to volunteer information about these subjects, which are probably far more common factors in the histories of child and adolescent mental health patients than they are generally acknowledged to be.

Use of Drugs and Alcohol

To the informant's knowledge, has the patient used any substances? Ask specifically about alcohol, marijuana, cocaine, opioids, sedatives, hallucinogens, inhalants (especially popular among younger children), and central nervous system stimulants. For any positive answer, try to ascertain amounts, age at which use has occurred, duration of use, effects, consequences (medical, loss of control, personal and interpersonal, school or job, legal, financial), and attempts at treatment.

EXAMINER: Do you take PCP, LSD, heroin, cocaine, speed?

KEVIN: No.

EXAMINER: Not this year? Last year? Any year? Never tried it?

KEVIN: [Shakes his head in response to each question.] I tried crank [methamphetamine] before.

EXAMINER: How many times?

KEVIN: Once.

EXAMINER: When was that?

KEVIN: About a year ago.

EXAMINER: And just one time?

KEVIN: Just one time.

EXAMINER: Did it cause any problems, like medical?

Suicide Ideas and Attempts

Has this patient ever shown evidence of thoughts about self-harm? Most obvious is an actual attempt, but more likely are wishes for death or relief from mental or physical pain. Any such behavior or statement is especially likely in a patient who has been depressed, abused, rejected, or involved with drugs or alcohol. Statements such as "Nobody cares about me," or "I want to give my dog to my friend Joe," or "A friend told me that he al-

On which axis can we code a suicide attempt? Except as it pertains to diagnostic criteria, DSM-IV is silent on the subject; however, the behavior is so important that it should be flagged, especially if it seems likely to be repeated. If you say something like "Suicide attempt" into your hospital's dictation system, the coding staff will probably put it on Axis I and assign it a multi-purpose number (300.9). You can then put any physical effects of the attempt (e.g., wrist laceration) on Axis III. However, because suicidal behavior is not a disorder but a symptom, we prefer to record it on Axis IV. Although suicide attempts are not environmental problems, they are psychosocial problems that affect a patient's management. Use as many words as necessary to convey a complete, accurate message about this patient.

most got run over by a car" are sometimes indirect clues to the suicidal ideation of a young child.

Violence and Delinquency

Especially for an older child or adolescent, inquire about any history of violence, such as excessive fighting, destruction of property, or cruelty to animals. Also ask about any involvement with the legal system, including truancy, running away, theft, and other legal difficulties. What were the offenses and outcomes? Do the informants know of any other illegal behaviors for which the patient was not apprehended?

Sexual and Physical Abuse

Because of its exquisite sensitivity, abuse is perhaps the topic about which it is most difficult to gather information comfortably. Yet abuse is distressingly common, and not just in the lives of inner-city children. A gentle but direct approach may produce the least resistance from informants.

In the case of sexual abuse, you might ask, "Is there any possibility of sexual activity?" or "To your knowledge, has [the patient] ever been approached for sex by a peer or by an adult?" A positive answer must be explored carefully for details: What actually happened? Was there physical contact? How many times did it happen? At what ages? Who was the perpetrator? Was this a blood relative? How did the patient react? How did the parents find out? How did they react? How have these incidents affected the patient and family since?

In the case of physical abuse, you might ask, "Do you ever feel you get spanked [punished] too hard?" Once again, you will need to follow up all the pertinent details.

Legislatures and parliaments in many parts of the world have mandated the reporting of child abuse. However, what must be reported, to whom, and within what time frame varies depending on the jurisdiction. Even where law is lacking or unclear, medical and mental health professionals (as well as teachers, case workers, the clergy, and even laypeople) have an ethical duty to protect children from physical and mental harm. Clinicians everywhere must acquaint themselves with the requirements that pertain to them and determine how to balance the requirements of the law against the need to maintain confidentiality.

Some clinicians would forewarn all clients about reporting abuse; others would only mention it if the suspicion of abuse arose. We favor being as open and honest as possible, using statements such as, "When I find out this kind of information, I am required by law to report it. Reporting does not imply guilt, it only triggers an investigation, which is really for everyone's safety." However, few would routinely inform children in the absence of any suspicion.

Medical History

What were the facts about the mother's pregnancy with this child? How was her health during pregnancy? Was the delivery vaginal or cesarean? Did the baby breathe right away? Was there jaundice? If so, why—was this an Rh-positive baby? Was a transfusion required? Were mother and child discharged together?

Next, have the informant describe the physical health of the patient since birth, including operations, hospitalizations, allergies, and both current and past medications (for mental and physical conditions). For each medication, what is (or was) the dose and frequency?

Family History

What sort of people are the parents? (If your only information about one of them is from the other, be aware that it may be colored by the feelings surrounding a divorce or interparental strife.) And do the parents or any other relatives have a history of mental disorder? To learn of any mental health difficulties in family members, you may have to bend your rule about asking long questions (although it is far better to ask short, single-answer questions about each of the difficulties):

> "Has anyone related by blood had nervousness, nervous breakdown, psychosis or schizophrenia, depression, problems from drug or alcohol abuse, suicide or suicide attempts, delinquency, arrests or other trouble with the police, hypochondriasis, mental hospitalization, or treatment for mental disease? By *relative,* I mean to include parents, brothers, sisters, grandparents, uncles, aunts, cousins, nieces or nephews."

Depending on the informant's level of sophistication, you may need to define some of these terms.

Mental Status Examination

In many respects, the mental status examination of a juvenile and of an adult have much in common. However, a number of factors distinguish the evaluation of mental status in young patients, especially preadolescent children, from that of adults.

- Because young patients vary in age and developmental stage, the examiner must be familiar with the spectrum of normal behaviors at all ages (see Chapter 3, Table 3.1).
- The examiner must have materials available for eliciting age-appropriate behaviors.
- The evaluation of a young child is usually carried out in part with other family members present, in part with the child alone.
- Depending on the age of the child, toys of varying complexity or other age-appropriate projective material can be used to facilitate the communication.

At the conclusion of the evaluation, the clinician organizes the interactions and observations of behavior with the child and family into a coherent mental status report. The categories of the mental status examination usually include appearance, speech and language, motor activity, sensory capacities, affect and mood, thinking, intelligence, attention, orientation, and relationship with the examiner and with other significant participants.

| Structuring the First Interview
with the Young Patient

An adult who appears for a mental health evaluation usually knows more or less what to expect. The clinician invites the patient into the office; both patient and clinician get comfortable in their chairs; and the interview begins. The patient then describes a set of symptoms or problems in a language that is familiar to the clinician, who listens to content, observes behavior, and evaluates mood and affect. All of this is in the service of establishing rapport and trust, and thus of obtaining reliable information, which can be integrated into a diagnostic formulation with a differential diagnosis and a plan for further evaluation and/or treatment.

Clinicians who evaluate juvenile patients have the same end in mind, but they must use methods carefully tailored to each individual child or adolescent. After all, their patients may not be able to understand the purpose of the evaluation or to use the subtleties of speech that convey meaning adequately. Diagnostic impressions often must be inferred. How rapid, how thorough, how abstract the interview can be will depend on a patient's chronological age, developmental stage, and cognitive capacities. Of course, rapport between the young patient and the interviewer is just as important as with the adult patient.

SETTING UP THE FIRST INTERVIEW

Although adults usually understand why they have been referred for a mental health evaluation, this is not the case for most children and some adolescents referred to mental health professionals. Because the behavior under review may have been viewed by the parents or school as "being bad," young children especially may believe that the evaluation is a form of punishment. Or, when told they are "going to the doctor," young children may expect a physical examination or a "shot." Many children receive no information at all about the visit and come totally unprepared. Inadequate preparation, or none at all, makes the initial contact more difficult. And though parents may understand the reason for the evaluation, they too often have misguided expectations of what will take place or what will happen as a result. Helping young patients and their parents understand what to expect—and helping them to expect the same things—can greatly facilitate the gathering of information. Usually this means that the clinician educates parents and gives them instructions about what to pass along to their child.

All family members involved should know that this appointment will be different from a visit to other health care professionals—that the emphasis will be on feelings and behavior, not physical well-being, and that the professional person will need to understand the nature of these problems so as to be able to help. A patient's parents should be instructed that the clinician will talk with them and their child both together and separately. For a younger child, the parents could suggest which toys and play the mental health professional might use to help understand the problem. Depending upon the age of the child, specifics of the evaluation should be reviewed in advance. For example, young children should be made aware of planned formal psychological testing, play techniques, family interviewing, or separation from their parents. They should be told that the initial visit should take a certain length of time, that they are not being taken to see the clinician as a punishment, and that they will be returning home after the visit (unless the evaluation is for inpatient or residential care). Young children should also be reassured that the professional will not hurt them, although if a physical examination is a possibility, this too should be made clear.

Communicating these difficult concepts is an immediate, practical task. Parents should be helped to select language and phrases that are appropriate to their children's age, level of development, and level of cognitive comprehension. In an initial phone interview, a parent can be asked what words and phrases a young child uses, and then can be encouraged to couch the description of the evaluation in the child's own language. It is often useful in opening the session to ascertain a young patient's understanding of and expectations for the evaluation. This question can be followed up with one about what the patient knows about the problems that are of concern.

THE FIRST CONTACT

A youngster may be reluctant to talk directly about symptoms or problems, and may be frightened by the strange professional and unfamiliar surroundings. Like adults, children become anxious in the doctor's office. Thus a typical concrete response by a young child to the more adult-appropriate question "What brought you here today?" is "My mother." Similarly, "How are you feeling [doing] today?" is usually answered, "Fine."

What type of first interview should you use? Clinicians disagree, perhaps in part because young people and situations can differ so greatly. Controlled studies do not help in choosing one mode over the other, so you should choose an initial interview style that is based on what you already know about a patient from the referral source, the patient's age, and your own interviewing experiences and preferences. Sometimes the structure of the initial evaluation will derive from external circumstances, such as an insurance plan's number of authorized visits. It is more important to attempt to establish a positive therapeutic alliance with the patient and family from the first moment of contact than it is to follow a rigid scenario for an initial evaluation. Structured and semistructured interviews—which follow a schedule of questions, sometimes with branching questions, even "twigs" and "leaves"—may assure coverage of all aspects of mental health, but they are less successful in eliciting affects and unusual items of historical material.

The adults who schedule the interview may be able to help determine how the first interview should be structured. Do they feel that they can speak freely in the young patient's presence? Will the patient's behavior be too distracting? Parents should usually be present for a part of the initial interview, so that you can observe the parent–child interaction. At the time of the initial referral call, emphasize that both parents should attend the first session if at all possible; however, if only one parent shows up (as is often the case), reemphasize the importance of meeting later with the other parent or other family members involved in the care of the child. A good rule of thumb for a young child is to divide the first interview so you see the parent and child together for the first part, then ask the parent to leave while you continue to interview the child alone. You can reverse this order for an adolescent.

Sometimes a child or adolescent is brought for evaluation as the identified patient, but you recognize that the problem is more pervasive. The young person may be reacting with symptomatic behavior to other problems more prominent elsewhere in the family. Often no one openly acknowledges these other problems. You will need to observe sensitively, using your own clinical experience to evaluate the multiple sources of stress and dysfunction.

ESTABLISHING RAPPORT

An initial evaluation has three components that proceed simultaneously: establishing a positive therapeutic alliance, information gathering, and (to a lesser extent) therapeutic intervention. Your first task is to establish a working relationship with the young patient and the family. This takes flexibility, a good working knowledge of children's capacities at different developmental stages, and lots of patience and good will. More than one session may be necessary. With a young child, you will often use toys or play materials to break the ice (see "The Play Interview," below). Conversations about topics that are familiar to a child or adolescent can also help develop rapport. To draw young patients into participation, you might try questions about familiar TV programs, movies, sports events, computer games, or other relevant, age-appropriate activities that capture their interests. Your ability to make a young patient feel comfortable and relaxed, avoiding condescension or manipulation, is crucial to building a trusting relationship.

INTERVIEW STYLE

Young children respond more openly when using spontaneous recall than when being questioned directly. Therefore, in general, the younger the child, the more nondirective and inferential the evaluation needs to be. (See the material on directive interviewing in Chapter 1.) Whereas adolescents are often able and willing to answer questions directly and to elaborate on feelings, preadolescent children are more likely to express feelings and portray conflict through themes that emerge in play. You will also need to observe how the interview develops over time. For example, does the shy, recalcitrant child warm up and engage during the course of the session? Does the anxious, scattered, hyperactive child settle down as the interview proceeds?

CONFIDENTIALITY AND SAFETY

In every case, the participants need to be assured about confidentiality. Of course, you must explain to both child and adolescent patients that you will have to share with the appropriate responsible adults any information about situations potentially harmful to the patients' health or well-being. The issue of confidentiality should be discussed with all children older than about 7 years of age. You might tell an adolescent,

"What we talk about alone will stay confidential with me. I won't tell your parents or anyone else. An exception to that rule is if I am worried that you are doing something that is dangerous to yourself or others. Then the law says I must tell your parents. I won't do that without telling you first. And, if at all possible, I will talk about you only when you are in the room."

With a younger child, you might have this to say:

"What we talk about in here is only for us. Once in a while, I may want your mom and dad to come into the room with you so we can all talk together. But unless you're there, I won't talk about what we do in this office. When your mom has some worries about you, I will want her to tell me when you're present, so you can hear them too."

In the presence of the child or adolescent, you might tell a parent,

"Whatever I learn in our sessions, I will keep confidential unless I am worried about [the patient's] safety or well-being. Then I will ask you to join us, and we can discuss what worries me. Similarly, I will keep to myself what you tell me in confidence about yourself or your family."

Although you will usually want to watch a young patient interact with at least one parent, you must first protect the patient from information that is potentially harmful—parental love affairs, an impending divorce or lawsuit, the possibility of a parent's job loss. Any of these may eventually become known to the patient, but if so, this should occur at a time and place better suited for it than the first interview. Some parents will report just about everything while their children sit listening; others seem reluctant to mention anything potentially anxiety-provoking in the presence of their children. Either extreme suggests patterns of family interaction that are important to understand. Over time, experience will indicate what information is appropriate to be imparted to young patients, based on its nature, the parents' observed sensitivity, and the patients' developmental stage.

THE PLAY INTERVIEW

Rationale and Materials

Why do clinicians so often use play? Young children frequently tell a story through play as they make believe that events happen to dolls or imaginary human figures. In a play interview, the interviewer is a participant–observer, following the lead of the child in choosing the direction of play. Play provides the child with the safety of distance from the emotions created by the problem. It also serves as a natural bridge for communication between the child and the adult. Because children are familiar with play at home and with their peers, it helps decrease their anxiety in strange surroundings. Play can also mirror situations and behavior a child experiences in real life, and can provide an opportunity to experience mastery of various physical and intellectual tasks.

Play materials should allow for fantasy production. Human and animal figures that can be constructed into family constellations are popular, as are materials with which to draw or build. We especially like *transformers*—that is, colorful action toys that a child can manipulate to create a variety of forms. Remember that the more structured the games and toys, the less personalized they are. Board games such as checkers and Candy Land, and card games such as Old Maid or Black Jack, may elicit interest and cooperation from the child, but they rarely yield much clinically useful information. At best, they indicate whether a child can understand and follow the principles of rule-bound games. (Most adolescents prefer to talk about their problems, but some require a game of basketball, a walk outdoors, a computer game, or a soda to break the ice and facilitate interaction.) During the preparatory phone call, you might ask the parent which play materials might be most suitable for this particular child.

Clinical experience demonstrates that an adult professional who gets down on the floor at the same level as a child who is seated on the floor, or lower than a child who is seated in a chair, is less intimidating and often more successful in eliciting engagement. If a parent and child enter an interview room that provides an appropriate selection of play materials, it is often helpful for the clinician to sit at the level of the child, either on the floor or at a play table. The parent, who is familiar and nonthreatening, can sit in a chair or wherever it is comfortable.

Conducting the Play Interview

Invite the child to explore the play materials. As the child begins to verbalize action or ideas related to the play materials, ask for elaboration: "What shall we call this guy?" "Is he a good guy or bad guy?" "What are we going to do with him next?" As the theme develops, it will often reflect the child's concerns. Through make-believe, as noted above, children can distance themselves from the powerful emotions they may be experiencing.

Sometimes resistance may appear in the form of play disruption. The play seems to be going smoothly, and the child appears intensely involved; suddenly the child shifts the focus of interest to another game or breaks up a previous construction. Such play disruptions should be noted, but, like themes of conflict, their interpretation should be saved for a time when you have become better acquainted with both child and family.

Although play sessions will usually involve only you and a child, it is sometimes useful to allow a parent's presence in the room, or even to involve the parent in the play. The parent's response as a participant or interpreter of the play may provide useful additional information about the parent–child relationship.

Interactional Engagement Strategies

A skillful interviewer employs a number of interactional engagement strategies in play interviews. In the chapters that follow, we will present examples of these strategies, many of which are also applicable outside the play context.

Engagement refers to a clinician's strategies for building a respectful, interactive relationship. Some of these have been previously mentioned. Examples include letting the child set the pace of the interview; sitting at the child's level; keeping the child informed of what will be happening; and listening to and following in play, rather than directing it.

Exploration attempts to elicit information about both positive and negative aspects of the lives of the child and family. Getting the child and parent to relate their separate versions of events, asking the child to elaborate on a play theme with questions that maintain the "imaginary" mask of distance ("How do you suppose Jack [a doll] should handle this?"), and using an interactive style that puts the child at ease are examples of this strategy. It is usually more productive to ask children what they understand about an event or topic than to ask them to explain this event or topic.

Continuity/deepening allows the clinician to expand a child's thematic play or dialogue to elicit additional information related to a particular problem behavior. Commenting on the child's drawings, or whatever the child is playing with, works better than asking the child to discuss a particular topic or to elaborate on feelings in the abstract.

Remembering-in-play (interpretation) acknowledges reenactments of behaviors of which the child has been unaware, possibly because they occurred at a developmental stage prior to the onset of verbal language. Such interpretations should be few in number and parsimonious in presentation, and they should usually occur later rather than earlier in therapy; thus, as a rule, they are generally not appropriate in an initial evaluation.

Limit setting requires a clinician's intervention to maintain boundaries. A basic rule in interviewing children is to set the fewest limits and controls possible, but hurting the therapist or another person and purposefully destroying play materials or office equipment must be prohibited early and consistently. However, interviewers must also define their own "comfort zones" for acceptable behavior. Averting temptation is far better than repeatedly telling a child not to use something because it makes a mess; arranging the office or playroom before a session in a way that will minimize the need for limit setting may be the key. Obviously, an office that contains a scattering of fine lamps and small art objects is not the place to evaluate a child known to be "hyperactive and destructive." Similarly, if it is important to keep the office neat, clay, paints, or sand and water should not be provided as play materials.

SPECIAL ISSUES

There is no easy formula that will make every interview simple and successful. If a child or adolescent is going to receive ongoing treatment after the initial evaluation, then establishing rapport and gaining compliance are much more important goals of early meetings than obtaining reliable or valid information; information can always be gathered from additional sources. Clinical experience, an appreciation of the young patient's developmental stage, and an empathic approach to the patient's problems within the context of family, friends, and school should facilitate the establishment of rapport. Nevertheless, because they have experienced significant trauma and disappointments, many children and adolescents referred to mental health professionals have lost their ability to trust. Only a safe, accepting, and consistent therapeutic milieu can rebuild their ability to harbor nurturing relationships. In the remainder of this chapter, we consider questions that may arise in the course of interviewing such patients.

How should I deal with strong negative emotions, such as "I hate my father"?

Children and adolescents often exhibit strong negative emotions, such as hatred for a parent or the wish to kill a sibling. Recognizing that frequently these are projections of self-hatred or suicidal feelings, the therapist needs to tolerate such negative emotions. Sometimes, however, these feelings reflect the reality that a young patient is being abused; in such a case, the patient must be protected. Whatever their meaning, the clinician must accept such expressions of negative affect and attempt to understand them.

How should I respond to a child or adolescent who habitually responds, "I don't know"?

Of course, if a young patient genuinely doesn't comprehend, rephrasing questions is appropriate. Sometimes, however, "I don't know" means a fear of answering; perhaps the child has been warned by a parent not to reveal certain information. Assurances of confidentiality may succeed with older children or adolescents, but clinicians must guard against making promises they cannot keep. For example, an admission of physical or sexual abuse may not, by law, be held confidential by a therapist.

A clinician may suspect abuse or harsh treatment from the themes expressed in play. A child who persistently examines the genitals of a doll, causes animal figures to mount one another, or hits at a doll and calls it "bad" may be demonstrating the likely source of the problem. Observing such play and making comments, such as "Why is the dog being hit all the time? I think he is trying to be a good dog," will elicit further information. For example, a child may reply, "No, he's being bad. He's always messing up the house." The interviewer can then respond, "I bet he tries to be good, but the daddy dog doesn't believe him."

In working with a young patient, a clinician must constantly balance the adult, neutral, professional self who is observing the patient with the self who is engaging the patient in interaction. The participating self—the clinician's "inner child"—can react in a benevolent way to the negative expressions of affect emanating from the patient, whereas the adult, observing self can note the interactions and the progressive deepening of their meanings.

When is it permissible to touch a young patient? When not?

The same general rules that apply to touching adult patients apply to children and adolescents. For some young patients, a touch is provocative—a potential sexual advance or physical assault. For others, a touch is a sign of undeserved familiarity or being treated like "a baby." The clinician must walk the line between social appropriateness (shaking hands, patting someone on the back for a job well done) and condescension or overfamiliarity. Each situation merits individual therapeutic scrutiny. Transference and countertransference issues are as important in the treatment of children and adolescents as they are in the treatment of adults.

That said, sometimes young patients—especially younger children—need to be held. When a child is out of control and destructive, it is appropriate for the clinician to contain the child in a safe embrace. Some young children express extreme anxiety in certain situations. It is perfectly acceptable for a clinician to ask a child whether being held will provide comfort. Or a child may ask to sit in a clinician's lap during times of extreme stress. Such gestures of comfort and support are always appropriate within the boundaries of the clinician's asking permission and the child's granting it. It is also important to obtain a parent's permission.

How should I respond to a child or adolescent who lies?

Whereas children and adolescents are often evasive, withholding, or vague ("I don't know," "I don't remember," "Maybe and maybe not"), it is unusual for a young patient flatly to lie in the course of an interview. Of course, to escape the consequences of their behavior, some patients, usually those who are older and engaging in delinquent activities, will say, "I didn't do it—he did." Although assurances of confidentiality may yield the truth, these can backfire, as when a clinician must warn parents of life-endangering activities. A direct confrontation early in the course of a relationship with a child and adolescent will usually engender only ill will; the best approach is prevention. One strategy is to explain how confusing lies can be to clinicians and how they can get in the way of what young patients want (e.g., release from the hospital), and then to offer an alternative: "If you don't want to talk about something, it's better to say, 'I don't want to talk about that.' " Sometimes *not* learning every detail of an event or behavior early in the therapeutic relationship may reduce the likelihood of a lie. Of course, if the information seems critical to an accurate diagnosis or an appropriate treatment plan, questions should be asked. However, if it can be obtained from other sources or is not immediately necessary, then delaying until more trust is established will reduce the necessity to lie.

How can I engage a child who neither talks nor plays?

Some children may refuse to talk, play, or interact in any other way with a clinician. In such cases, neurological disorders, Mental Retardation, and pervasive developmental disorders must be ruled out. Children who present with Selective Mutism may also refuse to engage. Usually the history from other sources is helpful in differentiating these sources. If such behavior emerges in a child who has previously interacted, it usually relates to significant new trauma in the child's life or to a change in attitude about the clinician or the therapy. Communication with family members about the changed behavior is important. Of course, it is important not to take the behavior personally. Instead of coaxing or threatening attempts to engage the child, detached, patient observation is required.

Should I use a structured interview with children or adolescents?

Structured interviews for children and adolescents were developed to improve the quality of information obtained from mental health interviews. They also allow lay interviewers with instrument-specific training to obtain such information in a way that has adequate validity and reliability for research purposes. Child mental health clinicians have available several such interviews; all provide guidelines for their administration and cover a variety of symptoms, behaviors, and situations. These interviews differ in the flexibility they allow in administration. The most highly structured specify the exact wording, order, and coding allowed, and minimize the role of clinical inference by the interviewer. Semistructured interviews are designed to be administered by clinically sophisticated interviewers who have received extensive training in their use; these interviews are less prescriptive and allow greater latitude for clinical decision making. Although we have listed some of these interviewing tools in Appendix 1, we believe that the most relevant clinical information will be obtained by an empathic clinician with experience in the science and art of interviewing young people.

CHAPTER 3 | An Introduction to Development

This book is not the place to present the full details of child and adolescent development. However, because both interview technique and diagnostic acumen in child and adolescent psychiatry require a firm grounding in the stages of development and the achievement of developmental milestones, some review of these is appropriate. Table 3.1 summarizes some of the more significant milestones. We intend this chapter as an introduction to the importance of developmental concepts and the precepts needed to evaluate young patients at all their varying developmental stages. We will touch on some of the changes that characterize development from earliest infancy to young adulthood.

Development flows seamlessly from one stage to the next; there are no sharp demarcations. An individual's capabilities evolve continually over time. Moreover, changes involve not only the unfolding of biological maturation, but the effects of environmental influences. Height and weight, for example, result from the interactions of genetic programming with nutritional intake. Most of the environmental advances affecting our current generation of children and their parents were unknown 100 years ago. In practice, the following material, so tidily contained in sections and paragraphs, is tightly interwoven.

We also caution readers to remember that there are tremendous variations from one child to another in the rate of normal development. In one actual example, twin A of a pair of boys learned to read at age 3½, just after twin B learned to swim. Twin A did not learn to swim or twin B to read until nearly 2 years later, but as teenagers both twins swam and read well. The ages we report here are either averages or the consensus of experts yet, as with the twins, the expected range within a normal population will be broad.

INFANCY (BIRTH TO 1 YEAR)

The period from birth to the first birthday encompasses the greatest changes in any year of development. It spans the time from total dependence to the first signs of autonomy, from dyadic regulation to the beginnings of self-regulation. This period witnesses the development of the social bond that ties the infant to adult human beings.

In the past 20 years, much has been learned about the remarkable capacities of a newborn infant. As recently as the 1940s, most developmental psychologists believed that infants were, in the words of William James, "buzzing, blooming beds of confusion." Because infants were perceived as sleeping most of the day and as only feeding when awake, their exquisite sensory capacities were relatively unknown. However, sophisticated new methods of infant assessment, combined with the observational skills honed by animal behavior ethologists, have revealed that infant brains are prewired to recognize human signals almost from birth. There is rapid development of visual acuity, from 20/200 at 2 weeks of age to 20/70 at 5 months to 20/20 vision at 5 years. One-week-old infants can discriminate their mothers' odor from that of an unfamiliar lactating female. They can also distinguish their mothers' faces visually and the mothers' voices acoustically. These sensory preferences assist infants in bonding to their parents, and thus launch the process of attachment.

Without adequate caregiving in early life, human infants will die. The attachment system ensures survival by providing infants with a balance between security/safety and curiosity/exploration. Infants who do not have a sensitive, consistent adult devoted to their care often do not become securely attached to any one adult and are less socially sensitive. Some are less likely to smile, vocalize, laugh, or approach adults; others are "promiscuous" in the constant search for attention, moving from adult to adult without any special

A special note on birth order seems called for here. More than 80% of U.S. children have one or more siblings, who can influence a child's personality development. Parents tend to be more involved with and attentive to their firstborn children. In the absence of other children, firstborns receive more stimulation, but the expectations and demands placed upon them are also greater. For these reasons, firstborns tend to identify more closely than younger siblings with their parents (and with authority in general), and to conform more closely to their values and expectations. They are also more strongly motivated toward school achievement, more conscientious, more prone to guilt feelings, and less aggressive than those born later. Perhaps because of these traits, many eminent scientists and scholars have been firstborns. But firstborns also tend to be less receptive to ideas that challenge a popular ideological or theoretical position.

TABLE 3.1. Developmental Milestones of Childhood and Early Adolescence

Age	Gross motor movements	Fine motor movements	Affect/mood	Language/speech	Relationships	Intellectual/symbolic capacity
1 mo.	Raises head slightly when lying face down			Small noises in throat	Can identify mother by sight	
2 mo.	Head control when held seated	Will grip an object placed in hand	Smiles (reflex)	Spontaneous babbling	Responds more to mother than to others	
3 mo.				Responsive cooing		
4 mo.	Can clasp hands together, hold rattle	Will look for an object that has vanished from gaze	Smiles at others (social smile)			Grasps objects
5 mo.	Rolls over; plays with own foot	Will reach for an object and grip it	Will laugh, show excitement; displeased if toy is removed			Explores objects with mouth
6 mo.	Remains seated when placed in position; good head control	Will shift an object from one hand to the other				
7 mo.	Can hold two toys at the same time		Beginning to show stranger anxiety	Definite syllables, such as *ma* and *da*		
8 mo.	Pulls to seated position; feeds self a cookie			Comprehends *no*; says *dada* and *mama*, but not as specific names		
9 mo.	Crawls on hands and knees; holds own bottle	Will hit two objects together		Uses *Dada* and *Mama* as names; will look at an object when its name is said	Plays "where's baby?" and other games	
10 mo.	"Walks" if both hands are held	Will pinch an object between forefinger and thumb to hold it	Will express several emotions, such as affection, anger, anxiety, sadness	Can say at least one word other than *dada* and *mama*	Will wave "bye-bye"	Prefers certain toys
11 mo.	Walks by holding on to furniture	Will remove the cover from a box		Understands about 10 words	Will offer toy to image in mirror	
12 mo.	First steps alone; will help with dressing (e.g., push foot into shoe)		May show separation anxiety			
13 mo.	Crawls up stairs			Can say five or six words other than *dada* and *mama*		Can find an object screened from view

TABLE 3.1 (continued)

Age	Gross motor movements	Fine motor movements	Affect/mood	Language/ speech	Relationships	Intellectual/sym- bolic capacity
14 mo.	Walks alone	Will scribble			Gives teddy bear a kiss	Imitates behaviors of parents
15 mo.		Will use spoon to feed self		Points to wanted objects	Returns a hug; likes to please parents	Likes to play with adult possessions
18 mo.	Can throw a ball; climbs up onto chair; walks up and down stairs unaided	Will imitate a single stroke with a crayon	Onset of negativism	Can say 10–50 words; points to own body parts; follows easy directions; points to pictures of common objects	Seeks loving attention; hugs doll or teddy bear with affection	Likes to explore closets and cabinets
21 mo.	Can squat and return to standing position	Can manipulate a spoon to eat		Can use two- or three-word sentences (usually verb + noun); uses words to ask for things	Possessive of toys	Recognizes self in a mirror
24 mo.	Runs well; can walk backward	Can draw circles		Can say up to 250 words; uses three-word sentences; uses *I, me, you*; calls self by name	Play is mostly solitary (parallel play), though will show interest in others' play	Onset of fantasy play (e.g., with dolls); can remember one or two pieces of information (e.g., numbers or words)
30 mo.	Can jump a few inches to the floor; achieving control of bowels and bladder	Can hold a crayon between fingers and imitate vertical, horizontal lines	Expresses pride in own accomplishments	Can identify five to seven objects or pictures; uses full (four- to six-word) sentences with pronouns; names six or more body parts	Plays at helping with housework; relates to members of own family	
3 yr.	Pedals tricycle; can hop on one foot; can feed self without spilling; grooms self; can throw overhand; begins to show hand preference	Can manipulate small objects skillfully; imitates plus (+) sign; can build tower (up to 10 blocks)	Decline of negativism; enjoys showing off	Has a working vocabulary of ~1,000 words; can state use for objects (ball, pen)	Plays with other children; interested in sex differences	Comprehends meaning of two or three of an item; can compare sizes (big vs. small); can state own gender; uses objects to represent people in play; can state own full name
4 yr.	Can jump forward; can dress self with supervision; can walk upstairs, left–right–left	Can draw a person with a face and arms or legs; can copy a square from a picture	May attempt to control emotions (e.g., crying)	Can name at least three colors	Will take a role in play with others	Can make and honor an agreement

(continued)

TABLE 3.1 (continued)

Age	Gross motor movements	Fine motor movements	Affect/mood	Language/ speech	Relationships	Intellectual/symbolic capacity
5 yr.	Can skip on alternate feet	Can copy a triangle from a model; draws a person with head, body, extremities		Can define simple nouns; can tell a story	Can follow rules of simple games	Beginning sense of values (right vs. wrong, what's fair); can evaluate own capabilities with some accuracy; counts to 10
6 yr.	Can bounce a ball on floor several times; can ride a bicycle	Can tie a bow or shoelaces; can print letters		Can tell left from right; corrects own grammar		Begins to develop ability to regulate own behavior (ability to wait, check aggression)
7–8 yr.	Can hop, jump, run, skip, throw	Can copy a diamond; capability for cursive writing develops	Moods more stable; beginning capacity for empathy, worry	Verbally expresses fantasies, needs, wishes	Develops peer and best-friend relationships	Increasing curiosity, morality emerging; is concerned about opinions of others; recognizes that the whole comprises its parts
9–10 yr.	Increasing strength; individual and team sports			Expresses ideas with complex relationships between elements		
11–12 yr.			May develop animal phobias			Can reason about hypothetical events
15 yr.						Can hold in short-term memory seven or eight independent units (e.g., numbers or words)

Note. This table generally lists those behaviors and accomplishments that a parent or a teacher might ordinarily perceive in the course of ordinary interactions with a child, or that simple testing procedures would reveal. Many other accomplishments and attributes, including those in the areas of ethics, memory, sexual development, and development of attachment to parents, may be determined by in-depth interview or special testing.

It should also be noted that authorities don't always agree on the ages at which specific tasks are first accomplished. The possible reasons for this include data from different populations or different eras, or perhaps dependence on impressions rather than data. The variability should warn us not to take any set of norms too literally, but to regard them as guidelines rather than standards.

preference. Such behavior has been observed in children raised in relatively impersonal institutional surroundings and in monkeys reared in isolation.

The characteristics of the attachment relationship can be measured in a laboratory paradigm, the Ainsworth Strange Situation, when an infant is 1 year old. The Strange Situation involves a series of separations and reunions with a parent (usually the mother), both in the presence of a stranger and with the 1-year-old left alone in an unfamiliar room. A child who shows only moderate distress when the mother leaves, seeks her upon her return, and is easily comforted by her is assumed to be *securely attached*. By contrast, a child may be *insecurely attached* in one of two ways. A child who does not notice the mother's departure, plays uninterruptedly while she is gone, and seems to ignore her when she returns is termed *avoidant,* whereas a child who becomes extremely upset when the mother leaves, resists her soothing when she returns, and is difficult to calm down is termed *resistant*. About 65% of U.S. children tested are classed as securely attached, 20% as avoidant, and 15% as resistant. All else being equal, it is believed that those children who demonstrate a secure attachment during the first 2 years of life are likely to remain more emotionally secure and to be more socially outgoing later in childhood than those who are insecurely attached. Although the data are not incontrovertible, it is felt that insecurely attached children are probably at heightened risk for social or emotional problems later in childhood.

Aspects of Development

Development doesn't happen in a vacuum. The sum (in terms of complexity of function) is greater than the simple addition of increase in size, maturation of the nervous system, and the vicissitudes of the environment. The intersection of the child's innate potentials with parental influences has been referred to as *dyadic regulation*—an emotional process that is most obvious during the first year of life.

Physiology

A major task of the first year is to move from parental regulation of eating and sleeping to self-regulation. New parents are often astonished at the degree to which their household becomes organized around the needs of their infant. The young baby sleeps a majority of the day and night—as much as three-fourths of the time—and does not distinguish between daylight and night hours. During the first few months after birth, the struggle between the baby's innate sleeping schedule and that of the caregiving adults is ultimately resolved in favor of the demands of socialization. The adult pattern of sleep—throughout the night, rather than in 4-hour increments—is established by the end of the first year.

Even young babies have keen senses. As determined by the direction of head turning, an infant can distinguish the odor of the mother's breast pad from that of another lactating woman, can visually discriminate the mother's face, and can distinguish her voice by the age of only 1 week. (Researchers have even suggested that some familiar sounds are heard before birth.) Of course, throughout the early years of childhood, these early memory associations are reinforced many times over.

Temperament

How rapidly and how well the baby settles into the rhythms of life depends in part on the fit between the child's and the parents' temperaments. *Temperament* can be defined as those innate characteristics that color an individual's character. That temperament is inherent and to some extent biologically determined was demonstrated by Stella Chess and Alexander Thomas in the 1960s. They described nine basic dimensions of temperament: activity level; rhythmicity of biological functions; approach versus withdrawal to novel stimuli; adaptability; sensory threshold of responsiveness to stimuli; intensity of reaction; mood quality; distractibility; and attention span/persistence. Chess and Thomas characterized an "easy" child as one who is adaptable, readily approaches new stimuli, has regular (rhythmic) biological functions, and has a positive mood of moderate intensity. It is obvious to what degree an easy baby can help to facilitate the task of parenting. A "difficult" child (10% of their sample) has irregular biological functions, withdraws from stimuli, is slowly or poorly adaptable, and has a mood that is intense and often negative. They also describe the "slow-to-warm-up child" as one whose responses to new situations are mildly negative and whose adaptability is low, even with repeated contact. However, individual temperamental characteristics observed in babies don't necessarily predict later behavior accurately.

Motor Behavior

The first organized motor behavior, present even before birth and necessary for survival, is sucking. Next, very early in life, babies control their heads so as to select stimuli that interest them. This immediately suggests the importance of parental stimulation as a determinant of the speed and extent of motor development. Motor control proceeds from head to foot and from proximal to distal (shoulder to arm to hand to finger). There is a gradual progression from instinctive behavior (grasping an object placed in the hand) to reaching for an object to manipulation of objects for a purpose (e.g., the child learns to assist with feeding by holding first a bottle and, a little later, a cup and spoon). Note again the parents' opportunity for influencing development by verbal and nonverbal encouragement (smiles and applause). The supply of materials for exploration can also promote development of fine motor coordination as the baby progressively practices grasping, transfers, and pointing.

Affective Behavior

As early as 8 weeks, the baby's smile fosters interaction and bonding with the parents. By 10 months, children have selectively attached themselves to a few other people—parents, siblings, sitters. Fear of strangers appears by 8–12 months, characterized by wariness when an unfamiliar person attempts to interact with a child. Separation anxiety begins a few months later and can be observed when a parent leaves. The child may fuss at the departure even when left with another familiar person. Also at about this age, the child begins to share emotional experiences with parents and to be influenced by the feelings of others nearby. This is known as *social referencing.*

Once mobility has been enhanced by crawling, the child can begin to explore the environment. Crawling to the parent upon request helps foster the bond between parent and child. The developmental sequence is from a recumbent, dependent position to an upright, "moving away" position. The attachment relationship (a basic survival mechanism, as noted above) fosters a balance between comfort and proximity during stress on the one hand, and exploration and curiosity during times of well-being on the other.

The development of attachment also relates to the process of differentiation of self from other nearby objects and people. Babies explore the world first by visually following the movements of others, and later by reaching for objects and exploring them with their mouths. Self-stimulation begins by the fourth month and becomes a genuine part of play by the eighth month.

Communication

Infants smile, babble, and coo, capturing the attention of their parents. These early social stimuli elicit positive interactions centering around caregiving and play. There is little relationship, however, between the sounds produced during infancy and the amount or quality of speech produced by a child at age 2. Development of speech depends on the maturing brain, as well as on a child's exposure to speech and cognitive stimulation through interaction with adults. Vocalization progresses from crying through cooing and random sounds to the beginnings of meaningful speech. When only 3 months old, the baby begins to vocalize in response to human speech; this leads to approval from parents, which reinforces the child's efforts to communicate through more speech.

Obtaining Information

Of course, in the usual sense of the term, no one ever truly interviews a tiny baby. Much of the information is obtained from the parent who has brought the infant to the session. You can obtain a great deal of information from the adult directly, as well as from observing the infant in interaction with the adult. Infant evaluations should always be carried out with at least the infant and parent present at the same time.

Here are some questions of special interest in the evaluation of an infant: Was this a planned child? Was the pregnancy uneventful? How irritable has this baby been? How easy to soothe? How regular in feeding and sleeping schedules? How have the parents dealt with abnormalities such as premature birth or a physical anomaly, either suspected or real? Do they accept the child's condition, or do they feel guilty and regard the problem as evidence of parenting failure? Are the parents' expectations of this child age-appropriate and realistic, or is this child at risk for eventual feelings of inferiority and guilt as a result of repeated failures?

Most of the information you can derive directly from an infant will come from observing the baby's interactions with others and from performing developmentally appropriate motor, sensory, and cognitive examinations. Often the infant responds most positively when sitting in the parent's lap. You should check for mutuality of gaze behavior, capacity for visual fixation and following, auditory responsiveness, and social (smiling, avoidant, crying) responsiveness. Note aspects of general development: Does the baby appear normal and healthy, or is there evidence of arrested development or failure to thrive? Are there any obvious physical characteristics, such as the classic stigmata of Down's syndrome? Does the older baby (or toddler) enthusiastically enter into simple games, such as peek-a-boo? Separation of the infant/child from the parent constitutes part of the standard evaluation of any young child. How does the child respond—with a brief whimper and a ready response to distraction, with inconsolable wails, or with indifference?

Finally, note that because very young children tire quickly, more than one session may be necessary for the initial evaluation.

Symptoms

A number of characteristics, some of which may turn out to be symptoms, can appear even during the first year of life. Of course, most of them can also be manifested at later stages of development.

- Failure to gain weight and length (failure to thrive)
- Poor social responsiveness (paucity of smiles, failure to hold out arms to be picked up)
- Problems with eating (fussiness about new foods, multiple food allergies, irritability when feeding, frequent regurgitation/rechewing of food, eating material that is not food)
- Problems with sleep regulation (failure to establish a diurnal rhythm, excessive sleep during the day, excessive wakefulness at night)
- Relative lack of vocalization
- Response to strangers that is excessively fearful, intense, or prolonged, or failure to appreciate differences between strangers and familiar caregivers

DSM-IV Diagnoses Most Likely to Be Made First at This Age

The diagnoses listed below typically first appear at about this age. See Appendix 2 for a more complete listing of diagnoses and ages at which they typically are encountered throughout childhood and adolescence.

- Mental Retardation: nonspecific but Severe or Profound, or specific syndromes (e.g., Down's syndrome) of any severity
- Rumination Disorder
- Feeding Disorder of Infancy or Early Childhood (failure to thrive)
- Reactive Attachment Disorder of Infancy or Early Childhood
- Parent–Child Relational Problem (V-code)

TODDLERHOOD (1–3 YEARS)

No sooner do children begin to form a social bond with caregiving adults than they start a decades-long struggle for independence. Even through young adulthood, as they establish families and careers themselves, young people strive for significant autonomy—a sense of self. The toddler period is the stage of the "terrible twos," the first "no," even the first lie ("Who spilled that milk?" "Not me!"). These are important and positive first developmental indicators of being separate, individual, unique.

Aspects of Development

This is also a period of tremendous curiosity and joy in the discovery of what is possible. Expressing feelings is important, but so is accepting limits; thus parents need to foster the balance between exploration and consistent discipline. Toddlers need to be protected from violence and harm and to learn about safety—avoiding light sockets, busy streets, and anything that is hot. During these years, children develop the beginnings of self-discipline (e.g., leaving items on the shelves in the store, looking at but not touching a Christmas tree).

Babies and young toddlers are almost entirely egocentric. One challenge that parents face during this period is to help their toddlers learn about sharing, taking turns, and waiting patiently. Toddlers begin to discriminate self from nonself. As they near their second birthday, they come to recognize themselves in a mirror, and can point to their own images and those of other persons. They also become fascinated by other children. During this time, a toddler may acquire a new sibling; this offers the prospect of a built-in playmate and the opportunity to become a big brother or sister, but it also sets the stage for withdrawal of parental attention. Toddlers also acquire a fuller complement of affects. Nuances of mood and moodiness develop (lightning-quick changes, sadness, tantrums, and whining); the response to limit setting may be negativity.

During these 2 years, language acquisition progresses at the rate of several new words per day, while vocabulary increases from 1 or 2 words to about 1,000. At the same time, the use of language develops from single words to full sentences that embody the rudiments of correct grammar. By the end of this period, most children have learned to substitute verbal requests for pointing and crying.

Parallel to language acquisition, toddlers' motor activity progresses from uncertain, unsteady steps through climbing stairs to running, hopping, and pedaling a tricycle. With developing motor skills come the beginnings of self-care. Young toddlers will help to undress and dress themselves (e.g., pushing a foot into a sock), learn to choose foods, and begin to feed themselves with a spoon and cup. The perception of grown-up behavior and the desire for proficiency drive much of this progress, which ushers in fantasy play as a rehearsal for grown-up behavior. By the end of toddlerhood, a toy begins to represent some object perceived as important in the grown-up world, instead of just an object to be manipulated.

Obtaining Information

Toddlerhood is (another) difficult age at which to obtain reliable information from a child; again, multiple, brief diagnostic sessions may be necessary. As with infants, all historical information comes from the parents, whose descriptions and concerns must be taken seriously. In the office, many children will not exhibit the symptomatic behaviors that are of concern to their parents (a generic warning that applies to patients well into their teens—and sometimes beyond). Repeated office visits to foster comfort and familiarity, or visits to the home or to the day care center (where the symptoms are purported to occur), may be necessary. Sometimes bringing a child to the office with the opposite-sex parent or even the entire family is illuminating.

As with an infant, it is important to observe a toddler's interactions with a parent and then to note the child's reaction when the parent briefly leaves the room. During this absence you can attempt to engage the child in play; observe relatedness, exploration of new toys, and apprehension with a stranger. How would you characterize the reunion once the parent returns? Assessing separation anxiety, which is normal at this age, should be part of every evaluation. A child who has previously experienced illness, hospitalization, or other separation may vigorously resist being interviewed alone. Early in the relationship, it may not be possible to interview the child at all unless the parent is present.

It is hard to sustain a conversation with toddlers, who need more verbal probes and structure in play than do older children. In posing questions or in proposing play, offer multiple choices, which increase the options for response. Even relatively nonverbal children may be able to respond to queries that relate directly to the play sequence they have just completed: "Is that the way it is [in this sort of situation] at your house?" However, it is extremely important not to play into the suggestibility of young children; they are eager for the approval of adults and may say "yes" to just about anything. Observe a toddler's ability to use language (vocabulary, complexity of sentence structure) and affect (type, range, and appropriateness). Evaluate fine motor skills by drawing figures, squares, and diamonds. Assess handedness and footedness by catching, throwing, and kicking a ball.

Excessive shyness or excessive lack of inhibition may be apparent. How much control does the child require in the playroom setting—a simple "no" or repeated physical interventions?

Symptoms

Most of the same symptoms first identified in infancy can still be issues a year or two later. In addition, new symptoms may worry parents:

- Aphasia
- Disturbed consciousness (abrupt onset of inability to focus or sustain attention)
- Excessive crying, night waking, or refusal to go to bed at night
- Extreme misbehavior: temper tantrums, lying, refusal to cooperate, destruction of toys, cruelty, violence
- Extreme shyness, presenting as withdrawal and apathy
- Inadequate social interaction (poor eye contact, body language, sharing of interests or enjoyment, inadequate fantasy play, or inability to sustain a conversation)
- Inflexible adherence to routine
- Language delay (e.g., no language use by 18 months or no use of phrases by 30–36 months)
- Motor hyperactivity, which tends to subsume many problems or disorders
- Refusal to separate from parents or stay with sitters, a desperate need for attention, "being spoiled"
- Stereotyped movements
- Struggles over toilet training or new foods
- Testing limits, "being a devil," getting into everything, being "just like Dad or Uncle Ernie"

DSM-IV Diagnoses Most Likely to Be Made First at This Age

- Mild or Moderate Mental Retardation
- Autistic Disorder
- Rett's Disorder
- Reactive Attachment Disorder of Infancy or Early Childhood
- Delirium
- Parent–Child Relational Problem (V-code)

PRESCHOOL AGE (3–6 YEARS)

During the next 3 years of life, children begin to develop the ability to observe, to think, and mentally to manipulate formed constructs in a way that will be used later during school as they equip themselves for life as adults. These abilities form the basis for the existence of a private self within a child—one that is not readily discernible to the parents.

Aspects of Development

As development proceeds, children realize that there are adults other than parents and grandparents. Whereas relationships with parents were initially the main focus for interaction and for need fulfillment, children at this age gradually grow more interested in friends their own age—playmates at the playground, in day care, and in the neighborhood. They begin to attend birthday parties and other multiple-family events. Play, which becomes increasingly complex and symbolic, serves as a vehicle for wider socialization. Play relieves tension, works out problems, and helps children build a sense of identity and mastery over conflict. Differences between the sexes become especially pronounced in social situations. As same-sex friendships begin, activities tend to become gender-specific—dolls for girls, adventure toys for boys—though there has recently been a trend toward some degree of blended play.

By the end of the preschool years, all the elements of basic communication skills are in place. The child can converse in complete sentences that are logical and grammatically correct; eye–hand coordination allows printing and writing; and the basics of numbers, colors, and drawing are in place.

Locomotion becomes smooth, and all gross motor movements are better coordinated. These children have boundless energy and curiosity, but their judgment is limited, so parents still need to guard against various types of accidents. Toward the end of this age, there is a gradual reduction of impulsiveness.

As they near school age, children begin to adopt moral values. At first, these are strict and lacking in subtlety—a sense of right and wrong, good and bad, and fair play. They also begin to demonstrate a capacity for empathy for the distress of friends and parents. Children of this age want to please; as a result, loving discipline increasingly serves to keep order. At the same time, the children develop a capacity for jealousy and rivalry, and are fascinated by secrets.

Obtaining Information

A preschool child can provide some verbal information of diagnostic use, but most of your information will still come from nonverbal facial and body language and from the quality of the child's interactions with you. Verbal interviews most often focus on the here and now, and children's responses consist of one-word or short-phrase replies to questions. Because of their age and inexperience, these children cannot supply much of the material vital to their own histories (especially family history and parental strife), but they may show surprising insight into the functioning of their nuclear families.

Start the interview not by discussing problems, but by asking confidence-building questions a child can answer easily—the child's own age, where the child lives, and with whom. Preschool children need encouragements to keep them going. Wait until rapport is established to ask what a child's feelings are about a parent or sibling. To address the child's wishes, body image, living situation, self-assessment, and other features, ask, "What would you like to change about yourself?" (An answer of "Everything" may indicate severe depression.) The child's sense of the future and aspirations can be addressed by asking direct questions or by beginning a story that the child completes: "Once upon a time there was a little boy named Billy, and what he always wanted to do was . . . " To assess mood, present the child with a simple scale: "How do you feel most of the time? Really sad, sad, sort of in the middle, happy, or really happy?" But unless you have formed a trusting relationship with the child, the response may be a clumsy attempt to please or to keep back information: "Really happy," the child may state in a subdued voice, while failing to make eye contact.

Young children also enjoy play interviews, which are used to obtain information that the children may not otherwise divulge (because direct questions are seen as a threat). You can interact directly with a child and/or observe the child's spontaneous play (with peers, on the playground, etc.). Carefully observe the child in interaction with others for the assumption of social roles (leader vs. follower, gregarious vs. isolated individual). In play, evaluate the child's choice of toys, affect regulation, activity level (normal exploratory curiosity vs. destructive, driven, reckless hyperactivity), concentration, frustration tolerance, mastery motivation, and persistence at a task.

Symptoms

- Anxiety symptoms (may be shown in play or dreams)
- Anxiety upon separation from parents
- Elimination problems or genital complaints: enuresis, encopresis, pain, repeated genital touching/masturbation, self-exposure (the latter complaints in particular may indicate sexual abuse)
- Extreme jealousy of a new sibling
- Few or no friends
- Impulsiveness of a self-destructive nature (running in the street, grabbing knives, attempting suicide, ingesting medications or other substances)
- Multiple fears (which may be manifested as excessively shy, withdrawn behavior)
- Nightmares, fear of the dark
- Refusal to follow directions
- Risk taking (recklessness, inappropriate fearlessness)
- Somatization of grief or stress (loss) reactions in stomachaches, headaches, "not feeling well"
- Speech that is difficult to understand, stuttering
- Temper tantrums or aggressive outbursts

DSM-IV Diagnoses Most Likely to Be Made First at This Age

- Expressive and Mixed Receptive–Expressive Language Disorders
- Phonological Disorder
- Stuttering
- Childhood Disintegrative Disorder

- Pica
- Specific Phobia
- Breathing-Related Sleep Disorder
- Sleep Terror Disorder
- Physical Abuse of Child, Sexual Abuse of Child, Neglect of Child (V-codes)

SCHOOL AGE (6–12 YEARS)

Social relationships with peers become dominant as the child moves outside the family for interpersonal contact and reinforcement.

Aspects of Development

By the early grades of elementary school, preference for playmates of the same sex becomes dominant, with differentiation of styles of play and behavior by gender. Boys favor rough-and-tumble play in larger groups, oriented around shared experiences; they play away from the immediate confines of home, exploring the environment. Girls tend to play indoors or near home in smaller groups, oriented around shared confidences. For many children, socialization proceeds through group identification (such as Scouts and soccer). Games and play become much more rule-oriented. Activities at first occur close to home (Cub Scouts, Brownies), but take older children farther afield for hikes, overnight camping trips, and "away" sporting matches.

Although this age has been called the *latency period,* these children have significant developmental tasks to master. Indeed, *mastery* and *competition* are two of the watchwords of these years. A child's focus moves outside the family to include schoolwork, which provides practice that lays the foundations for later, life-sustaining work. Of course, mastering basic educational skills (reading, writing, math) occupies much of the child's attention. At least as important are developing good study skills and feeling positive about learning—experiences that are balanced by the competing demands of games and other play, entertainment, and hobbies.

For the first time, a child may shift allegiances to a new authority figure, the teacher, often forcing a reevaluation of the parents' values (especially about education). School-age children become progressively able to keep reality and fantasy distinct, and in general to view the world from the perspective of increasing experience and judgment. Before the age of 8, children describe others in terms of physical appearance; later they will use more abstract terms. They develop the verbal ability to express complex ideas and relationships between elements (cause and effect), and to show off their improving use of language with plays on words.

Children at this age have an increasing ability to retain and operate on information (e.g., to keep a string of digits in mind). At first rigid and moralistic, children may express feelings of guilt or remorse when they fail to attain a given standard. (Not until the late teenage years, if ever, may they accept a lesser standard of performance in themselves.) During this period, they also become able to modulate their own affects and to show emotions different from what they feel inwardly. Moreover, they experience completion of the development of gross motor skills: running, jumping, and throwing, with accuracy and increasing strength.

Obtaining Information

Although it is still necessary to speak with parents and teachers first, you can obtain considerable historical information from school-age children. It is important to be clear when explaining the reasons for the evaluation. Straightforward, simple communication about expectations and confidentiality usually works the best. Although some (older) children can talk about themselves nearly as well as adults can, play is still a useful facilitator of communication, especially in the grade school years. Studies have demonstrated that behavior in play reflects a child's everyday activities and concerns. Games and drawing may also facilitate communication. Sometimes moving the interview away from the office by walking or sitting outdoors makes a child feel more at ease.

Each evaluation should begin with some preliminaries—perhaps asking whether the child knows the reason for the interview. A little explanation of the process can help allay the anxiety that many younger children will feel when confronted by a new environment and a strange adult who asks a lot of questions. Above all, a child should experience any clinical interview as both nonjudgmental and nonthreatening. Use smiles, eye contact, and other physical signs of welcome and ease to communicate comfort and the feeling that it is safe to reveal information.

Allowing the child to lead the interview (especially in play) gives the child a sense of control, which tends to facilitate communication. Sparing use of humor can help build rapport. At the same time, avoid being excessively friendly; you want to learn how the child forms a new relationship with an average person. "Tell me about your family" isn't likely to net you much; instead, ask the child to describe a typical activity, such as washing dishes—who directs, who dries. Try using a just-reported scenario to learn how the child might respond in other circumstances: "Instead of [a circumstance the child has just related], what if . . . ?" Asking the child to state "three wishes" can help reveal aspects of the child's fantasy life and view of the future.

Children tend to be more accurate in reporting facts (what actually happened), but less accurate in reporting judgments (whether an event or behavior was good or bad, whether it occurred frequently or infrequently). Therefore, you aren't likely to learn much from asking "why" questions, which may only make a child feel incompetent, puzzled, or threatened. The "why" of things is deduced gradually from the accretion of evidence obtained from other informants, patient interviews, and testing. In play or in verbal interaction, it is important to gauge both the spontaneity and the logical, goal-oriented nature of the communication. Young children will recall more accurately if open-ended questions are used, but their information won't be as complete as that provided by older children. Children under the age of 10 report their fears (but not much else) accurately, if they are only asked yes–no questions. If a child does not answer a question, you will need to shift topics or get the answer in play.

Speech and language symptoms, such as articulation defects or problems with understanding, can be evaluated by direct observation during the initial interview. Samples of writing and reading should be obtained as a further assessment of language proficiency. You can test spelling and writing by asking the child to label a just-completed drawing of family members. What do you observe about the child's thought progression and logic? Of course, much of *any* interview is nonverbal, so observe the child's temperament, frustration tolerance, and ability to relate to you.

Depressed affect, with tearfulness and feelings of worthlessness, can be expressed verbally or in play. A child's moods will be reported better by the child than by parents, but contemporary diagnosis of depression and other negative affects requires more than cross-sectional observations. Historical and behavioral data are also needed from parents and other informants.

Various writers have suggested methods for dealing with the threat that negative feelings pose for children:

- Suggest that many other children feel the same.
- Present two or more acceptable constructs: "Do you like school pretty well, or would you rather not go?"

- Express the assumption that *all* children sometimes engage in negative behavior (such as fights with siblings).
- Adduce an acceptable reason for bad behavior: "Maybe you ran away because you needed to show someone how you felt."

Throughout an interview, though you may not agree with a child, it is important to respect the child's defense mechanisms. This is especially true of younger children, whose need for approval can be both intense and immediate.

Play can be used in three ways with children of this age. First, it can be used as a therapeutic tool whereby a child plays imaginatively, engaged in fantasies that project conflicts and their resolution. Second, play can be used as a topic of dialogue. Third, while you and the patient engage in conversation, toys or games can be used to ease tension. Most often, you will find yourself using combinations of all three—straight play, straight talk, and talk facilitated by play—to keep the momentum of a session going. It is usually not difficult to decide which technique(s) should be used. At first, try all three to see how the child responds, then proceed with whichever seems easiest for the child. If one method works for a while but then becomes cumbersome, try another.

Try to use as few rules as possible, but enforce them consistently. If behavior becomes unruly, you may need to protect the child as well as the environment. You can say, "I won't let you hurt me or destroy toys [objects] in the office." When behaviors get out of control and the child's attention cannot be diverted, the child can be physically held or the session can be stopped. It is important to set the limits clearly in advance and to define the parameters of intervention. (Be sure to inform the parents of these limits and the methods available to enforce them.) If you suspect that a session may end prematurely, be sure that a parent is available to take charge of the child.

The important themes to watch for in play are little different from what an older adolescent or young adult might talk about as trauma or conflict. Loss and grief, anger, fears, feeling unloved, low self-esteem, isolation, and alienation all commonly appear in play. These can be manifested in specific play scenarios with animal or human figures; in drawings, they may be indicated by the choice of colors, shapes, and sizes, by order versus chaos, and by the presence or absence of key figures. Often children tell as much by what they leave out or avoid in play as they do through inclusion. Normal children have a variety of themes, affects, and play preferences, and share their interactions and experiences easily in play interviews. Psychopathology in play is most evident in rigid, fixed themes, affects, and preferences, whereby the child excludes you or other participants entirely, or is inappropriately compliant, seductive, or combative. Watch for the affect. Bland themes may be as telling as violence or chaos.

Symptoms

In addition to the symptoms mentioned previously, watch for the following:

- Absence of speech in specific social situations
- Angry mood
- Anxiety in girls who physically develop prematurely
- Deliberately blaming others
- Depression
- Enuresis
- Hyperactivity, fidgeting, talking excessively
- Impulsiveness (inability to wait for turns, intrusiveness)
- Inability to focus attention during class
- Learning problems
- Loss of temper, arguing, defiance, spite
- Nightmares
- Panic attacks
- Repetitive motor behavior that is nonfunctional
- Rituals or magical beliefs associated with unreasonable fears
- School refusal
- Somatization
- Substance use
- Stuttering and other verbal fluency problems
- Temper outbursts
- Tics
- Trouble with reading, math, writing
- Withdrawal or isolation

DSM-IV Diagnoses Most Likely to Be Made First at This Age

- Learning disorders
- Asperger's Disorder
- Oppositional Defiant Disorder
- Conduct Disorder

- Attention-Deficit/Hyperactivity Disorder
- Tourette's Disorder
- Chronic Motor or Vocal Tic Disorder, Transient Tic Disorder
- Encopresis
- Enuresis
- Separation Anxiety Disorder
- Selective Mutism
- Obsessive–Compulsive Disorder
- Generalized Anxiety Disorder
- Factitious disorder by proxy (a proposed diagnosis—see Appendix B of DSM-IV)
- Sleepwalking Disorder

EARLY ADOLESCENCE (12–15 YEARS)

Although the drive to achieve independence from parents continues and even accelerates during early adolescence, the family remains a preeminent influence for adolescents, contrary to popular belief. Several recent studies have found that most adolescents have relatively few serious disagreements with their parents. Whereas adolescents and parents often disagree (sometimes sharply) on issues of contemporary social concern such as politics, drug use, and sexuality, these are mostly differences in the intensity of an attitude rather than its direction. Generation gulfs usually reflect different levels of support for the same position. In sum, there is not much evidence supporting the myth of adolescence as a period of storm and stress. Most teenagers continue their close and supportive relationships with their parents; in their relationships with peers, they tend to embody parental values rather than to oppose them.

The onset of adolescence is so variable that no exact age can be given. Early adolescence is marked by the onset of puberty, which can be as young as 10, in some girls. Mid-adolescence usually refers to a period that begins 2–3 years later, with late adolescence beginning another few years later. Typically, early adolescents will be 6th–8th graders, mid-adolescents will be 8th–10th graders, whereas late adolescents may be in the 11th grade through the first 2–3 years of college. Somewhat arbitrarily, we have chosen age 15 as the crossover point between early and late adolescence (we cannot make clear enough distinctions behaviorally and emotionally to distinguish a middle phase); in reality, the ages can vary by several years.

Aspects of Development

Adolescence is marked by the beginning of the shift from same-sex to opposite-sex preoccupations and activities. If this does not take place early during this period of development, it will occur in most cases within the next few years. An adolescent feels a powerful adherence to the peer group; cliques and clubs are critical to the sense of belonging, which also fosters a need to stay in touch with peers by phone, through after-school sports and other activities, and through social events. Getting ready to drive a car heightens the sense of moving away and belonging to a new group.

Sibling rivalry can sometimes become intense, especially if siblings are the same sex, are close in age, or have similar interests. Stepsiblings in blended families are especially at risk for rivalry and territoriality. Outside the family, competition intensifies in a variety of areas—athletics, attractiveness, and academic/intellectual pursuits. Preeminence in sports supersedes the mere development of skill.

Early adolescents experience a growth spurt. In boys, it begins at about age 12. In girls, growth accelerates a year earlier, with menarche occurring at about 12½ years (3 years earlier than was the case a century ago). Early-maturing adolescent boys are typically better adjusted than those who mature later; they have more favorable interactions with peers and adults. For females, however, the teasing and self-consciousness associated with early maturation can produce psychosocial trauma.

By the midteens, intellectual development is nearly on a par with that of adults. Children of this age can define complex scientific terms and reason about theoretical events or constructs. Despite increasing prominence of moral distinctions and a sense of what is right or good in others (particularly their parents), adolescents' judgment about their own behavior is often their downfall. The typical adolescent illusion of invulnerability promotes risk taking, which so often leads to experimentation with drugs, sexuality, or illegal behavior as to constitute almost a rite of passage for young people.

Obtaining Information

Early adolescence is the youngest age at which information from a patient becomes predominant. Adolescent patients know more of their own histories and can communicate in an interview on a more nearly equal footing than younger children can. Usually the patient should be interviewed first; the subsequent parent interview is often best accomplished when the teenager is present.

Developing trust and rapport with a teen is critical. At the outset, it is especially important to explain about confidentiality and its limits. Try to establish a trusting relationship that will increase the likelihood of obtaining trustworthy data and set the stage for future therapy. It is often useful to balance the need for trust against the need for truth with a statement such as this: "Don't tell me what you don't want to, but don't lie. If you can't tell the truth about something, just ask me to move on to another topic." Sometimes adolescents will talk about experiences that their friends have had, while denying (falsely) that they themselves have been involved.

In an interview with a teen, you should be friendly and interested, but respectful of the age difference. It is helpful to be reasonably knowledgeable about cult heroes, athletes, and rock stars. Beware, however, of being overly friendly or of trying to act too "hip"—teenagers can see through artifice like a windowpane. You will especially need to assess the following:

- The family situation, from the dual perspectives of adolescent and parents; presence or lack of support in the primary family system
- Sexual knowledge, including sexual experiences, both heterosexual and homosexual; pregnancy; use of safe-sex practices
- Use of tobacco, illicit or prescription drugs, and alcohol
- Delinquency, truancy, and participation in gangs
- Friendship patterns and activities with peers
- Issues of dependence–independence; developmental readiness to meet the demands of society
- Identity formation ("Who am I? What will be my place in the world?")
- Self-esteem—a big concern for the preadolescent and adolescent
- Empathy (how sorry does the adolescent feel when a sibling or friend has a problem?)
- Conscience ("What would you do if . . . ?")

As with an adult, try to end your interview with a teen by giving some sort of a summing up. As positively as possible, state your initial impressions. What do you propose for treatment? For future meetings? What will you tell the parents?

Symptoms

- Adherence to fads of food, clothes, and style, including hair dyeing and body piercing
- Anxiety symptoms in boys or girls who experience late onset of puberty

- Impulsiveness
- Loneliness, sadness, suicidal ideation
- Overt aggression, destruction of property, theft, rule violation
- Poor school attendance (either truant or avoidant)
- Rebellion against authority (at its highest during these years)
- Somatic complaints

DSM-IV Diagnoses Most Likely to Be Made First at This Age

- Tourette's Disorder
- Chronic Motor or Vocal Tic Disorder, Transient Tic Disorder
- Generalized Anxiety Disorder
- Body Dysmorphic Disorder
- Pathological Gambling
- Circadian Rhythm Sleep Disorder, Delayed Sleep Phase Type

LATE ADOLESCENCE (15–21 YEARS)

Although we have stated the limit for late adolescence as age 21, in reality it can last much longer; the final leg of the march to independent life often extends through college and a graduate degree or two. But by that age (more or less), the personality of the adolescent has been established, and the inclination toward marriage and the bearing and rearing of children has been determined.

Aspects of Development

As adolescents move toward the completion of their education, they increasingly take on adult responsibilities and viewpoints. Of course, the exact time and sequence of these events can vary widely; about a third of young people are late bloomers. Depending on social milieu and parental mores, dating usually begins early in this time period; sexual activity is the norm by the end of the teen years. The young adult develops the capacity for mature love. Judgment improves, and as the end of the teens looms, the typical adolescent becomes serious about work or further education.

Obtaining Information

Older adolescents may present themselves for evaluation, without the immediate prospect of information from outside resources. As for any other patient, collateral information should be sought and evaluated whenever possible. The material covered, including the mental status examination, will be essentially the same as for an adult.

Symptoms

- Concerns about masturbation, other sexual behaviors
- Onset of realization of homosexuality (earlier for males than for females)

DSM-IV Diagnoses Most Likely to Be Made First at This Age

- All adult Axis I diagnoses except Dementia of the Alzheimer's Type and amnestic disorders
- Most personality disorders (Antisocial Personality Disorder is first diagnosable at age 18)

*A Variety of Interviews
with Children and Adolescents*

CHAPTER 4 | The Infant/Toddler Interview

PURPOSES AND GOALS OF THE INFANT/ TODDLER INTERVIEW

Most infants and toddlers referred for mental health evaluation *won't* meet criteria for a DSM-IV diagnosis (exceptions include the pervasive developmental disorders and some Mental Retardation syndromes). Yet clinicians need to feel comfortable and competent in evaluating these very young children, in order (1) to institute treatment early enough to avert permanent damage to a growing child, (2) to assess the potential risk of similar conditions in siblings and other children in a household, and (3) to identify problems in parents. Of course, infants and toddlers can only receive an adequate evaluation in the presence of their primary caregivers.

Most often, the primary caregivers interviewed will be one or both parents, grandparents, or foster parents. (As in other chapters, however, we use the term *parents* here for all primary caregivers.) Usually they are concerned about lack of developmental progress or a disturbance of regulation— significant problems with sleeping (the most common of all), crying, feeding, or limit setting. Many clinicians feel that such abnormalities foreshadow anxiety disorders, disorders of attachment, and pervasive developmental disorders. Clinicians need to help parents differentiate normal variances in development from more significant disturbances and disorders that can benefit from an intervention. It is also important to distinguish among the regulatory disorders (e.g., to differentiate autism from failure to thrive).

A mental health clinician evaluates an infant and parent with three goals in mind. One is to develop rapport with the parent; another is to obtain a clear picture of the nature of the symptoms and concerns. The third is to observe a variety of clues to the nature of interactions between the infant and parent:

- Does the infant clearly signal either pleasure or distress, making it easy for the parent to understand the communication?
- How sensitively and consistently does the parent respond to the infant's signals and bids for attention, as well as to expressions of pleasure and satisfaction?
- How does the parent handle the infant's expressions of frustration or lack of interest that may result from the interactions?
- When the infant cries, is the reason clear?
- Does the infant smile readily? Is the infant easily consolable?
- Will the infant engage the examiner?
- Does the infant show clear preferences for certain individuals and toys?
- Does the infant seem hypersensitive to loud noises, bright lights, or rapid transitions?
- Does the infant seem to have the temperamental characteristics of an "easy" baby, "difficult" baby, or "slow-to-warm up" baby (see the discussion of infant temperament in Chapter 3)?

The following interview with a toddler demonstrates many of these points. The material in **boldface** indicates some of the areas the interviewer tried to evaluate in this brief interview.

JOAN

Joan is a 14-month-old child who is just beginning to toddle. Her pediatrician has referred her because her mother is worried that she is excessively shy, especially with strangers. The referral note indicates no history of important problems during the pregnancy (poor nutrition, illnesses, use of drugs or alcohol) or perinatal period (postpartum depression, single-parent status, low family income).

Once they enter the examination room, the examiner sits on the floor and points to a set of toys placed nearby on the floor. Following this lead, the mother also sits on the floor. At the beginning of the interview, Joan sits quietly on her mother's lap, looking about cautiously; after a few moments, she allows herself to be placed on the floor. At first, the interviewer does not attempt to engage Joan directly, but stacks some blocks and observes her from a slight distance. Joan will be permitted to join in at her own pace.

INTERVIEWER: Hello, I'm Dr. V. You must be Ms. T. And this must be Joan. She is all dressed up for her outing. Let's begin by seeing how Joan is doing these days in terms of her development. It looks like she's walking.

*In an initial attempt to establish rapport and to indicate that observations are an important part of the interview, the interviewer acknowledges that Ms. T. has made a special effort in preparing her infant. The interviewer notes that Joan's **general development** is that of a normal, healthy-appearing child who shows no evidence of arrested development or failure to thrive. Neither does she have the **physical characteristics** of some Mental Retardation syndromes (such as Down's syndrome), or hand flapping or other unusual behaviors that could suggest a pervasive developmental disorder. Although shy at the outset, Joan is definitely engaged in the process. During this earliest part of the interview, the interviewer observes how secure Joan seems to feel while still on her mother's lap and how much stimulation her mother provides.*

MOTHER: She's started to walk, but she's afraid to let go. She's been cruising [i.e., walking while holding on to furniture] for a long time, but she won't just get up and walk. If you distract her, she'll sometimes take a few steps on her own, but even then she tries to hang on.

The mother immediately expresses a concern about Joan's developmental progress. Her anxiety is evident, both in the care she has taken with Joan's dress and in this initial expression of concern.

INTERVIEWER: She seems to be able to pull herself to a stand. So physically, she's right on schedule?

MOTHER: Yes.

*The interviewer observes and underscores Joan's developmentally appropriate behavior and strengths, commenting on the normal **motor development** (walking at a developmentally expected age, absence of hyperactivity). This strategy is an attempt to reassure the mother and to foster the therapeutic alliance, thereby shifting her focus from developmental failure and pathology to normality and progression.*

INTERVIEWER: And how about her schedule—does she sleep and awaken at regular times?

MOTHER: She eats regularly. She sleeps through the night, but sometimes she'll nap and sometimes she won't. The most she'll do is two naps about an hour and a half each, and most nights she screams when you put her to bed. She'll fall asleep, but she always screams.

In response to questions about her infant's routines, the mother, as before, emphasizes potential problems, not strengths. For the time being, the interviewer again steers away from possible pathology to focus on what the child is doing well. Note the following bridge to another topic, using the mother's own words. Questions about **eating** *and* **elimination** *form a part of every infant/toddler interview.*

INTERVIEWER: Tell me about her eating regularly.

MOTHER: She has cereal in the morning and a bottle and juice. She eats almost anything.

INTERVIEWER: Anything?

MOTHER: Pretty much anything that is finely chopped.

INTERVIEWER: Cookies?

MOTHER: I try not to give her any, but if I do, she likes them.

INTERVIEWER: Candy? [Meanwhile, Joan has pulled herself to a standing position, but still clings to her mother's shoulder and avoids eye contact with the interviewer. She has not begun to explore the age-appropriate toys on the floor.]

The interviewer is trying to see what limits the mother may be setting for the child. In the evaluation of any infant, there is the possibility that at least a part of the problem may relate to the nature of the **dyadic relationship** *between the child and parent. What is their quality of shared attention and intimacy? How well can the adult tolerate tension while skillfully returning the infant to a state of comfort?*

MOTHER: She doesn't get very much of it, but for Halloween she started chewing on the bowl of Halloween candy.

INTERVIEWER: How would you describe her temperamentally? Is she an easy child, or is she difficult?

MOTHER: I think she's a little bit of a mixture, because she's very intense and she's very stubborn. Her emotions are very intense.

INTERVIEWER: So when she cries, she really cries?

MOTHER: And if something happens that she doesn't like—like the other day she was trying to push the buttons on the TV, and she couldn't get them to do what she wanted—she just started screaming. She's not easily soothed. She's really happy except when she gets mad.

The interviewer notes the two adjectives stubborn *and* intense. *They may prove important to the assessment of Joan's* **temperament.** *But her mother quickly notes that Joan's* **basic mood** *is neither depressed nor anxious, but happy. It is important to determine whether infants can communicate their needs and feeling states clearly. Through her intense emotions, Joan seems to communicate readily; however, these intense emotions are viewed by her mother as a difficulty. Infants who are difficult to comfort often challenge the competence of their parents and trigger feelings of inadequacy.*

INTERVIEWER: Today she's cautious in a strange situation, but when she's at home, she's out there exploring?

MOTHER: At home, she's constantly exploring and moving around. She loves music; she'll start dancing.

INTERVIEWER: Really! Does she watch TV?

In a child so young, a formal assessment of intelligence will be pretty unreliable. Instead, the interviewer asks about such qualities as curiosity, persistence, attention, and task mastery, which may give clues to Joan's **cognitive development.**

MOTHER: Yes, there's a morning show for children. She'll stop whatever she's doing and watch.

INTERVIEWER: How is she at home? Does she play with toys?

MOTHER: Her favorite thing is to mess up the house. She'll take all the clothes out of the drawers and all the pots out of the cabinets and rummage through the trash, if she can.

INTERVIEWER: [To Joan] You're so curious at home, all the time playing and exploring things. What do you think I'm playing with here? Do you want to play with me? [At last, Joan timidly takes a block and puts it into a cup, imitating the interviewer. She seems about to engage. Almost immediately, her mother moves back, first a few inches. Then, over the next few minutes, she retreats further; she eventually gets up from the floor and sits in a nearby chair.]

Such interactions can provide an opportunity to evaluate how very young children play with toys, as well as how they respond to strangers, to direct gaze, and perhaps to being picked up. Engagement, mood, "leading versus following," creativity, spontaneity, motor skills, and attention span can all be assessed in the course of simple games. In play, the interviewer follows Joan's lead, placing blocks in a cup. This type of parallel play is less threatening for an inhibited, anxious child, such as Joan is reported to be. However, the mother's early, somewhat rapid withdrawal poses a potential threat. So the interviewer tries to maintain the tie to the mother by continuing to question her, which also serves to take the pressure of direct engagement off the child.

INTERVIEWER: Does she like books?

MOTHER: She loves books. She'll let me read a book to her at almost any time.

JOAN: [Babbles.]

INTERVIEWER: [To Joan] Everything is interesting to look at. [To the mother] Does she speak words yet?

The interviewer has observed Joan beginning to explore and, for the first time, comments directly to her from a slight distance, rather than interacting and possibly driving her away. Her babbling prompts questions about speech development. Even in a preverbal child, an interviewer should look for early evidence of **language difficulties,** *such as slow onset of speech sounds or (later) problems with pronunciation.*

MOTHER: Just a few—*Mama* and *dog.* She loves the dog. She fights with the dog for the same toys.

INTERVIEWER: Can I have that?

Now the interviewer attempts to interact with Joan by asking her for an object. The play engagement proceeds slowly, however, suggesting shyness and inhibition. If these are temperamental traits, these qualities may be strengths, even though the mother may view them as problems. However, if the infant's inhibitions reflect the mother's overcontrolling, anxious interactions, they probably reflect a relationship problem. A third possibility is that a strange, unfamiliar setting such as the clinician's office produces appropri-

ate caution. In this case, the infant should slowly begin to "warm up." The interviewer's task is to attempt to differentiate the several possible sources of Joan's caution.

INTERVIEWER: Do you think she'd play here all day?

This suggestion that Joan is beginning to enjoy herself is designed to reassure the mother; it may also reassure the infant through their mutual nonverbal social referencing.

MOTHER: She might.

INTERVIEWER: Is she in day care?

MOTHER: No, she's at home with her nanny.

INTERVIEWER: [To Joan] Well, let's see if you can put these blocks in the cup. [Beginning to interact with Joan more directly, the interviewer intentionally shifts positions to block Joan's view of her mother. Joan experiences the anxiety of separation and at once begins to cry vigorously, even though her mother remains seated nearby.]

Perhaps the interviewer has moved too quickly. However, evaluation sessions are usually time-limited, and some observation of "separation," even in a parent's presence, is important.

INTERVIEWER: She's been holding it in.

The interviewer comments that Joan has been a reluctant participant, holding in her anxiety about the evaluation. She has not fully engaged with the interviewer, bravely trying, but in fact beginning to cry almost immediately after the interviewer starts to interact with her directly. On the positive side, Joan's ability to **discriminate significant figures** *can be in no doubt.*

JOAN: [Cries loudly and inconsolably.]

MOTHER: Joan! It's OK, honey, you can play.

INTERVIEWER: As long as she is playing by herself, she's fine.

JOAN: [Ignores the sound of her name and continues to cry. Her mother holds her, tries to reassure her, and finally picks her up and rocks her, all to no avail.]

So far, the most striking features of this interview are the intensity of Joan's crying and, as her mother has described previously, her inconsolability. An older child of 2 or 3 might be testing limits by indicating behaviorally, "No, I won't listen." At Joan's 14 months, her selective attention and reluctance to engage suggest not defiance, but a need to control her separation anxiety by shutting out all novel stimuli and other sources of comfort, focusing exclusively on her mother.

MOTHER: It's OK, honey, it's OK. [The Mother continues rapidly rocking Joan, who cries harder and begins to kick and arch away, clearly resisting being comforted.]

At this point, the mother might excuse herself from the interview for a moment and comfort Joan in private. She might also comment on how difficult the interview is for Joan, or for both of them. Rather, eager to please the interviewer, she continues to rock mechanically and answer questions, seemingly oblivious to the child's needs. As a result, Joan's crying escalates.

Caregiver response to a very young child's needs is a core characteristic for any clinician evaluating an infant or toddler to observe. In this case, the mother seems almost agitated in her need to soothe Joan. At this developmental stage, stress with new settings, experiences, and strangers can be expected. But Joan's distress seems to be, at least in part, a response to her mother's affective signals.

INTERVIEWER: If you have strangers in your home, how is she?

MOTHER: It depends on who's there. She loves women about my age and other little kids. If she's with relatives she hasn't seen in a while, she's very slow to warm up, but if I'm there it's OK, and once she gets used to them she's OK.

Some infant symptoms are transient and often present only with a specific caregiver. When the other parent or a grandparent is present, an evaluator may see a different picture. In evaluations of infants and toddlers, the critical issue is to determine which behaviors are age-appropriate and normal (and thus represent transient parental concerns) and which are likely to cause significant future problems. For this reason, the interviewer wants to learn whether Joan's behavior occurs in multiple contexts and social situations. Despite the child's almost constant clinging and refusal to explore and engage, it is not clear how far these behaviors generalize to other settings. Later the interviewer will need to ask about Joan's interactions with her nanny.

INTERVIEWER: What about going into a grocery store—do you think she does OK then? [The interviewer begins playing with the blocks, clinking them together, but Joan continues to whimper. Although she has finally stopped crying, Joan is obviously not happy to return to the play.]

It is important to ask what the child's behaviors—and **parents' expecta-tions**—*are like in different settings. Even shopping in a grocery store can become an overstimulating outing. If parents expect behaviors that are not age-appropriate, they will judge a child's actions as inadequate.*

MOTHER: People come up to us and it doesn't bother her. I think she doesn't like women in their 70s with lots of makeup on. I think they scare her. She'll start crying. She's used to going out to stores, though.

INTERVIEWER: Ah, good. Well, perhaps we've done enough for today.

A brief session is often dictated by the limited attention span of a very young child who has tired. Several sessions over a period of weeks or longer may be needed for infants and toddlers, whereas a single session is often sufficient to evaluate older children and adolescents.

MOTHER: What do you think is wrong with her?

INTERVIEWER: I understand your concern about the intensity of her emotional responses. We saw that here today. We also saw how difficult she can be to soothe and how stubborn she can be, but I'm not sure yet that there is any-thing fundamentally wrong with Joan. Of course, we'll need to evaluate her some more to see how she acts in other settings and with other people. But there will be a few things we can talk about that could help you with her. [Mother and child get ready to leave. Joan brightens at the prospect. Despite her mother's encouragement, she refuses to wave goodbye.]

Although such a preliminary conclusion may bring relief to some parents, others may disagree with the clinician as to the seriousness of the behavior they observe in their infant or toddler. A parent should help determine whether a more extensive evaluation is indicated. Such an evaluation might include a home visit, a visit with the infant and father, and a talk with both parents without the infant. Often parents have different views of a child's problem and different approaches to resolving the behavior. The clinician should always listen attentively to parental concerns. For parents who do not wish a complete evaluation, reassurance should be framed in the context that they can come back in a few months if they are still concerned. In any event, time may yet prove this mother correct: Extremely shy young children often grow into older children who have anxiety disorders.

CHAPTER 5 | Play Interview with a 6-Year-Old Girl

As we have described in Chapter 2, examiners interviewing young children frequently use play material to enhance interaction; to observe the children's physical, emotional, and cognitive capacities; and to elicit areas of conflict or trauma. Providing distance from anxiety-provoking situations, play allows a child to communicate indirectly. Feelings can be expressed without direct verbal acknowledgment, though the interviewer needs to confirm suspected play communications with direct questions. However, when a child has been playing comfortably, it is likely that pretend feelings or experiences will match those the child actually experiences. Play sessions like the one presented here are most helpful in evaluating school-age (latency-age) children. However, toddlers, some early adolescents, and children of any age with developmental delays also respond positively to play techniques.

Some children move right in and begin to explore; others require time (or a nearby parent) to warm up to the interview situation. In either case, an amount of time suited to a child's own interactive style should be allowed for engagement.

At age 6, Susan was brought for evaluation because her teacher was concerned that she was bossy at school with her friends. The teacher was also concerned that Susan did not pay attention appropriately for her age, at times seeming lost in her own fantasy world. Susan's mother was also concerned about excessive sibling rivalry.

INTERVIEWER: Hi, you must be Susan. My name is Dr. Q. Did your mother tell you why you are here today? [Susan nods affirmatively.] What did she tell you?

SUSAN: That you could help me with my problem.

INTERVIEWER: What kind of problem do you have?

SUSAN: My mom says I don't get along with my sister, but I don't think so.

INTERVIEWER: Well, I hope I can help in understanding whether or not there is a problem. I like to play with children. It helps me to understand the problem. Do you like to draw?

Throughout, the interviewer uses smiles, eye contact, and other nonverbal signs (difficult to depict on the page) to communicate concern for Susan's comfort and well-being. Above all, a child should experience any clinical interview as both nonjudgmental and nonthreatening.

SUSAN: Yeah.

INTERVIEWER: Well, I've got some Magic Markers here. I'd like you to draw a picture of your family. Do you understand?

SUSAN: OK. [Using bright colors, Susan begins to draw figures, neatly and appropriately proportioned for her age. The interviewer observes and says little, except to ask who the figures represent and the names of the siblings and dog. Susan proudly shows off her spelling and writing abilities by printing the names boldly next to the figures.]

Younger children often don't really understand the meaning of the word understand. *To ascertain a child's understanding, an interviewer can ask for a repetition of the task. Susan, however, seems to have no such problem. (If Susan were an older child, the floor plan of where she lives might serve as an icebreaker.)*

INTERVIEWER: That's really excellent. Who taught you how to spell like that?

SUSAN: My mommy.

INTERVIEWER: Really? And who's this?

SUSAN: My dad.

INTERVIEWER: And who's that?

SUSAN: My sister, Denny, and my baby brother, Isaac.

INTERVIEWER: How do you spell Denny?

SUSAN: D-E-N-N-Y.

INTERVIEWER: How old are the three of you? Can you write your ages? [Susan writes the ages above the child figures in the drawing: 6 above her own name, 4 above Denny, and 6 months above baby Isaac.]

Here and in the next few moments, the interviewer tests several aspects of Susan's development by asking her to spell, to write, and to talk about her family.

INTERVIEWER: You have very good writing. And this is your dog? What kind of dog is Roscoe?

SUSAN: A yellow Lab.

INTERVIEWER: How old is Roscoe?

SUSAN: She's 4 or 5.

INTERVIEWER: Where does she sleep?

SUSAN: She's an outside dog—she stays in the back yard.

Names of siblings, friends, and animals provide anchor points to help to focus later discussions; they also help to make those discussions more real for the child. Information about relationships with animals often provides an indication of the child's capacity for empathy.

[All this while, Susan has been finishing her drawing, filling in colors and details of clothing. The interviewer has been observing, praising her skills and asking questions about her picture. Susan has readily answered.]

INTERVIEWER: I see you've put sunglasses on Denny.

SUSAN: 'Cause she likes them.

INTERVIEWER: She likes them? [Instead of offering more information about these sunglasses, Susan takes a new piece of paper and begins to draw more people.]

INTERVIEWER: And these are your friends?

SUSAN: Uh-huh.

INTERVIEWER: What are their names?

SUSAN: Melody, Vanessa, Johnny, Mara—these are twins.

INTERVIEWER: So there's one boy, Johnny?

SUSAN: Johnny and Mara are twins.

INTERVIEWER: Do any of them live near you? [Susan nods while continuing to draw.] They all live by you? [She nods again.] And do you go over to their house to play with them?

SUSAN: They come and play with me. And sometimes I go to their house.

INTERVIEWER: Can you draw a picture of your house?

SUSAN: Yeah.

INTERVIEWER: Has it been raining a lot at your house?

The interview is taking place during a time of local flooding; the interviewer is assessing Susan's awareness of current events.

SUSAN: Yeah.

INTERVIEWER: Have you had any flooding?

SUSAN: No.

INTERVIEWER: It looks like you like to draw. Do you draw in school, too?

SUSAN: Yeah.

INTERVIEWER: You're a good artist. Who else in your family draws?

SUSAN: Denny.

Using this medium, in just a few minutes the interviewer has obtained a lot of information about Susan's experience of her family, friends, and home environment.

INTERVIEWER: Do you get your own room, or are you sharing it?

SUSAN: I have to share my room with Denny and hear her snoring at night.

INTERVIEWER: And hear her snoring at night?

SUSAN: Yeah.

INTERVIEWER: Oh, my. What time does Denny go to bed?

SUSAN: The same time I do, 7:30.

INTERVIEWER: Then she falls asleep and starts snoring, and you can't get to sleep?

SUSAN: She starts snoring in the middle of the night and wakes me up.

INTERVIEWER: Do you guys have bunk beds, or are the beds next to each other?

SUSAN: Bunk beds.

INTERVIEWER: Who's on top?

SUSAN: Me.

The actual facts about who sleeps where and when are less important than ascertaining the overall thematic structure of the household and flavor of personal relationships. Note that the interviewer uses a number of closed-ended questions in this interview. Of course, by allowing a child to respond from the universe of personal experience, open-ended questions will yield information that is more valid; however, young children will give less information in free recall than will be the case with older children and adolescents.

INTERVIEWER: Where does Isaac sleep?

SUSAN: In the room next to ours. He has his own room.

INTERVIEWER: You said Roscoe sleeps outside. You never let her in the house?

SUSAN: No, never.

INTERVIEWER: And your mom and dad have a big bedroom. Is it next to yours?

SUSAN: It's next to Isaac's.

INTERVIEWER: [Pointing] What's that—a fence?

SUSAN: That's to keep Roscoe in the yard.

INTERVIEWER: If she gets out of the yard, does she run away?

SUSAN: Yeah. Then we have to try and catch her. We have to call her a thousand times.

INTERVIEWER: You said you have bunk beds—tell me more about your room.

The interviewer begins to explore the sibling relationship with Denny, who "lives" in the bed below and who snores. Asking Susan to describe her room helps the interviewer obtain a feeling for her surroundings.

SUSAN: Yeah.

INTERVIEWER: Do you have your own dresser and your own clothes? [Susan nods "yes."] And what about your toys? Where do you keep them?

SUSAN: In our cupboard. We share them.

INTERVIEWER: You share?

SUSAN: Our room is always a mess.

INTERVIEWER: Messy? And does your mom say, "Clean up your room, girls"?

SUSAN: Yeah.

INTERVIEWER: And who cleans it up.

SUSAN: Me! Denny starts playing a game and I say "No, Denny, we have to clean up, not play." And *she* says, "But I want to play, not clean up."

INTERVIEWER: She doesn't obey you very well, does she?

The interviewer repeatedly comments on what Susan says. Such comments show children that they can talk to adult professionals about what bothers them and that they will be listened to.

SUSAN: No, she doesn't.

INTERVIEWER: Do you ever beat her up a little bit?

SUSAN: No.

INTERVIEWER: No. Does she ever hit you?

SUSAN: Yeah, a lot.

INTERVIEWER: She hits you and takes things away from you?

SUSAN: Uh-huh.

INTERVIEWER: How does that make you feel?

The interviewer already knows much of this material, but studies have shown that children themselves are the most accurate reporters of their own feelings, moods, and inner experiences. On the other hand, parents and teachers give more accurate reports of children's behavior.

SUSAN: I don't know, kinda mad. But maybe, not very . . .

INTERVIEWER: Since you're the oldest, I guess you have to set a good example. You have to behave yourself and not get into any trouble?

By framing the question as "I guess," the interviewer provides an opportunity for Susan to answer negatively.

SUSAN: I do get in trouble.

INTERVIEWER: What happens?

SUSAN: I keep yelling at her if she doesn't mind me. She *never* stops playing.

INTERVIEWER: And then do you get in trouble, or does she get into trouble?

SUSAN: We both get into trouble.

INTERVIEWER: Well, here's an idea. Pretend like this is your sister and I'm going to be you, OK? I'm going to be playing with these toys here and behaving myself and just having a little tea party here, and what does your sister do? [While continuing to talk, the interviewer sets two teacups on saucers and pours pretend tea into the cups. Susan immediately takes her assigned role as little sister.]

Giving Susan the opportunity to play-act Denny may indicate how "pesky" and unmanageable her sister really is. Roll-playing, often with dolls or hand puppets is often useful to help children divulge material that they cannot or will not express in other ways. In this case, the interviewer uses information obtained earlier to set up themes of play.

SUSAN: Oh, I want to play with you, too.

INTERVIEWER: No, go away. I want to play with my . . . Hey, you can't hit me. What are you doing? I might just hit you right back. Now you behave yourself. Do you hear me?

In the role of the younger sister, Denny, Susan immediately becomes combative. The interviewer, in the role of the older sister, threatens justifiable retaliation (Susan has previously said that she never hits Denny). The interaction, however, suggests two possibilities: (1) Denny is quite provocative and immediately invokes physical altercation; (2) Susan carries a significant amount of pent-up anger toward her sister. Of course, these possibilities may coexist.

SUSAN: Who cares?

INTERVIEWER: Who cares? *I* care. I'm having a tea party here. You want a cup of tea?

Susan continues in the role of the bratty younger sister. The interviewer switches gears from threats to an opportunity for joining in. The switch allows "Denny" to start playing cooperatively. Does Susan's version of Denny have this capacity?

SUSAN: Yeah.

INTERVIEWER: OK. Here. But clean up after yourself. Don't make a mess.

SUSAN: Uh-oh, I spilled my tea. Can you go get me a washcloth?

"Denny" does indeed switch, but the interviewer immediately throws out a challenge, which "Denny" creatively meets with another immediate provocation.

INTERVIEWER: Why don't you go get your own washcloth?

SUSAN: 'Cause I don't know where Mom hides them.

INTERVIEWER: OK, here's a washcloth. Clean up your mess. Thank you very much, now go away and stop bothering me.

SUSAN: OK. [Giggles.]

Susan is obviously involved and enjoying the game, which may well reflect real-life interactions with her younger sister.

INTERVIEWER: You want another cup of tea?

SUSAN: Yeah. I'm going to play Barbies, though.

INTERVIEWER: But they're *my* Barbies. I don't want you to play with my Barbies.

SUSAN: I have my own under my bed.

INTERVIEWER: Well, don't play with mine, all right?

SUSAN: OK.

Notice how Susan has now taken control of the theme. The interviewer has suggested the tea party, but Susan wants to play with dolls. The interviewer has tried to generate a conflict between the sisters, but Susan has deflected an argument by stating that she has her own dolls. As the game progresses, the interviewer will notice whether Susan insists on maintaining control or is willing to share.

INTERVIEWER: [In an adult voice] Do you want to play with a girl Barbie or a boy Barbie?

In the written transcript, it is hard to keep in mind who is playing whom, but as Susan and the interviewer get into their respective roles, their play is likely to reflect the everyday interactions of these two sisters. The interviewer changes to an adult voice to provide distance momentarily from the pretend situation. This is an attempt to realign the play roles according to Susan's preference.

SUSAN: Will you play with my Barbies with me, please, please?

INTERVIEWER: Oh, you are such a pest, Denny, but I will play with you a little while, all right? Oh, this is a lovely Barbie. Let's play house.

SUSAN: I'm the mommy.

Now Susan changes from the role of Denny to that of Mommy. In three words, the interviewer makes the transition.

INTERVIEWER: I'm the sister.

SUSAN: [As Mommy] You go clean up your room!

INTERVIEWER: [As Denny] Do I have to, Mommy?

"Mommy" becomes a little bossy, both in tone and in direction. The interviewer's "Denny" pouts and acts resistant.

SUSAN: Yeah. Now.

INTERVIEWER: How come? Can't I just play a little while longer? I'll do it later, all right?

SUSAN: An hour longer. In an hour you've got to take a bath.

INTERVIEWER: I hate baths.

SUSAN: You got dirty in the mud yesterday.

INTERVIEWER: Yeah, but I'll take a bath tomorrow.

SUSAN: You still need to make your bed—now!

INTERVIEWER: Well, if I make my bed all muddy, Susan will clean it up for me.

SUSAN: She won't have to clean it up. She's going to school.

INTERVIEWER: No! I don't want her to go to school. I want her to play with me.

The theme is control, with the interviewer playing the role of the resistant, entitled baby sister, attempting to evaluate the kinds of reprisal that "Mommy" might invoke. We note that "Mommy" and "Susan" appear understanding, patient, and benevolent. From this play interaction, compromise and resolution, rather than physical punishment and yelling, seem the preferred modes of interaction in this household.

SUSAN: I'm sorry, she must go to school. Goodbye.

INTERVIEWER: Goodbye, Susan, have a nice day at school.

SUSAN: Now you go play and take a bath.

INTERVIEWER: Oh, boy! I love this bathtub. I'm going to make a big mess in here. I'm going to splash around and make a mess.

SUSAN: Did I hear you say *mess*?

INTERVIEWER: Nope.

SUSAN: You're going to clean that up.

INTERVIEWER: I'm not going to clean it up, 'cause I'm having too much fun playing in here.

SUSAN: Your brother's coming in to take a bath with you.

Again, "Mommy" is not provoked into an argument by "Denny's" challenges, but shifts focus by introducing the baby brother. In this way, she avoids a confrontation over "Denny's" mess.

INTERVIEWER: OK, but I don't like him. He's such a baby. He put soap in my mouth.

SUSAN: You can behave, or *I'm* going to put soap in your mouth.

Here, for the first time, "Mommy" threatens retaliation if any harm comes to the baby.

INTERVIEWER: No, I'm behaving, but he's bothering me.

SUSAN: He's doing nothing except playing there in the tub.

INTERVIEWER: He's crying, he's screaming, he's bothering me.

SUSAN: You get out now. Get out now!

INTERVIEWER: OK, Mommy.

The theme of Susan's younger siblings being irritating and provocative is constant, fueled by the interviewer's role playing that supports sibling rivalry. However, Susan as Mommy (previously as Denny) could have changed themes or tone. At the end, "Mommy" finally becomes firm and insistent.

INTERVIEWER: Mom?

"Denny" starts again. The interviewer and Susan are really involved in a life drama. The interviewer is trying to push the limits, so as to observe Susan's responses as she play-acts them through the behavior of her younger sister.

SUSAN: What?

INTERVIEWER: I'm hungry.

SUSAN: You already had dinner. No more snacks.

INTERVIEWER: Oh, please?

SUSAN: No.

INTERVIEWER: Couldn't I have a little snack?

SUSAN: No.

INTERVIEWER: Please? I'm hungry. How about a cookie?

SUSAN: You can have carrots.

Another demonstration of patience and compromise.

INTERVIEWER: No, I don't want carrots. I hate carrots. I want cookies.

SUSAN: No sweets after dinner!

INTERVIEWER: Oh, please? I promise to brush my teeth.

SUSAN: You'll have to brush 'em 14 times.

INTERVIEWER: Fourteen? OK, just give me one cookie and a little milk.

SUSAN: Here you go.

INTERVIEWER: You threw my cookie in the bath. It's all wet. Help! Let me out of here. I'm clean. Help! Help!

SUSAN: OK, you can get out. Go to bed—you're being mean.

INTERVIEWER: But I'm not tired. You told me I could stay up late tonight.

SUSAN: Well, it's 9:00.

INTERVIEWER: No, I want to watch TV. One more program.

SUSAN: OK, but that's it.

> *The foregoing drama reflects conflict and resolution, provocation and compromise—interactions typical of everyday family life. Struggles centering around eating, bedtimes, and cleanliness are universal and often serve as a focus for play interactions. In more disturbed children, violence becomes a fixed theme early in the play. Profanity, sexualized interaction, catastrophic accidents, and risk-taking behaviors are more ominous signs of serious psychopathology.*

INTERVIEWER: I don't want to go to bed. You know why?

SUSAN: Why?

INTERVIEWER: Because my sister snores.

SUSAN: Susan?

INTERVIEWER: Yeah, Susan. She snores and I don't want to go in there.

> *In reality, Denny snores, but Susan accepts the switch and continues to respond as Mommy.*

SUSAN: I'll set you up in the baby's room.

INTERVIEWER: Thank you very much, but I won't go in there, either.

SUSAN: All right.

INTERVIEWER: I'd like to come in your room, Mommy.

SUSAN: OK. Bedtime.

INTERVIEWER: Guess we'll sleep next to each other.

SUSAN: [Makes a snoring sound.]

INTERVIEWER: Oh, gosh! I can't sleep here. There's so much noise. Stop snoring!

SUSAN: Sorry, that's the only thing I can do to sleep.

INTERVIEWER: I'm scared. It's like a thunderstorm.

SUSAN: I'm not a thunderstorm.

INTERVIEWER: You *are* a thunderstorm! [Changes to an adult voice.] When you snore, do you know what that means?

SUSAN: What?

INTERVIEWER: Sometimes it means that you have a stuffy nose. And sometimes it means that when you sleep, you breathe through your mouth instead of your nose.

SUSAN: Children, put your stuff away.

Either the interviewer's educational intervention is premature or the play is too much fun. Susan switches to cleaning up, rather than going to sleep.

INTERVIEWER: Mom, you do it. We don't want to clean up. You clean up.

SUSAN: I'm gonna call Dad in on this.

INTERVIEWER: [As Dad] You kids clean that up and stop fighting.

The interviewer takes on the role of Dad, who speaks in an authoritative tone. By bringing Dad into the play, Susan has expanded the cast of characters, and the interviewer jumps on board to see whether any new information can be obtained. Such expansions and switches are common with children who have active imaginations and can maintain their orientation and focus. Such flexibility is not usually characteristic of retarded, psychotic, or severely anxious or depressed children.

INTERVIEWER: Here, have a cookie. Do you want some juice?

SUSAN: Yeah.

INTERVIEWER: Well, here's your juice. Now you kids turn the light off and go to sleep. I'm not coming in here again. You hear me?

SUSAN: OK.

INTERVIEWER: Good night. And no snoring!

SUSAN: [Makes snoring sounds.]

INTERVIEWER: What did I say? No snoring!

SUSAN: Sorry, Dad, I just couldn't help it.

INTERVIEWER: Denny, I'm telling you. You stop snoring, or you're gonna have to sleep outside with Roscoe.

SUSAN: Susan did it.

> *By accepting blame, is Susan here being protective of her sister, who is being threatened by "Dad," or is she showing how Denny shifts blame upon her? Notice the fluidity of the role playing as Susan and the interviewer move in and out of all four family member roles.*

INTERVIEWER: Are you snoring, Susan?

SUSAN: Yes, but I'll try not to. Can I stay up a little later?

INTERVIEWER: No, it's a school night. You've got to go to school tomorrow, and you need your sleep.

SUSAN: Who says I can't?

INTERVIEWER: Dad says you can't. You want to fight with Dad?

SUSAN: I'm going to go get Mom.

INTERVIEWER: [As Mom] Who's calling me? What's the matter, Susan?

SUSAN: Go get Dad and tell him I want to stay up a little later.

INTERVIEWER: [As Mom] She wants to stay up a little later. [As Dad] Well, I said she has to go to bed. Now, who's the boss? [As Mom] I told her earlier that she could stay up a little later. [As Dad] All right.

SUSAN: Thanks, Mom.

INTERVIEWER: You can stay up a little later, but just a few minutes.

SUSAN: A few minutes. OK, Mom. I want a cookie. Where are they?

INTERVIEWER: It's too late for cookies now, honey. No more snacks now. It's time to get ready for bed.

SUSAN: Now?

INTERVIEWER: Is that all right?

SUSAN: OK.

INTERVIEWER: Good night, girls. No snoring. I'll see you in the morning, and sleep well. I'll give you each a kiss good night.

As with the other play sequences, bedtime has ended with everyone consoled and asleep. Negotiation and compromise have largely resolved the control and limit-setting issues. Susan recognizes the end of the sequence, but wants to continue to play.

SUSAN: Let's play something else.

INTERVIEWER: OK. Now, let's play school. What's your teacher's name?

SUSAN: Mrs. G.

INTERVIEWER: Mrs. G.? This is Mrs. G. [Takes another doll and plays the role of the teacher with yet another voice.] Well, good morning, Susan. It's nice to see you.

SUSAN: [Yawns.]

INTERVIEWER: Ooooh. You're very tired. I bet you stayed up late last night, huh? You're supposed to go to bed early.

The interviewer maintains an authoritarian demeanor. Susan attempts to stand up for herself, but the interviewer persists. Ultimately, as before, she retreats from confrontation.

SUSAN: I'm not tired.

INTERVIEWER: You were taking a nap. I'll have to tell your mom to get you to bed earlier. Did you do your homework?

SUSAN: Unh-unh. I was sleeping.

INTERVIEWER: Well, we're having a spelling test today. Are you ready for a spelling test?

SUSAN: I think so.

INTERVIEWER: I'm going to pick a hard word. How do you spell *father*?

The interviewer is attempting to assess some of Susan's cognitive skills; with young children, this is often best done in a play context. The chosen word may be too hard for most 6-year-olds, though some children memorize it early.

SUSAN: F-A-T-H-E-R.

INTERVIEWER: You get an A. Very good.

SUSAN: [Pleased] Ooooh!

INTERVIEWER: Now we're going to have math.

SUSAN: M-A-T-H. [Giggles.]

INTERVIEWER: Do you know what 7 plus 6 is?

SUSAN: No.

INTERVIEWER: Do you know what 3 plus 1 is?

The interviewer starts with a task that is difficult, then follows with a more age- and grade-appropriate problem. Other clinicians might start with easier problems to build confidence.

SUSAN: Four.

INTERVIEWER: Do you know what 6 plus 2 is?

SUSAN: Eight.

INTERVIEWER: Very good. Do you want to learn how to play Squiggles? If I make a squiggle like that, can you make a picture with my squiggle?

The Squiggles game, first described by David Winnicott, is an attempt at projective testing with young children who like to draw. The child or the examiner draws a squiggly line or shape; the other adds to it, making it a meaningful drawing. After a few turns each, the child is asked to "tell a story" linking the squiggles together. If possible, the examiner's completed squiggles should try to reflect some of the child's presenting conflict areas.

INTERVIEWER: Great. A flower. Now you make a squiggle and I'll draw a picture. [Susan complies.] You made a hard one. [The interviewer turns the paper on which her squiggle is drawn around and around, trying to visualize a completed drawing, then completes the squiggle.]

Like most children, Susan has grasped the concept easily and appears to enjoy the game.

SUSAN: What's that?

INTERVIEWER: I drew a horse. So what do we have? A flower, then a horse. Now it's my turn. [In all, Susan and the interviewer draw a flower, a horse, a tree, a lady with curly hair, diamonds, and a house with smoke coming out of the chimney. Susan's mother enters the room before they get to the storytelling part of the game.]

INTERVIEWER: Well, Susan, I see we've run out of time. We have to stop playing. Thank you for coming. Goodbye.

CHAPTER 6 | Play Interview with a 7-Year-Old Boy

It is especially challenging to obtain meaningful information from a child who has a disturbance of emotion or behavior. It requires simultaneously following the child's lead; trying to establish and maintain meaningful engagement; and obtaining information that relates to distractibility versus attentiveness, focus versus impulsiveness, cooperation versus control, curiosity versus inhibition, rigidity versus flexibility, and engagement versus isolation. The use of age-appropriate play materials often facilitates the process.

The play interview that follows illustrates the great difficulty even an experienced interviewer can have in maintaining a relationship with a challenging patient. In the comments, we note in **boldface** 10 important qualities that should be observed in any child interview: activity level; attention span and distractibility; communication facility; coordination; frustration tolerance; impulsiveness; mannerisms and other peculiarities of physical motion; mood state; response to limit setting; and response to praise.

Norman is a 7-year-old boy who has been a patient in a day treatment program for over 2 years. Initially, following his parents' divorce, he experienced irrational fears that he would be abandoned. The present referral has stemmed from tics, hyperactivity, distractibility, and aggression not adequately managed by Ritalin. His working diagnosis is Attention-Deficit/Hyperactivity Disorder comorbid with Tourette's Disorder.

Curious and extremely active, Norman enters the examination room unaccompanied. (Neither parent is present, since he has come from his day treatment classroom.) On the floor is a bucket of toys, which immediately attracts his attention. At first, he darts from toy to toy and explores the room.

INTERVIEWER: Hi, Norman. I'm Dr. S. Come and look at some of the things I've got here.

The interviewer, noting Norman's high **activity level** *at once, begins with a smile and an invitation to explore and play with the play materials. These are efforts to put the child at ease.*

NORMAN: What's this—costumes?

INTERVIEWER: I'll show you. This one is a puppet.

NORMAN: What?

INTERVIEWER: Put your hand in it.

NORMAN: [Sniffs the puppet.] Smells funny. What's this? [He removes a doll from the toy pail.]

INTERVIEWER: It does?

NORMAN: Yes.

Norman does not take to the puppet in the usual way. Rather, he sniffs it (a mannerism?) and immediately goes to another toy. The interviewer is unable to sustain his interest and thus shifts with Norman to the next object.

INTERVIEWER: What does he look like?

NORMAN: Looks like a Barbie doll.

INTERVIEWER: Except he's lost a shoe. [Norman drops the doll and keeps moving on to new toys. He asks a barrage of questions about each of the items he has handled: "What's this?" "What does this do?" "How do you use this?" However, he doesn't really listen to the responses of the interviewer. Finally, Norman impulsively picks up a camera, then darts to the videotaping microphone and pulls at the wires. Now the interviewer sets limits and asks Norman not to touch the microphone. Norman responds by expressing his desire to leave the session. After the interviewer urges him "to play for a little while longer because I want to play with you," Norman returns to the toy box but remains focused on the microphone.]

Norman's **impulsiveness** *and* **short attention span** *are plainly evident in this sequence of events, along with his need for (and resistance to)* **limit setting.**

NORMAN: What's the microphone for?

INTERVIEWER: So that people can hear what we're saying when they watch the movie. Didn't your teacher take a movie of you? Don't touch it, please. No, you have to leave it.

NORMAN: Yeah.

INTERVIEWER: Was it a videotape?

NORMAN: [Turns his attention back to the toy camera.] I wish there was film in here. How to you open this?

INTERVIEWER: Do you like cameras?

NORMAN: Yeah. How do you open it?

INTERVIEWER: Here. [Opens back of camera.]

NORMAN: I like cameras. Ready? [He snaps the shutter and then runs to the microphone mounted on the wall, bends down, and shouts into it.] Are you ready?

INTERVIEWER: [Attempts to distract Norman from the microphone.] There's no film in the camera. Do you like to draw? Do you like to draw pictures?

NORMAN: No film? Well, let's get some film.

INTERVIEWER: Well, we can't right now. We could get some film some other time. Please leave the microphone. Let's see what we've got here.

NORMAN: We can talk in this. Are you ready? [Shouts into the microphone.] I'm going to go back to my class now.

INTERVIEWER: Well, I just wanted to play with you for a little while. Look at all these things. [The interviewer dumps the container of toys onto the floor.]

Norman's **distractibility** *is shown in his attraction to the recording equipment. He resists interacting directly with the interviewer and repeatedly threatens to end the session and return to the classroom. The interviewer keeps trying to engage him with toys.*

INTERVIEWER: Let's see, a doctor and a nurse. What else do we have here?

NORMAN: Why are they so mad?

INTERVIEWER: Are they mad?

NORMAN: Uh-huh. [Whispers something.]

INTERVIEWER: Well, we'll go back in a few minutes, all right? I want to play with you for a little while.

Several times now, Norman has made it clear that he wants to go back to his class. It is not unusual for a child to show resistance early in an interview; some children become frozen with anxiety, whereas others will cry and refuse to let go of a parent's hand. Persistence and considerable ingenuity may be needed to keep a child in the room long enough to become engaged.

Norman's question about the neutral doll's being mad may be an indication of **affect***. Is he annoyed that there is no film in the camera? That he can't touch the microphone wires? That he can't leave the playroom to return to his classroom? Before the interviewer can respond further, Norman veers off in yet another direction.*

NORMAN: What's this?

INTERVIEWER: Oh, it's one of those things that doctors use. What do you call it?

NORMAN: A needle. Why do people have to have a shot?

INTERVIEWER: Because they're sick. Norman, did you ever get a shot?

NORMAN: Ready? [He turns off the light.]

INTERVIEWER: No, leave the light on. Can you put it back on? Can you put it back on, please?

NORMAN: We don't need a light.

INTERVIEWER: Yes, we need the light. [Firmly] Please turn the lights back on for me! Thank you.

Questions about medical interventions fail to engage Norman, who now runs off and begins to turn the light switch on and off. Despite the goal of allowing a child relatively wide behavioral latitude as a diagnostic measure, it happens with some frequency that **limits** *must be firmly set—even to the point of physically restraining a child who hits or damages furniture or equipment.*

INTERVIEWER: [Turns back to the dolls.] They're sick. You're going to have to give them a shot. All right? Do you want to do it? You want to be the doctor? I hope he doesn't cry. Don't cry, little boy, because you're sick. Where should I give it to him, in his arm?

NORMAN: I'll take his picture.

INTERVIEWER: Oh, you're going to take a picture?

NORMAN: Yep. See?

INTERVIEWER: Take another one! I'd better take his clothes off.

NORMAN: He's sick?

INTERVIEWER: I have to find his arm. Where . . .

NORMAN: How do you know he's sick?

INTERVIEWER: I don't know. Let's make up a story. What's wrong with him? [By this time, the interviewer is lying almost full length on the floor, trying to engage the child in play.]

The interviewer again suggests "illness" in an attempt to solicit identification from Norman and possibly to gauge his capacity for empathy.

NORMAN: I don't know. [Norman now takes up a transformer (see Chapter 2, p. 42), which he manipulates into its several identities.]

INTERVIEWER: Norman, what's that?

NORMAN: What is it? I don't know. What is it?

NORMAN: How does it work?

INTERVIEWER: Can you make it change shape?

NORMAN: Yeah.

INTERVIEWER: Oh, you're good, Norman. You know how that works?

NORMAN: I know how it works.

INTERVIEWER: Great! Can you show me?

NORMAN: [Does so, and continues to play with the transformer.]

Part of an experienced interviewer's "stock in trade" is allowing a child to demonstrate expertise at operating a piece of equipment, which promotes a sense of mastery and boosts the child's ego. The technique also works well when the child brings in a show-and-tell item, embodying a scientific princi-ple or historical event that can be "taught" to the interviewer. **Responding to praise,** *for the first time Norman begins to answer questions, all the time forming and reforming the transformer.*

INTERVIEWER: Norman, how do you feel today?

NORMAN: Um, fine.

INTERVIEWER: Are you happy?

NORMAN: Yeah.

INTERVIEWER: Good. Do you feel sad?

NORMAN: Yeah.

INTERVIEWER: Do you feel sad today?

NORMAN: I don't feel sad today. I feel happy because . . .

INTERVIEWER: Because what? Because you're here?

The interviewer suspects that Norman may not be pleased to be involved in the interview, so attempts to elicit a negative reaction, but is surprised to get a positive one.

NORMAN: Yeah.

INTERVIEWER: Did you want to come here yesterday?

NORMAN: Yeah.

INTERVIEWER: Yeah! Hey, you're doing great with that transformer. [After considerable discussion about the transformer, yielding much praise, the interviewer attempts to draw Norman's attention to some more meaningful human figures—doll figures in the doll house—but is once again rebuffed. Ultimately, a pair of scissors and a folded piece of paper turn the trick.]

INTERVIEWER: Do you know how to cut with these scissors? I was going to make a pattern.

NORMAN: Yeah.

INTERVIEWER: You know about the Mario Brothers?

NORMAN: Is that what you're making? Is that Mario?

INTERVIEWER: Yeah.

NORMAN: Where's his legs?

INTERVIEWER: What's the other guy's name? Uh, do you remember what his name is? The other guy? I'll make him, too. [The interviewer creates patterns in the folded piece of paper with the scissors and shows the patterns to Norman. Over the next several minutes, their play centers around the theme of various Nintendo characters—Mario, Luigi, and the Princess.]

Child mental health professionals must remain current in children's popular games, music, and cult heroes.

INTERVIEWER: What do you think?

NORMAN: I don't know. Is he happy?

INTERVIEWER: He's a little angry.

The interviewer is attempting to match Norman's feelings.

NORMAN: Why?

INTERVIEWER: I don't know. Somebody isn't doing what he wants to do.

NORMAN: Why?

INTERVIEWER: And they don't want to play with him.

NORMAN: They don't want to play with him?

INTERVIEWER: Yeah. But the Princess, now, she wants to play with him. [While the interviewer cuts the Princess out of the paper, Norman continues to play with the transformer. But he is engaged in the play theme.]

INTERVIEWER: This is a very fancy Princess.

NORMAN: Is she happy?

INTERVIEWER: Yes. But not Mario and not his brother, Cuomo. I think his brother's name is Cuomo.

NORMAN: I think it's Luigi.

INTERVIEWER: Luigi! That's his name, not Cuomo!

NORMAN: Yeah, Luigi.

INTERVIEWER: What a good memory you have, Norman. Mario and Luigi are not going to play with the Princess. What level is she locked up on?

NORMAN: The Dragon level.

INTERVIEWER: Yeah, the Dragon level. And . . .

NORMAN: Why is she locked up on the Dragon level?

INTERVIEWER: Ah, because somebody evil has kidnapped her.

The interviewer is pushing the themes of good and evil, of anger, and of separation and reunion. Norman finally seems actively engaged in this plot. The Nintendo figures are well known to him.

NORMAN: Yeah?

INTERVIEWER: And locked her up.

NORMAN: Yeah.

INTERVIEWER: And Mario and Cuomo—what's his name?

NORMAN: Luigi.

INTERVIEWER: Mario and Luigi have to rescue her. But there's a lot of enemies in the way. Right?

NORMAN: Right.

INTERVIEWER: I think there's all those things that try to come down and shoot them and bomb them. Can you help to get the Princess out?

NORMAN: Yeah

INTERVIEWER: And save her? You cut it out. I can't do it.

NORMAN: You can do it.

INTERVIEWER: I can't do it. I did it crooked. You do it. Just do this side.

NORMAN: I'll try.

INTERVIEWER: Try to save her. [Norman finally takes the scissors and begins to cut the paper.]

INTERVIEWER: Yeah, you're a good cutter. The Princess is great! [The interviewer puts the cutout Princess into the doll house. Norman crawls over to the table on which the doll house is standing and stands up. Each takes a toy figure.]

The interviewer finally has Norman playing in an unstructured, fantasy mode. Now Norman introduces a theme.

NORMAN: Yeah! I'll be the kid.

INTERVIEWER: You be the kid. And I'll be what?

NORMAN: The teacher. Time to get up for school!

INTERVIEWER: What's the kid's name?

NORMAN: Johnny. But there's something flying up in the sky!

INTERVIEWER: What is it? What is it Johnny. What's flying?

NORMAN: A space ship. [He reintroduces the transformer into the play, zooming it around.]

INTERVIEWER: Ah! Is it a friendly one?

NORMAN: Yeah.

INTERVIEWER: Oh, good. Then he can come into our house. [Taking the part of the mother, the interviewer now talks in a play-act voice. Norman is actively engaged in playing with the doll house.]

NORMAN: What's the spaceman called?

INTERVIEWER: Zorro.

NORMAN: I am a nice robot. [He talks in a mechanical, spaceman voice.]

INTERVIEWER: Thank you for coming into our house. Did you bring anything with you from outer space, Zorro?

NORMAN: Yeah. A race car.

INTERVIEWER: A race car?

NORMAN: That's right.

INTERVIEWER: What's the matter, Zorro?

NORMAN: Something happened to me.

INTERVIEWER: Are you broken?

NORMAN: Broken? I'm turning myself into a spaceship.

INTERVIEWER: Oh.

NORMAN: I'm getting him into a spaceship. You can help me.

INTERVIEWER: I'll try. Do you want to make a rocket ship like that?

NORMAN: Could you fix him?

INTERVIEWER: Oh, I'll try. You know, this is so hard for me to do. You're very good at it—I don't know how to exactly do it. It goes right in here, doesn't it?

Although Norman is now involved, mechanical manipulation of the transformer, in a manner inappropriate for his age, dominates his interest. His verbal responses are generally limited to brief, single sentences; clearly, his **ability to communicate** *is restricted. It is noteworthy that for the first time, he has asked for help. However, with time running out, the interviewer tries to switch to information gathering. This is met with some (albeit limited) cooperation from Norman.*

INTERVIEWER: Do you remember my name?

NORMAN: Yeah, you're Dr. S. [He turns the transformer back into his rocket ship.]

Two activities are going on simultaneously as the interviewer attempts to persuade Norman to cooperate in further tests of cognitive and motor skills.

INTERVIEWER: Do you remember Dr. C.?

NORMAN: Yeah, I do. Do you? I have to leave now. I'm going to space. Bye.

INTERVIEWER: Oh, please don't go. Come back again.

NORMAN: I will, I promise. After supper.

INTERVIEWER: [To doll] Johnny, Zorro went away. Now it's time to get into the school bus and go to school.

NORMAN: I have to go back now.

INTERVIEWER: Oh, I'm going to miss you. Are you going back to outer space?

NORMAN: We're there now.

INTERVIEWER: Oh, Johnny, we're going to miss Zorro so much. [Norman is flying the spaceship around the room, but is actively playing with the interviewer.]

The theme of leaving and reunion remains prominent. Norman has picked up on the interviewer's cue that the time of the session is nearing an end.

INTERVIEWER: You're back. Are you back from outer space?

NORMAN: Yep.

INTERVIEWER: Hooray! Zorro's back!

NORMAN: Can I go back?

INTERVIEWER: Go back where?

NORMAN: My class.

INTERVIEWER: OK. Can you do one thing for me? Do you know how to jump? Can you jump off this?

NORMAN: No.

INTERVIEWER: Try it.

NORMAN: No. I'd just like to go back. [He begins to fly the transformer back into space.]

INTERVIEWER: Just give it a try for me. [The interviewer puts away the materials, then gets up onto the first step of the stair climber and jumps down.]

*In this and subsequent tests, Norman's **physical development and coordination** appear to be at a level a year or two younger than his chronological age of 7.*

NORMAN: OK.

INTERVIEWER: Oh, you're going to do it from the top step. Oh, boy, you're a good jumper. OK, wait a minute. Do this. Can you hop on one foot like that?

NORMAN: I'll do it from up here.

INTERVIEWER: No, just do it down here. Good. Now do the other foot.

NORMAN: Ah, I can't do that one.

INTERVIEWER: Oh, you can't?

NORMAN: If I jump on that foot [pointing to his left], can I hold on to something?

INTERVIEWER: Here, hold onto me. OK, can you catch? Here comes the ball. Put the transformer down for a minute. Now throw it to me.

NORMAN: [Misses the ball and picks it up.]

INTERVIEWER: Good. Try it again. You've got it. Do it again. Whoa, here comes one. Oh good, you catch great. And you throw great. Once more.

NORMAN: [Drops it.] We're all done.

INTERVIEWER: All right. We're all done. Do you know what I'm going to do, Norman?

NORMAN: What?

INTERVIEWER: I'm going to get some film, and I'll bring my camera back and let you take some pictures. But we have to stop now.

NORMAN: Yeah.

INTERVIEWER: OK? Let's go see what your class is doing.

NORMAN: No, I want to stay here.

INTERVIEWER: Not now. We have to stop.

NORMAN: We can't stop right now, 'cause we're playing.

INTERVIEWER: I know, but I need to stop now because we don't have any more time. But you did a good job.

NORMAN: No, no, no, no.

INTERVIEWER: Come on.

NORMAN: Let go of my hand.

INTERVIEWER: Thank you for coming. [Exits, with Norman in tow.]

In the space of an hour, the interviewer has managed to engage reluctant Norman's interest to the point that he now wants to stay and play. All of Norman's presenting problems are evident in this play interview: anxiety and distractibility, inability to become involved with a toy or with the interviewer, continual disruption of the session, and preoccupation with mechanical toys in preference to animal or human figures. There has been no real opportunity to observe Norman's **frustration tolerance.**

| Interview
with a 9-Year-Old Girl

Julia comes for an evaluation because her mother feels that she has too few friends and spends too much time alone daydreaming. She is a mature, bright child who easily answers all of the questions put to her. Two interviewers are involved—a graduate student, who uses drawings to facilitate a question-and-answer interview, and a faculty member, who continues the interview using play techniques. Nine-year-old children are on the borderline between using play techniques and responding to direct questions. The interview demonstrates that a child of this age still enjoys play and can share her fantasies through this medium.

TRAINEE: Hello, my name is Dale. I would like to get to know you a little. Do you mind chatting with me?

JULIA: No.

Most interviewers usually state more about themselves and give some idea of the interview's purpose. There is some controversy about use of first names versus surnames. Teachers at school are rarely addressed by their first names; the same is true of pediatricians and family doctors. There probably is no right or wrong, but this trainee might say, "My name is [Dr., Mr., Ms.] Smith, but it might be easier for you to call me by my first name, Dale. Have you been told why you are here today?"

[The trainee and Julia both sit on the floor amidst some soft pillows and toys. The interview proceeds for some minutes, the trainee asking a great number of questions that are mostly closed-ended. In brief answers that she does not amplify, Julia reveals that she is a 9-year-old third-grader who likes recess the best at school, though she won't say why. She has friends (though not in her class), and two brothers, one older, one younger than she. Finally, the trainee asks whether Julia likes to draw. A nodded "yes" leads to proffered paper and Magic Markers.]

TRAINEE: Why don't you draw a picture of your family?

[While Julia is drawing, the trainee continues the questioning, asking whether she has her own room, what colors it is painted, and whether she has privacy there. Julia's mostly one-word answers reveal that her older brother does not play with her, but teases her a lot. She feels closer to her younger brother; however, she spends a lot of time in her room listening to her CD player. Her family has only lived in this area for the past year.]

TRAINEE: Did you move because of somebody's job?

JULIA: Dad's.

TRAINEE: Did you have trouble making friends here?

JULIA: No, I have better friends here.

TRAINEE: How did that happen?

JULIA: I don't know. It just did.

TRAINEE: How do you get to school?

[Julia states that she walks to school. It appears from her replies to subsequent questions that she prefers this school because it is less structured. She previously attended a private school where teachers were strict and children didn't misbehave. There is some confusion: She doesn't exactly acknowledge that children in her current school misbehave, but she expresses some concern about disruption and lack of teacher control in the new school. She also reveals that her mother is at home after school, and that she has fewer friends to play with than at her former home.]

Julia's tedious, meticulous focus on her drawing may help her avoid fuller responses to questions. It is often better to let a child finish drawing before continuing with an interview—a principle that applies to play of all sorts. When a therapist and child are engaged in a play activity—either structured, such as a game of checkers, or unstructured, such as doll play—it should be the focus of the therapist's attention, as it is of the child's. The therapist should be involved fully. If more specific information is needed, a clinician might say, "Let's stop playing now so that I can ask you some questions." Like a bridge between topics in an adult interview, such an intervention focuses mutual attention on the questions to follow.

Although playing and questioning at the same time should generally be avoided, this principle has its exceptions. Occasionally a child may answer questions more reliably and feel more relaxed and comfortable with a minor distraction, such as fiddling with a transformer.

INSTRUCTOR: Hi. Can I join you? Are you working on a picture of your family? [Julia nods.] Let's see, who is that? And that? [Julia writes names over the brightly colored figures of her mother, father, and two brothers.]

The interviewing instructor, who had been observing from a slight distance, joins the two on the floor and refocuses on the drawing. As should be done with all drawings done by children, the instructor carefully notes the colors, sizes, and shapes of objects, and their positions on the page. Drawings may be used to assess age-appropriate skill levels, but, more importantly, may be used as a projective technique to elicit thematic material.

INSTRUCTOR: Is your older brother really that tall? He looks almost as big as your father.

JULIA: No, he's not really that big.

INSTRUCTOR: You said that you moved here from another school. [Julia nods.] How do you like this school?

JULIA: Some things are good, and some things are bad. [Stops drawing.]

INSTRUCTOR: Tell me more about that.

This is an exploratory, nondirective question. Once the instructor begins to ask questions, the drawing stops. Julia tries to please the interviewer by answering with more detail, but the conversation remains bland.

JULIA: Well, there are better climbing structures here, and there are no bugs or ants here.

INSTRUCTOR: Do bugs make you nervous? [Julia shakes her head.] What's the matter with ants?

JULIA: They make me itch.

INSTRUCTOR: What about the kids?

JULIA: There are some really mean kids in the school. Also, when it rains, the water comes inside the classroom.

INSTRUCTOR: Do you have to wear a raincoat and boots in the room? [At this smiling attempt at humor, Julia returns the smile and shakes her head "no."] What happened in your old school if some kids were mean?

JULIA: Well, the teacher would call the parents and tell them that they had to stop, and the kids would not be mean any more.

INSTRUCTOR: And what happens here?

JULIA: There aren't any mean kids here.

> *Julia is reluctant to engage in emotionally charged, potentially upsetting dialogue. Pursuing more specific questions only makes her more defensive. The instructor takes the cue and, in the next exchange, changes topics, learning that the family's move a year ago may be a source of Julia's current problem. Getting the name of a best friend in the old school, and then learning that she has had no contact with her past friends, strengthen this hypothesis.*

INSTRUCTOR: You mentioned that you had a best friend in your old school. What's her name?

JULIA: Erin.

INSTRUCTOR: Have you visited her since you moved here? [Julia shakes her head.] Have your written or called her? [Another denial.] You haven't called her? How come?

JULIA: Well, I tried calling her once, but she didn't call me back. And I wrote her five letters, but she never wrote back.

INSTRUCTOR: What do you think happened?

JULIA: [Dejectedly] She doesn't know my address.

INSTRUCTOR: What a shame. Maybe something can be done to help get you guys together.

> *The instructor attempts to be helpful, not really believing that her best friend couldn't contact Julia if she really wanted to remain in contact. This statement needs further exploration in the future. By conveying warmth and the possibility of help in the future, the instructor attempts to establish a positive therapeutic alliance.*

INSTRUCTOR: [Takes up a spider hand puppet.] Do you want to play with some of my toys? I've got some puppets here. Hi, I'm a friendly spider. Do you want to be my friend?

[Selecting a turtle, Julia eagerly takes to the hand puppets. Adopting a different voice from normal in playing the spider, the instructor approaches the turtle, waving one of the spider's many arms.]

INSTRUCTOR: Ms. Turtle, I'm going to be moving away and I wanted to come by and say goodbye. I will miss you a lot. Will you write me a letter? I don't want to move away. Do you promise to stay my friend?

The instructor sets the tone of the interaction as a follow-up to the previous discussion. It is important in fantasy play to seek as much distance from the source of trauma as possible without losing sight of the core issue. Toys, especially puppets, dolls, and animal family figures, are ideal stimuli for evoking imaginary material. Pretend voices help in the distancing; playful, childlike antics also often break the ice. When play content turns serious, however, the clinician should also become serious. Children deserve respect for their painful material, just as adults do.

JULIA: [Also using a pretend voice.] What's your name?

INSTRUCTOR: My name is Ms. Spider.

JULIA: OK, I won't forget your name. Goodbye, I'll miss you too.

INSTRUCTOR: Could I give you a little kiss goodbye?

JULIA: No, not a kiss. You can shake my hand. Bye-bye.

Ms. Spider has moved in to give Ms. Turtle a farewell kiss, but even in play Julia clearly defines her boundaries: no kissing, just friendly handshakes.

INSTRUCTOR: Hey, Ms. Turtle, how come you didn't write me? You moved away a month ago and I've not gotten a single letter from you, and that makes me sad. [Ms. Turtle immediately hands Ms. Spider the picture she has been drawing.] Oh, you have sent me a letter. What a pretty picture. This is your family. I like getting it. Can you write again? [Ms. Turtle immediately draws a picture of a sunrise and hands it to Ms. Spider.]

This immediate compliance suggests that Julia wants to close down the painful feelings of separation. Even in play, Julia's need to deny painful experiences is obvious. The instructor respects Julia's defenses and avoids premature interpretations.

INSTRUCTOR: Ms. Turtle, I don't like my new house. Can I come back and visit you in our old neighborhood?

JULIA: OK.

INSTRUCTOR: It's so nice to be back here. I don't ever want to go to my new house again. Will you write my parents a letter for me and tell them that I don't want to go back?

Using clinical intuition, the instructor pursues the theme of separation. Though the instructor is now doing most of the scene directing and setting up the themes, once Julia begins to take the initiative, the instructor can begin to follow her lead.

JULIA: [Starts to write, but then takes an alligator puppet from the toy bag and speaks with a gruff voice.] You have to come home.

INSTRUCTOR: Who are you, Alligator?

JULIA: I'm the dad.

INSTRUCTOR: Hi, Dad. Can I stay with my friend Ms. Turtle for a couple of months?

JULIA: No, you have to come home immediately.

INSTRUCTOR: No, I won't go. I hate my new home.

JULIA: Well, you have to go home right now.

INSTRUCTOR: No. [To Ms. Turtle] Please hide me. Where can I hide?

JULIA: [As Ms. Turtle] Hide under the bed.

Although Julia has taken the lead by introducing Dad into the play and giving him the role he took in real life (i.e., forcing the family to move), the instructor attempts to explore the depth of Julia's feelings about the move by being extremely resistant to the move (to the point of hiding from Dad) and confrontational.

[Now a chase sequence begins in which the alligator chases Ms. Spider all over the house. Finally the alligator grabs Ms. Spider in his mouth and carts her off.]

INSTRUCTOR: I'm hungry. Do you have anything to eat?

JULIA: [Takes a bunny puppet.] Would you like to go on a picnic?

INSTRUCTOR: Who are you, Bunny?

Children can easily play-act multiple roles, keeping them straight. Sometimes the interviewer as well is required to play more than one role. It is appropriate for the interviewer to interrupt the play from time to time, if confusion arises, by using a natural adult voice and to ask for clarification. "Wait a minute. I thought I was the little girl. Who are you right now?" The principal issue is for the interviewer to get in touch with the "inner child" and let that child play with the patient while observing the interaction from the perspective of the adult. These are the two roles that all child therapists must entertain simultaneously.

JULIA: I'm the mommy. Do you want to go on a picnic?

INSTRUCTOR: Oh, yes. Thank you, Mommy.

JULIA: We have to make some sandwiches.

INSTRUCTOR: I love peanut butter sandwiches. And can we bring marshmallows?

JULIA: Sure!

INSTRUCTOR: Ooooooh, I love picnics, but I hope we don't run into any ants on this picnic. I don't like ants.

JULIA: Sometimes you can't help it when ants come.

The instructor reacts positively to the idea of a picnic, but sets the tone for a little trouble. Earlier in the interview, Julia has stated that she doesn't like her new school because of "bugs and ants." By introducing the abstract construct of ants at the picnic, the interviewer provides a bridge to learn what may be wrong with the new school. In other words, the picnic may become a metaphor for her new school. It appears that Julia may understand the ant analogy.

INSTRUCTOR: [Begins to fly by with a toy helicopter and carries on with the game.] The ant copter's coming with ants.

JULIA: [Begins to populate the picnic area with toy figures as she sets up the play theme.]

INSTRUCTOR: Who are these guys? Do they get to come to the picnic?

JULIA: These are my mom, my dad, and my brother. They can come on the picnic.

INSTRUCTOR: I'm comin' with more ants. [The instructor flies by with the helicopter, spraying ants all over the place. Julia, seeming to enjoy herself, vigorously brushes them away.] You can't stamp 'em out fast enough. You're gonna itch and itch, and it's gonna get into the picnic. [Julia grabs a dinosaur figure and begins to approach.] Uh-oh, here come the dinosaurs. I'm out of here. 'Bye. [The helicopter flies away.] Go away, Dinosaur. OK, you got me. No more ants. Hurray, the dinosaurs save the day! Now we can all play and have a wonderful picnic. Is the dinosaur gonna eat a marshmallow?

Earlier, Julia has described her response to ants as "They make me itch." Is this Julia's metaphor for stress and pain? Julia has resolved the problem of "itch" by calling into play a powerful force that drives the problem away. She also now reveals some of her heightened neediness.

JULIA: Since I got rid of the ants, I get to eat all the food.

INSTRUCTOR: Oh, a little greedy, aren't you, Mr. Dinosaur? I'm gonna have to take you on and bring some more ants around. Pssssssssssssssssssss. [The instructor returns with the helicopter and sprays ants all over the dinosaur.] That's what you get for eating all the food and not letting anybody else have any.

Here the instructor may be committing an error by confronting Julia's defense directly and attempting to label her hunger and neediness as greed. To counter this misinterpretation, Julia sets the source of her difficulty back on her father.

JULIA: I'm the dad. [She puts the dinosaur figure down and takes up the father figure.]

INSTRUCTOR: [Quickly shifts roles from helicopter pilot and ant spreader to hungry child.] I'm hungry. Can I have a marshmallow?

JULIA: No, you can't.

INSTRUCTOR: But I want some marshmallows, too. Please, Dad, can't I have a marshmallow?

JULIA: No, sweetheart, it's too much sugar for you.

INSTRUCTOR: Oh, come on, Dad. Don't be such a fussbudget!

JULIA: You can have a hot dog.

INSTRUCTOR: I don't want a hot dog. I want some marshmallows, Dad. Please!

JULIA: Well, you can't.

By this time there is some indication that one of the stresses at home may be struggles over limits. Dad is again portrayed as being strict and unbending.

INSTRUCTOR: Well, here comes the big bird. You think you're gonna take the marshmallow, mister? No way!

JULIA: Oh, yeah? [She enlists the help of another animal-monster figure.]

INSTRUCTOR: No way, it's mine! [They begin to struggle over the marshmallow.] Oops! Who's that? Are you the monster? Who are you?

JULIA: I'm the mother, and I say no fighting, you two.

INSTRUCTOR: Okay, Mom, you're the boss. [Then in a regular adult voice] I think our time is up and we will need to stop for today. Thanks for coming in.

At the end of this sequence, Mother has restored peace. Perhaps this is her usual role in this household. When the hour is up, a clinician often must end a session abruptly. It may be good to suggest that the play can continue next time (if so, the same toys and play setups should be available). If a child is in the midst of a drawing, it is important that the clinician keep the artwork for the next visit. In a therapeutic relationship that is going well, play themes may continue over many sessions.

CHAPTER 8 | The Adolescent Interview

An adolescent is neither a small adult nor a large child. By this age, toys and games have usually outlived their usefulness in an interview situation; however, an initial game of checkers or chess may help get some younger adolescents started. A snack or drink may also help facilitate dialogue (remember to ask parental permission first).

Depending on an adolescent's degree of maturity, most of the interview techniques that are used with adults can be applied to the adolescent interview. Regardless of age, an informant can help set the stage for the evaluation of a hospitalized patient. However, as with an adult outpatient, an adolescent office patient should usually be interviewed before information is obtained from the parents. At some point, you may want to follow up the individual interviews of adolescent and parents with a family interview to learn how the parents and their child interact.

As you will note in the interview presented in this chapter, the clinician spends much time trying to develop rapport. This is not unusual for an adolescent patient, who will not uncommonly require more time to develop trust in the clinician than will typically be necessary for either an adult or a younger child. To conserve space, we have summarized some passages of dialogue.

This interview takes place on an adolescent inpatient unit. (It is safe to assume that in this case it is not the patient who has initiated the evaluation—an issue that should be clarified at the beginning of any adolescent interview.) The interviewer has never met the patient before and does not have access to his prior history. Casey is dressed somewhat sloppily in baggy jeans, sweatshirt, and baseball cap turned backward. He lounges in his chair and pays as little attention as possible to the interviewer.

INTERVIEWER: Hello, my name is Mr. W. I want to thank you for agreeing to be interviewed today. Did your doctor tell you why I wanted to meet with you?

This rather formal introduction may seem foreign to some clinicians who treat adolescents. We feel it is important to find a middle ground between excessive formality and inappropriate familiarity. Adolescents need to feel that the adults in their world have the maturity and experience to handle their problems and to ensure their safety. Seductiveness, rampant informality, or attempts (usually unsuccessful) to dress or talk like teenagers can repel an adolescent patient as surely as condescension or lack of engagement can.

CASEY: Yeah . . .

INTERVIEWER: And why was that?

CASEY: I don't remember.

INTERVIEWER: Well, that's OK. Let me try and explain. I work with Dr. Z., and I would like to get to know you a little better so I can help Dr. Z. understand your problems better. Is that all right with you?

CASEY: [Long pause] Yeahhh . . .

INTERVIEWER: Could you tell me why you came here?

CASEY: I dunno. [Silence]

INTERVIEWER: What sort of problems were you having?

CASEY: Nuthin' . . .

INTERVIEWER: It sounds like you're not too keen to talk.

CASEY: [Prolonged silence]

The interviewer's good attempt at an open-ended beginning has been consistently rebuffed by a patient who is at best uninterested in talking. If possible, the interview must now be salvaged by closed-ended questions, with careful attention to opportunities to form some sort of relationship with Casey. First, the interviewer presents some ground rules.

INTERVIEWER: Let's talk a little bit about what we're trying to do here. You're here in the hospital when you don't want to be, and we're trying to learn what it will take to get you out. Dr. Z. has already heard something from your folks about why you're here; now we want to hear your side of it.

Anything you say that will help us may get you out of here more quickly. Do you understand?

CASEY: [Nods his head and steals a glance at the interviewer.] Uh-huh.

INTERVIEWER: We also need to agree on this: I'm going to try to be sensitive to your feelings, but I will have to ask a lot of questions. If I ask a question that you don't feel you can answer truthfully, just ask me to talk about something else. But don't just make something up. Any time you don't tell the truth, it will confuse us. And you could be here longer. OK?

CASEY: [Nods.]

INTERVIEWER: Still another thing: What you tell me I will treat as confidential. That means I won't tell anyone, without your permission. The only possible exception, I think you'll understand, is if you're planning to harm yourself or someone else. Then I'd have to make sure you and others are protected. OK?

CASEY: Sure.

With these statements, the interviewer has emphasized three important points: (1) a philosophy that the patient is not the entire problem, (2) the need for truth, and (3) the need for safety. These are fundamental to every adolescent interview; they may have to be stated more than once. In addition, the interviewer has addressed the adolescent's need for assurance that his possibly embarrassing thoughts and feelings will not be divulged without his express consent.

INTERVIEWER: How old are you?

CASEY: Fourteen.

INTERVIEWER: How long have you been in the hospital?

CASEY: This is my second week, I think.

INTERVIEWER: And you were an inpatient before at another hospital?

CASEY: Yeah.

INTERVIEWER: How long were you an inpatient?

CASEY: Nine days.

So far, the interviewer has been asking simple questions that this recalcitrant patient can answer in a word or two. The patient's slouched posture, brief answers, and initial refusal to cooperate all signal the absence of rapport.

INTERVIEWER: Was it helpful to you?

CASEY: No. I didn't like it. I thought it was just torture.

INTERVIEWER: Torture?

> *By repeating a word offered by the patient, the interviewer encourages an open-ended response. This technique is one of the most useful for guiding the direction of an interview while encouraging verbal output.*

CASEY: Yeah. They treated me like a criminal. Almost exactly the same as in juvenile hall.

INTERVIEWER: Have you been to juvenile hall?

> *A lapse: Instead of saying, "Tell me more," which would keep the dialogue open-ended, the interviewer asks a yes–no question.*

CASEY: I've seen it. Yes.

INTERVIEWER: From inside or outside?

CASEY: From inside.

INTERVIEWER: Boy, you've seen a lot of things! But you look kind of sad today.

> *The interviewer focuses on affect by making a statement ("You look sad") rather than by asking a question ("Do you feel sad?"). The statement avoids argument and reinforces the use of words to communicate (especially appropriate for younger children).*

CASEY: Well . . . yeah. Just today. I'm getting into trouble with Cherub. She is just provoking me until I say something to her, and she doesn't get into any trouble. They even notice it. I mean, she's calling me all these names.

INTERVIEWER: Do you feel they're picking on you?

CASEY: No, it's just really Cherub, and Johnny has done some stuff, too. He's thrown my dominoes out the window. I've seen him do that, and then he lies to me. And that makes me mad.

INTERVIEWER: I can understand that. Let me ask you this: Have you ever been in this place before?

> *The interviewer wants to move ahead, but an abrupt subject change may not be the best way to proceed, especially with a yes–no question.*

CASEY: No.

INTERVIEWER: How many times were you in juvenile hall?

CASEY: I wasn't in there.

INTERVIEWER: I thought you said you were?

CASEY: I saw it.

INTERVIEWER: From the outside?

CASEY: No, I was inside for a probation hearing.

> *Interviewer and patient are sparring, testing each other's veracity and trustworthiness. The patient continues to be guarded, but the interviewer responds with another attempt at open-ended questioning.*

INTERVIEWER: What were you doing on probation?

CASEY: I robbed this lady's house a couple of times. I went with someone the first time—an older guy. We took some cigarettes and some liquor and money.

INTERVIEWER: Uh-huh.

> *A barely uttered encouragement keeps the ball rolling without getting in the way of the patient's stream of thought. Adolescents often handle negative mood states (anger, anxiety, depression, guilt) through counterphobic acting out. Clinicians, like this interviewer, must be careful to respond with acceptance without appearing to condone the behavior in question. At the same time, they must dig beneath the behavior to search for its psychological underpinnings.*

CASEY: Well, it wasn't much. She lives a few blocks away from me, and we just walked in. The back door was open.

INTERVIEWER: [Waits in silence for many seconds until the patient, feeling the need to fill the void, begins to speak again.]

CASEY: He . . . he was my homeboy, and I just went along. It was a couple of months ago, beginning of the school year. He stole a car. I didn't steal the car, but I was in it. Now he's on probation. He—

INTERVIEWER: And when do you get *off* probation?

> *To keep the focus on the patient, the interviewer interrupts, but uses the patient's own word to make the transition.*

CASEY: I think it's going to be 3 years.

INTERVIEWER: And since then, have you been going to school regularly?

CASEY: Yes. Sometimes I ditch, but I've been going. Even if it's a lot of bullshit.

INTERVIEWER: Look, let's change our focus a bit. Tell me if there was ever a time in your life when you weren't getting into trouble. Were there happy times in your life, or has your life been kind of shitty all along?

This interviewer has obtained some information concerning Casey's relationship with his peers—an important topic for any evaluation of a teenager. The interviewer next tries to look for any past history of untroubled, positive family experiences. Although this transition is abrupt, it is announced ("let's change our focus") to let the patient know that they will be pursuing a different course and that the interviewer is assuming more control of the process. The mild vulgarity ("shitty") may be an attempt to use language the patient will relate to. Of course, it is important to speak so that the teen will understand, but an adult who tries to imitate teenagers' language too closely risks rejection. Clinicians sometimes feel that they must choose between relating to an adolescent patient as a peer and sounding like a censorious parent. In reality, a middle ground is almost always possible.

CASEY: Depressing, because of what happened at school. It was really one teacher, one bad teacher who started the whole thing.

INTERVIEWER: Uh-huh.

CASEY: This teacher—it was first grade—picked on me, and I had her all the way through sixth grade. She was a jerk. She'd pick three people out of each class, all these people she didn't like. Every time she came in, she'd make them sit outside just because she didn't like them. I was one of them.

INTERVIEWER: So it started in first grade, and it followed you because of that one teacher?

CASEY: Yeah.

INTERVIEWER: And you couldn't break the habit or change their minds?

Several summary statements verify that the interviewer understands.

CASEY: It wasn't that. It was the teacher. She was real mean. I accidentally broke a pencil once, and she got real mad at me and sent me down to the office. She says, "The school pays good money for these pencils, and you go around breaking them. You've got to go to the office." They did this stuff all the way through sixth grade.

INTERVIEWER: And then what happened?

Now the interview is moving along well, but the clinician is still concerned at the relative lack of affective material. It is fairly usual for an adolescent to portray all the problems as emanating from without. Denial of responsibility suggests character pathology in an adult, but may be normal for an adolescent.

[The patient relates more material about his progress through school.]

INTERVIEWER: When you started thinking about grade school, it seemed to me that you started to cry a little bit. Was it a hard time for you?

CASEY: I started to cry? What do you mean? I'm crying because of what's going on in that other room. [He gestures next door, where loud voices can be heard.]

Some facts have emerged about Casey's long-standing difficulties in school, but only a little rapport has developed. When the interviewer attempts to focus on affect, the patient shies away and returns to the present.

INTERVIEWER: You keep thinking about Cherub?

CASEY: And how I'm getting in trouble for things that she did.

INTERVIEWER: That's a pattern. People sort of pick on you, and you get into trouble. How come that happens to you?

Here the interviewer attempts an interpretation in the form of a question. In general, we agree with the conventional wisdom that it is best to avoid early interpretations. They are often wrong, and even when correct, they may prevent the revelation of more intimate material. In this case, however, the patient responds positively.

CASEY: It's because they know I'll get angry at them if they set me off, so they do.

INTERVIEWER: They try to set you off?

CASEY: They get me in trouble by doing that.

INTERVIEWER: So when you get angry, what happens? Do you hit them?

CASEY: No. Well, sometimes, but usually I start cussing at them and stuff. I did with Cherub and I got in trouble for it, even though Cherub was saying really disrespectful things, like "Oh, you have no friends." Stuff like that. She wasn't getting into trouble with that, and I'm really angry because I got in trouble.

INTERVIEWER: You got into trouble; she didn't. She got off free?

The interviewer is still trying to establish rapport with statements and questions that empathize with the patient's feelings of being scapegoated. This is a strategy that can backfire in the long run, because the patient surely understands on some level that he contributes to his own troublesome interactions. However, in this diagnostic interview, the interviewer still wants to develop reliable, diagnostically useful information. The information needs to include not only the symptoms of the illness and the facts of the past history, but also data about the patient's capacity for insight and for forming therapeutic relationships.

CASEY: Yeah. And she gets to leave the program today, and she barely goes to any of the groups. I go to the groups. I don't stay in my room and refuse to go to them.

INTERVIEWER: And she doesn't have to?

CASEY: No.

Some meaningful facts have been obtained, and some degree of understanding of this adolescent boy's minimal insight into his problems has been observed. The interview is proceeding smoothly, and much more information has been obtained from a reluctant patient than might be expected. By this time, the bridge to a different subject has been reduced to a single word, "Now."

INTERVIEWER: Now, how did you get yourself into the hospital here?

CASEY: I got really angry at school and spit at one of the teachers, and they suspended me, and my mom said, "That's it. You're going to a hospital."

INTERVIEWER: Do you think it's been helpful?

CASEY: I don't know, really. I'm *saying* it's been helpful because I want to get out of here, but I think it's just been torture.

INTERVIEWER: Do you have to take any medicine?

CASEY: I take lithium and Zoloft.

INTERVIEWER: How do they make you feel?

CASEY: Lithium makes me shake a lot, and Zoloft, I don't know.

INTERVIEWER: Do they help you control your temper?

CASEY: Sometimes, yeah, but when Cherub does that kind of stuff to me, I still get angry.

INTERVIEWER: When you're mad and get into fights, have you ever hurt anybody?

CASEY: Yeah. I don't fist-fight or anything too often, though.

INTERVIEWER: Give me an example of someone you hurt.

CASEY: This one kid at school, I whacked him across the face and hurt him really bad. I think I gave him a bloody nose, but that was all.

INTERVIEWER: Do you have friends in school?

CASEY: At B— High I was really popular, and I was hanging out with the popular students there. Then I got put in C— High, and I don't even know anyone there.

INTERVIEWER: What's C— High? Is that where the problem kids are?

CASEY: No. It's a really preppy school.

INTERVIEWER: Is it a private school?

CASEY: No. It seems really preppy, and I don't really like it.

INTERVIEWER: Why did you get put there?

CASEY: Because my mom felt that I was getting in too much trouble at B— High.

INTERVIEWER: Tell me about your family—your mom and dad.

Using a bridge supplied by the patient, the interviewer moves to another area.

CASEY: They're OK, I guess.

INTERVIEWER: Do they work?

CASEY: My dad does. He's an engineer.

INTERVIEWER: And your mom stays home?

CASEY: Yeah.

INTERVIEWER: Have you ever heard them fight?

CASEY: Yeah, I have, but they don't do it too often.

INTERVIEWER: So they get along pretty well?

CASEY: Yeah.

INTERVIEWER: Any brothers and sisters?

CASEY: I got a sister.

INTERVIEWER: Tell me about her.

CASEY: She's 12.

INTERVIEWER: Does she look up to you—try to do what you do?

CASEY: Not all the time. She doesn't smoke or anything, and if I smoke, she doesn't. I hope she doesn't copy me.

When talking about his sister and his family, Casey seems to soften, and even expresses the hope that the sister will not take after him. This may be evidence of a capacity for empathy—a subject that is very important to evaluate in any adolescent patient.

INTERVIEWER: When did you start smoking?

CASEY: This past summer.

INTERVIEWER: Did you start drinking then, too?

CASEY: I drank a little bit. I drank a lot of wine and stuff before that, but that's when I started drinking hard alcohol.

INTERVIEWER: Did you ever have any problems from drinking?

CASEY: What kind?

[After further questioning about possible academic, medical, and personal problems from smoking and drinking, followed by some questions about street drugs, the interviewer learns where Casey was born and why the family moved to the current location. Casey also discloses some facts about his grandparents.]

INTERVIEWER: Did you ever think about going back to D— to live?

CASEY: Yeah, I really want to go back to D—, but my mom says no.

INTERVIEWER: [Softly] It could be like a new start.

CASEY: Yeah. Everybody in my family wants to go back to D— except for my dad.

This has been Casey's first really enthusiastic response in the interview, and the interviewer builds on it. It is especially vital with an adolescent patient to project the clinician's genuine fondness for the patient. Because of Casey's initial hostility and resentment at hospitalization, it has taken much of the interview to get to this point.

INTERVIEWER: When your mom said no, did she mean she didn't want to, or she didn't want to because of your dad's job?

CASEY: She told me she did. She told me she'd like to move back to D—, but Dad's got a good job.

INTERVIEWER: So when you were 5, your family moved to this area, or did you move around a little bit?

CASEY: We moved here.

INTERVIEWER: You've had the same house that you've always had since you were 5?

CASEY: Yeah.

INTERVIEWER: Do you have any pets?

CASEY: Yeah, I have two cats.

INTERVIEWER: No dogs?

CASEY: I want a dog.

> *This is the second positive statement of the interview. The interviewer uses it as a springboard to the discussion of other positive feelings.*

INTERVIEWER: You do? A dog would be good for you. What kind of dog would you have?

CASEY: A golden retriever.

INTERVIEWER: Yeah, they're great. Say, do you think things are better between you and your mom and dad since you've been in the hospital?

CASEY: Yeah, and I haven't gotten yelled at by my dad.

INTERVIEWER: Are you mad at your dad?

CASEY: I get mad at him sometimes.

INTERVIEWER: Does he get mad at you? Does he hit you?

CASEY: Yes. Well, not hard.

INTERVIEWER: When you were smaller, did he hit you?

CASEY: No. Well, he spanked me.

INTERVIEWER: Did he—or anyone—really abuse you? Beat you up?

CASEY: No, nothing like that.

INTERVIEWER: Tell me a little bit about how a day is for you, when you're not in here. You said you're at C— High. What time do you have to be there?

CASEY: At 8:00.

INTERVIEWER: How do you get there?

CASEY: My mom drives me.

INTERVIEWER: Are you in school all day or half a day?

CASEY: All day.

INTERVIEWER: And how do you get home?

CASEY: My mom picks me up.

The interviewer now has a pretty good idea of Casey's relationship with his family; it is much more positive than might be expected of a troubled teenager. Learning how other family members interact with teens, and how independent the teens have managed (or want) to become, can be a difficult task for clinicians. Casey's evidence will still have to be evaluated against that of his parents.

INTERVIEWER: What do you do after school?

CASEY: I usually hang out with friends.

With more time, the interviewer would want to ask Casey to elaborate on his activities with his friends. What do they do? Where do they do it? Who is involved? Why does he like/admire certain friends? Some interviewers ask, "What would your best friend say if I asked [him or her] about you?" Children and younger adolescents can be asked, "What would you like to change about yourself?" (This is the equivalent of the classic question about "three wishes," asked of even younger children.) All such information provides a fuller picture of the more positive aspects of personality and interests, and the questions help cement the therapist–patient relationship by demonstrating an interest in the patient as a whole individual, much as do the questions about sports and hobbies that follow.

INTERVIEWER: Do you have a lot of homework?

CASEY: No.

INTERVIEWER: Are you on any kind of teams? Did you play soccer or anything like that?

CASEY: I did, but don't any more.

INTERVIEWER: Why not?

CASEY: Because I don't like soccer very much.

INTERVIEWER: Do you have any hobbies?

CASEY: Yeah, I bowl.

INTERVIEWER: You bowl? What's your score?

CASEY: My highest score is 147.

INTERVIEWER: That's pretty good. Better than me. What else? Does your family go camping or do anything like that?

CASEY: No, we don't go camping.

INTERVIEWER: You're from the East; you must like snow?

CASEY: Yeah, I like snow.

INTERVIEWER: Snowboarding? Do you have a skateboard?

CASEY: [Shakes his head "no" to each question.] I did, but someone stole it.

INTERVIEWER: Do you spend time on a bike?

CASEY: Sometimes.

INTERVIEWER: Mostly you just hang out with your buddies smoking and drinking?

CASEY: Yeah.

INTERVIEWER: Got a girlfriend?

CASEY: No.

INTERVIEWER: Have you had any girlfriends?

CASEY: I don't think so. Well, kind of. When I was in E— Hospital.

INTERVIEWER: Have you ever been really close to any girl?

CASEY: [Long pause] I don't think I want to talk about that.

INTERVIEWER: OK. I'm glad you told me. So E— Hospital was where you were an inpatient before?

Casey has complied with an earlier request of the interviewer, who will mark the area of sexual knowledge and experience as important to revisit later.

CASEY: Yeah.

INTERVIEWER: And what was that for?

CASEY: It was a couple of months ago. That was because I got into a fight with my dad.

INTERVIEWER: Do you remember what you were mad about?

CASEY: No, I don't.

INTERVIEWER: Besides that time in the hospital and this one, have you been in other times, too?

CASEY: No.

INTERVIEWER: Have you ever tried to hurt yourself or kill yourself?

CASEY: No. And I know what you're going to ask—I've never thought about it. Not seriously, anyway.

INTERVIEWER: Have you ever tried to hurt your parents or your sister with a knife or gun?

CASEY: I frightened my mom with a knife, but I wasn't going to hurt her. [Casey wipes his eyes.]

By now, the interviewer has addressed three areas that are vital to every patient assessment: sex, substance use, and suicidal ideas and violence. They have not been adequately evaluated yet (details of whatever suicidal thoughts Casey may have had should be explored in depth), but the interviewer feels that the patient is safe. And the ground has been prepared for further questioning later.

INTERVIEWER: You keep getting tearful. What are you sad about?

CASEY: I don't know just what's going on in there. [He points to the next room.]

INTERVIEWER: You can't let that go?

CASEY: It's hard to. I just get into trouble a lot when people do things to me.

INTERVIEWER: You're a nice kid, and you still get into trouble.

CASEY: I get into trouble.

INTERVIEWER: You try hard, and they don't appreciate you.

CASEY: Yeah.

INTERVIEWER: I don't understand that. I don't understand why they don't appreciate you. It's just that your temper gets out of control. They trigger something, and boom, you're gone. Is that the problem?

The interviewer now attempts again to form an alliance with the patient, and finally seems to be succeeding. The patient answers the next series of questions with more affect and conviction.

CASEY: Sort of.

INTERVIEWER: Sort of. Have you ever broken things, put your fist through the wall?

CASEY: I kicked a hole in the wall.

INTERVIEWER: What else? Broken windows?

CASEY: I broke my screen and jumped out the window.

INTERVIEWER: You mean to get out of the house? [Casey nods "yes."] Have you been involved in other stealing, besides breaking into that house those two times?

CASEY: I shoplifted a couple of times.

INTERVIEWER: And the car? Stealing the car.

CASEY: Yeah.

INTERVIEWER: Do you know how to drive?

CASEY: Yeah.

INTERVIEWER: Have you driven by yourself?

CASEY: Only with my friends.

INTERVIEWER: Do you like it? Are you a good driver?

CASEY: Yeah, I'm OK.

INTERVIEWER: Probably too fast.

CASEY: I'm too scared to go fast.

INTERVIEWER: I was going to ask you about that. Do you get scared?

A good transition to questions about his feelings.

CASEY: Yeah.

INTERVIEWER: What sorts of things scare you?

CASEY: Sometimes I get scared when I have to go to school. Some people, they came over and tried to beat me up and stuff, and they had a gun and stuff, and they were going to shoot me, and I get scared about that.

INTERVIEWER: Are these people in gangs?

CASEY: Yeah.

INTERVIEWER: Are you in one?

CASEY: No, I'm not.

INTERVIEWER: Now I need to ask you about some other feelings and experiences lots of people sometimes have. Do you ever get really scared, like when you go to high places, in elevators, or in crowds?

The interviewer signals another change of topic, and lets Casey know that these routine questions do not mean that he is suspected of having had such experiences.

CASEY: No. Well, when I get into big crowds and tight places, that scares me.

INTERVIEWER: Does your heart pound and you sweat?

CASEY: Yeah.

INTERVIEWER: You've had that? Tell me more.

CASEY: Sometimes I just begin to shake when I get scared. Then I can't breathe. I sweat a lot and my heart pounds.

INTERVIEWER: Does that happen very often?

CASEY: No, only once in a while when I'm in a panic. A bunch of guys are going to get me.

INTERVIEWER: Is it only when someone's trying to hurt you, or does it also happen when you're in tight places or crowds?

CASEY: Um, I guess just when I'm afraid of someone.

INTERVIEWER: Would you describe yourself as either especially neat or especially messy?

CASEY: I'm in the middle.

INTERVIEWER: But do you like everything in a certain order?

CASEY: No.

INTERVIEWER: What about voices? Do you ever hear voices that don't seem real?

CASEY: No.

INTERVIEWER: Do you ever see things other people don't see?

CASEY: No.

INTERVIEWER: What about high moods? Like you feel really terrific, *too* good, and there's no reason for it?

CASEY: No, unh-unh.

INTERVIEWER: Or been terribly overactive—maybe you didn't need to sleep much for days on end?

CASEY: No.

INTERVIEWER: Or have you ever felt so bad you had thoughts about harming yourself, killing yourself, maybe?

CASEY: Not really.

INTERVIEWER: What does that mean?

CASEY: You know, I guess lots of guys think about it. But I never *wanted* to or anything.

INTERVIEWER: OK. How's your appetite?

CASEY: It's good now. But sometimes it's bad.

INTERVIEWER: How long is it usually bad?

CASEY: I dunno. Just when I'm feeling lousy. Depressed, you know.

INTERVIEWER: Have you lost weight?

CASEY: I'm not sure. I don't think so.

INTERVIEWER: Are you about the right size, or are you small for your age?

CASEY: I'm small for my age.

INTERVIEWER: How do you feel about that?

CASEY: Bad and lonely, sometimes. But I do have some good friends.

INTERVIEWER: Do you talk to them about feeling lonely?

CASEY: I talk to them.

INTERVIEWER: When you're feeling depressed, how long does that last?

CASEY: I dunno—not long. Maybe a day or two.

> *The moods of adolescents tend to be short-lived and labile. When this fact is not appreciated, young patients sometimes get treated with medications and other unnecessary therapies. Clinicians need to evaluate possible mood disorders carefully, but must keep in mind that young patients typically lack perspective as to changes in their own moods. Repeated interviews across time are essential.*

INTERVIEWER: Our time is almost up, and I would like to ask you just a few more questions. They may seem boring, but I would appreciate it if you would try to answer as best you can. OK?

A complete, formal mental status exam (see Chapter 1, Table 1.1) is not necessary for every adolescent patient, any more than it is for every adult. Completeness is indicated whenever there is a question of severe mental pathology (e.g., cognitive, psychotic, mood, or substance use disorders), or when, for legal or other purposes, the record needs to reflect a complete baseline evaluation. Of course, the behavioral aspects of mental status should be noted for every patient—general appearance and behavior; mood; flow of thought—for these require no special set of questions. Questions necessary for much of the remainder—content of thought; insight and judgment; and aspects of the sensorium (memory, attention span, fund of information)— will come up as other matters are pursued. Note that in pursuing a formal assessment of Casey's mental status, this interviewer doesn't make the common mistake of describing the mental status tasks as "silly" or "dumb," which would convey the impression that they are not important.

CASEY: OK.

INTERVIEWER: What's the name of this hospital?

CASEY: F— Hospital.

INTERVIEWER: What day is it today?

CASEY: Thursday.

INTERVIEWER: Do you know the date?

CASEY: It's December.

INTERVIEWER: And the date?

CASEY: I don't remember.

INTERVIEWER: What year is it?

CASEY: [He states it correctly.]

INTERVIEWER: That's good. Do you remember my name?

CASEY: No.

INTERVIEWER: OK. What sort of work do I do?

CASEY: You're the consultant. You're supposed to help me get out of here.

INTERVIEWER: Good. Here's three words that I want you repeat back to me and then remember. *Apple, clock, mustang.* Can you repeat them for me right now?

CASEY: *Apple, clock, mustang.*

Before going ahead with the test of short-term memory, the interviewer ascertains that the patient has understood the items and that his immediate recall is intact. The interviewer does not alert Casey that he will be asked to repeat these items a few minutes later; that would invite rehearsal.

INTERVIEWER: Good. Here's a question: What's the same about an apple and an orange?

CASEY: I don't know. Nothing.

INTERVIEWER: Try to think about it a little bit more.

CASEY: You eat them.

INTERVIEWER: Sure! That's good! Anything else?

CASEY: No.

INTERVIEWER: How about a chair and a bed? What's the same about them?

CASEY: I can sleep in them both.

INTERVIEWER: [Chuckles.] I guess so! Anything else?

CASEY: Well, they're both furniture.

INTERVIEWER: Excellent! Here's a saying: "People who live in glass houses shouldn't throw stones." What does that mean to you?

CASEY: Stones break glass.

INTERVIEWER: Good. Anything else?

CASEY: No.

INTERVIEWER: OK. Do you remember those three things I told you to remember?

CASEY: I remember *apple,* but that's all.

INTERVIEWER: Are you sure? Try to recall the others.

CASEY: I can't.

INTERVIEWER: That's OK. You've done just fine. Now I want to go back to something we talked about earlier—the car theft. How would you deal with this now, if you were with your friend and he wanted to do it?

CASEY: You mean would I go along with it again?

INTERVIEWER: [Nods.]

CASEY: I dunno . . . I hope I'd say "No," but I dunno . . .

INTERVIEWER: Why "hope"?

CASEY: Well, it's sure caused me a lot of trouble.

INTERVIEWER: OK. Well, I really appreciate the time you've spent with me. Thank you.

Questions of the form "What would you do if . . . ?" serve as a check on judgment that may be somewhat more relevant to teenagers than asking them to state three wishes or to describe what they would do if they found a stamped letter. Such questions serve as a means of evaluating character and personality, and as a check on the congruence of an adolescent's values with those of mainstream adult society and culture. A similar sort of question, with many of the same advantages, takes the form "Tell me what you did in [a given situation]." This situation will usually describe an interpersonal problem the patient has already mentioned, though the interviewer may instead suggest a problem with a hypothetical relationship. Casey's responses to the last two questions asked of him address both insight and judgment.

| The Parent–Child
Initial Interview

A clinician often conducts an initial interview with a parent or both parents and the child together. Because children, especially young ones, are so responsive to their environment, it is rare for a child to be the only subject of distress. It is not unusual for a family, however, to identify only the child as the identified patient. A generation ago, the family assessment was usually carried out by a variety of professionals. A child psychiatrist might interview the child; a social worker might interview the parents; and a psychologist might use formal tests to assess the child's cognitive and emotional capacities.

More typically in recent years, a single professional completes the initial evaluation and makes referrals for specialized services only when indicated. Because children, parents, and teachers often tell different stories, it is especially important to obtain information from multiple sources. Interviewing a parent and child together, or the whole family when possible, provides an opportunity to reconcile discrepancies. It may also be therapeutically beneficial for each family member to hear the others' concerns. (For obvious reasons, a traditional family interview is contraindicated in cases of suspected physical or sexual abuse.)

GOALS OF THE PARENT–CHILD INTERVIEW

The family interview is not inherently superior to other types of interviews, but it has its advantages. It allows you to get different viewpoints about the problem and to meet all the players and observe them interact. The people the child talks about become real in your mind. When successful, a parent–child interview answers several questions:

1. What family dynamics can direct observation reveal? Some possibilities include the following:

   - Enmeshed relationships, where boundaries between family members are poorly defined, leading to a low degree of privacy and independence.
   - Disengaged relationships, in which there is little sharing of communication or lives.
   - Alliances between a child and the weaker of two parents.
   - Overprotection of a "sick" child.
   - Scapegoating of a "bad" child.

2. How does the family cope? Does it adapt by changing the alignments, boundaries, or distribution of power within the family to reflect altered family circumstances (e.g., entry or exit of a member, development of children into adolescence)?
3. How does the family work together to solve problems?
4. How do family members communicate with one another? Does each take a turn, respecting the rights of others to be heard? Does one member do most of the talking? Do all talk at once, seldom listening to what others are saying?
5. How can the family's decision-making process be characterized? It can run the gamut from authoritarian to democratic to permissive.
6. What cognitive distortions (inaccurate perceptions of any aspect of a child's conduct, character, or capabilities) bear on the relationships among family members?

Although a family interview elicits some information relevant to the mental status of the identified patient, individual interviews generally produce more detailed, high-quality information. This is easy to understand: The presence of other family members may inhibit the disclosure of certain types of sensitive material, even by a patient who is very young. When a family interview is desired as a part of the evaluation of an individual patient, it is often better to interview the family first. You will obtain information from the group more easily before you have developed an exclusive relationship with one individual.

CONDUCTING THE PARENT–CHILD INTERVIEW

Some clinicians like to begin the interview by introducing themselves by profession ("doctor," "social worker," "psychologist," "nurse") or by a more generic term ("counselor," "clinician," "therapist") who wants to get to know the child and the family in order to help with problems. Whatever introduction you use, make it clear that your job isn't to find someone to blame, but to "find out how your family works and help it work better."

You might start with an open-ended request, such as "Who would like to begin?" or "Who wants to tell us why we are all here today?" When the identified patient is a younger child, the person who begins will almost always be a parent, but you will have delivered the message that contributions are welcome from all. When talking with a parent, you should note the child's nonverbal as well as verbal communications. Ask whether the child agrees or disagrees with the parental rendition of a behavior, feeling, or sequence of events. As the interview proceeds, attempt to involve the child, continually balancing and integrating the child's and parent's contributions.

INTERVIEW WITH ERNEST MONAHAN AND HIS MOTHER

In the interview that follows, a family physician has referred Ms. Monahan and her 10-year-old son, Ernest, to evaluate his chronic physical complaints. Though tall for his age, Ernest is thin and slightly built. His mother is also tall, but overweight and somewhat overbearing. When invited to attend, Mr. Monahan has explained that he cannot be present but will participate in a subsequent interview.

In the dialogue, the *italicized comments* actually serve three functions. In some cases, they interpret the statements of Ernest and his mother. In others, they explain what the interviewer says or does. Finally, they sometimes serve to explain the interviewer's internal working speculations about family dynamics.

INTERVIEWER: So what brought the two of you?

The opening question is not "What is Ernest's problem?" or "What's wrong with Ernest?" Instead, the interviewer frames the problem as one affecting at least two people. Ms. Monahan provides the initial response.

MS. MONAHAN: We first figured out that Ernest was going to be sick for a long time

2 years ago, right at about March or April. We already knew that you [addressing her son] had been sick since maybe February. What happened was, right at Thanksgiving weekend, Ernest came down with what appeared to be a viral cold—headaches, fever, not a severe fever, 102, 103, a really bad sore throat, achy all over, no GI or gastric symptoms, just a bad cold. We thought, "Oh, great, our local cold for this winter." As we went into the second week, some of the symptoms got better, but he was still sick—feeling really bad, body hurt all the time. So about the end of the second week I said, "OK, this has gone on long enough, now let's go see the doctor," and she said, "Yep, it looks like one of those bad colds going around, just keep him home until he gets well." But by the end of the fifth week, we went back and said, "This isn't getting any better." Ernest had changed to the point where he was running periodic fevers up to 100, was in bed *exhausted*, and his body and throat hurt *all* the time, yet nothing was positive.

The very long run of speech allows the informant maximum scope to tell her story in her own words. There is a hint of dissatisfaction with the family physician. Also note that Ms. Monahan dominates the opening: She "tells" Ernest how he felt and what happened. At this point, Ernest sits passively, not interrupting.

INTERVIEWER: Mono?

MS. MONAHAN: Mono screen was negative.

ERNEST: I already had mono—

Ernest has been listening quietly and tries to interject. But his mother interrupts him and finishes for him.

MS. MONAHAN: Yeah, you'd had mono . . .

ERNEST: Second grade.

MS. MONAHAN: Second grade. And so, um . . .

INTERVIEWER: [To Ernest] Can you get mono more than once?

The interviewer wants to engage Ernest and ensure that his mother doesn't hold the floor too long, so responds to his interjection with a related question.

ERNEST: I don't think so.

INTERVIEWER: You're right. I was just testing.

ERNEST: Doesn't your body build up antibodies?

INTERVIEWER: Yep.

The interviewer maintains a relaxed, almost bantering style that might not be used if this interview were with the mother only. It serves to engage the patient, even though his mother provides most of the information.

MS. MONAHAN: So at this point people are throwing up their hands and saying, "What's wrong?" So the doctor had a leap of clinical intuition and had him tested for CM [cytomegalovirus]. His blood titer came back as positive, and he was spitting out a very high titer of live CM virus in his urine. So now we knew that he had a significant CM virus.

ERNEST: Mom, they did blood tests after I was sick a few months.

Ernest is still trying to tell his version. Although Ms. Monahan has dominated the interview, the interviewer chooses not to intercede. Ms. Monahan has made clear earlier that she becomes disappointed with physicians fairly readily, and the interviewer, content to watch the relationship unfold, is not threatened by being dominated.

MS. MONAHAN: The first time she picked it up, he had been sick about 2 months. At that point we knew that we couldn't treat him with anything. The only thing, since there weren't any antiviral drugs, was the old "Keep him comfortable, take him home, treat him well, feed him well, da da da da, and wait for it to go away; he will get better." It's now been 15 months.

Again, the mother's frustration with the medical profession is apparent.

ERNEST: But I'm so much better than I used to be, *so* much better!

MS. MONAHAN: Oh, yes, goodness. Anyway, we'd been home-schooling Ernest from Thanksgiving through March, but the stress was just too great, and he just wasn't getting well, and so we decided, "Screw it; we're just going to take him out of school, let him rest, really make this a therapeutic time." We brought in lots of funny movies; we brought in humor; we brought in—

INTERVIEWER: Had you read Norman Cousins?

The interviewer is assessing Ms. Monahan's health care knowledge. Cousins's book Anatomy of an Illness as Perceived by the Patient *(New York: Norton, 1979) is a best-selling autobiography of personal recovery from an unknown viral illness, similar to that described for Ernest. It is narrated with a strong antimedical bias.*

Ms. MONAHAN: I did. I'll tell you, I read everything I could get my hands on. We did humor; we did whole foods; we did fruits; I mean, we just—

INTERVIEWER: This was starting in March?

By now Ms. Monahan's circumstantiality has become apparent, so the interviewer cuts her off, feeling the need to be increasingly directive.

Ms. MONAHAN: Yeah, then as soon as he was strong enough, we started walking; the first time, he was just dragging. But he learned how to ride a bicycle that May.

ERNEST: No, I think it was, no—

Ms. MONAHAN: Maybe the beginning of May you started riding your bicycle?

ERNEST: The beginning of June.

Ms. MONAHAN: Beginning . . . So right before Bright Star you learned to ride your bicycle?

INTERVIEWER: What's Bright Star?

Ms. MONAHAN: That's a summer recreation day care program, and it starts the third week in June. School's out the 10th and it starts the week after, and we've been in it for years. So we just kept building towards this, and he kept getting better and better and better, but he'd have these days where he'd smack up against this wall [she emphasizes with a loud handclap], and you could just see him go whack and boom, and he would just sag and he'd be out for 2 or 3 days—what, about every 2 weeks?

ERNEST: Every once in a while.

Ms. MONAHAN: In the fall, we put him in several new schools, first one, then another—Crest View.

INTERVIEWER: Wait a minute, from Thanksgiving he wasn't in school, then Bright Star summer recreation, and now Crest View?

The interviewer makes a summary statement to clarify, and also to try to stay on track.

Ms. MONAHAN: Right, I'm sorry. Jimson Day. And let's see, this week you had an episode of weakness, Monday, Tuesday, and half of Wednesday, but I was trying to remember when your last episode was. It was about, what, 3 weeks ago, a month ago?

ERNEST: You mean when it lasted, like, 4 days?

Ms. Monahan: Yeah.

Ernest: But that was different, because I had a really bad cold.

Ms. Monahan: OK, I was thinking of the last time you were absent just for fatigue.

Ernest: Um, a couple days ago.

Ms. Monahan: Well, I mean before then.

Ernest: Oh, before that? Almost a month.

Mother and son again battle over clarity. Their inability to agree on events, and their inability to resolve discrepancy, reveal a significant power struggle. The mother is domineering and overwhelms Ernest (and the interviewer) with trivial detail. She controls Ernest and others around her with confrontation and obsessional thinking.

Ms. Monahan: Yeah, I think so. The episodes are getting farther and farther apart, so our attitude has been "OK, yes, we're getting better. Yes, this is slow, but at least we're getting better." So that's where we are today. He's back in school, but had one episode this week. What stimulated our visit was that, starting way back at the beginning of the process in March, April, May, I realized that we had a kid on our hands who is extraordinarily bright, has wonderful capabilities, and is now saddled with this chronic fatigue and pain.

Ernest: It's sad.

Ms. Monahan: And his throat hurts.

Interviewer: [To Ernest] What did you say?

Ernest: I just said "sad."

Interviewer: Sad.

Picking up on one word used by Ernest, the interviewer tries to change the direction of the interview, but the mother interferes.

Ms. Monahan: Sad, and you get sad, too. You feel really depressed during those times.

Ernest: No, I don't.

Ms. Monahan: OK.

Ernest: It just looks like it, since I'm in pain.

Ms. Monahan: Yeah, I think you're a little sad too, but, you know, it's not bad.

Once again the interviewer is excluded as mother and son try unsuccessfully to resolve their differences.

Interviewer: So did Ernest start in public school, then—

Ms. Monahan: We started, we had him in kindergarten and first grade, and just— it was horrible. The public school system, despite its reputation, is atrocious. In particular, the elementary schools are absolutely horrible. They were—

Interviewer: So second grade through—

Ms. Monahan: Second grade through the current grade, he's been in private schools. Second and third he was in Jimson Day; then he skipped fourth— we had him tested to skip fourth into fifth—and it was in that fifth grade, that Thanksgiving that he first got ill. So he missed that fifth grade. So he's now with his age group, which is so funny, because we just jumped through so many hoops to get him skipped, and—

Ms. Monahan is not only discontented with the medical system; in her view, Ernest's education has also been fraught with confrontation and disappointment. She tends to externalize, blaming others for the family's problems of living. The interviewer has begun to wonder whether Ernest's physical symptoms may be an expression of his frustration with satisfying his mother's need to control his education.

Interviewer: So you're back to where you started?

Ms. Monahan: Yeah.

Interviewer: [To Ernest] You're a fifth-grader?

Ernest: Yes.

Interviewer: And the reason to leave Jimson Day . . . ?

Ms. Monahan: Every time the teacher would walk out of the room, the kids were all over the place.

Ernest: You never did go in the room.

In contrast to his mother, Ernest tries to tell a balanced story.

Ms. Monahan: So then I learned about Crest View, which is for gifted children. You can't get in without testing. They have behavioral guidelines and expectations, and you have kids that are really interested in learning. You're not messing around with bums.

Ms. Monahan's message to Ernest is this: "Either you maintain a high standard of excellence or you are a bum." What alternative is there for him? To become sick and not compete? Although it is much too early to comment openly, the interviewer notes Ms. Monahan's apparent need for control as she lives vicariously through her son and denies her own inadequacies.

INTERVIEWER: You like it?

ERNEST: Yeah, I really enjoy the school.

MS. MONAHAN: Tell him about Mrs. Johnson.

Ms. Monahan continues to assert control over the interview, even as the interviewer tries to develop an alliance with Ernest.

ERNEST: My teacher, Mrs. Johnson, is 3 inches shorter than I am.

INTERVIEWER: You're pretty big for your age, aren't you?

ERNEST: Yeah, which makes me the tallest person in my class. And she's round and plump, and is always very stolid in front of parents and adults, but really loosens up when there are no other adults around.

The interviewer mentally files away Ernest's unusual (for his age) use of the word stolid, *as fodder for the mental status exam.*

INTERVIEWER: She's fun?

ERNEST: Yeah, she's really fun.

INTERVIEWER: What sort of courses are you taking this year?

ERNEST: Well, we're doing math—but, unfortunately, for the fifth grade they didn't have any sciences except computer science, which is really cool. So we have math, spelling, reading.

INTERVIEWER: What are you doing in math?

ERNEST: We just finished up proportions.

INTERVIEWER: Fractions?

ERNEST: Yeah, we're doing all sorts of stuff with fractions, and she's teaching us all the different uses of canceling numbers.

INTERVIEWER: Do they have a lot of homework?

ERNEST: Medium, but when it comes to reports and book reports—all different kinds of reports—and oral presentations, which we also have, it becomes a huge amount.

INTERVIEWER: And weekends?

ERNEST: On weekends if there're reports; otherwise, they're pretty easy on you.

The subject of schoolwork does not create conflict or threaten Ms. Monahan, who briefly falls silent. But the topic of weekends is more threatening—information about the family might be revealed—and, true to form, she now takes over. Her use of we *and* us *when talking about Ernest's homework suggests the exceptional degree to which she identifies with her son.*

MS. MONAHAN: One weekend we were accidentally trapped out of town because our car conked out. We fortunately had taken all his homework with us. We had 5 hours one day, just working on a state report.

ERNEST: And then 3 hours the next day.

INTERVIEWER: Let me go back to the pains and weakness. It seems like these episodes are spreading out a little bit. Do you feel like you're back to normal again?

ERNEST: Sometimes. But I'm almost always pretty tired, and once in a while I get sore but, other than that, between the episodes I'm feeling . . . [long pause]

INTERVIEWER: Pretty good.

The interviewer finishes up; this is not recommended as a rule, but here Ernest appears lost in thought. A better intervention might be to paraphrase his last few words: "Between the episodes you're feeling . . . "

ERNEST: Yeah.

INTERVIEWER: Do you have trouble sleeping?

The interviewer attempts to return with Ernest to the earlier reference to sadness and possible depression, but Ms. Monahan chimes in with her son.

BOTH: [Simultaneously] Yes.

INTERVIEWER: [Directly to Ernest] Can you tell me about that?

ERNEST: Well, it takes me a long time to get to sleep.

INTERVIEWER: Do you sleep in your own room?

ERNEST: Yeah.

INTERVIEWER: What time do you go to bed?

ERNEST: I have a deadline. I have to go to bed by 9:00. It's called "lights out." My parents just let me read to about 9:30, but then they just come in, and I close my book and turn off the light.

INTERVIEWER: But you're still not sleepy?

ERNEST: No, actually I'm sleepy, but I can't sleep.

INTERVIEWER: OK. And then what happens?

ERNEST: And then I . . . [long pause]

INTERVIEWER: Do you lie there awake in the dark?

ERNEST: I just kind of lay there until I go to sleep, and . . . [long pause]

The pauses suggest that there are topics Ernest may not wish to discuss in the presence of his mother. For now, the interviewer fills in to move the interview along, but will return to these subjects in a later private interview with Ernest.

INTERVIEWER: Do you have a sense of how long that is?

ERNEST: Yeah, sometimes I can be awake until 11:00.

MS. MONAHAN: And what I need to interject here is that I do research. And my business for the last 25 years has been illness patterns. And what I've noticed in him is that when he starts to have several late nights in a row where he'll say, "Oh, gosh, Mom, I just couldn't sleep last night," it will be just before one of his relapses.

Ms. Monahan now asserts her academic credentials. Not feeling threatened by her expertise, the interviewer respectfully asks her professional opinion, in order to maintain the alliance.

INTERVIEWER: Do you think that this is a biorhythm problem? Is his biological clock normal?

MS. MONAHAN: I don't know what's triggering it, but I know that one of the symptoms I watch for is several nights in a row where he is very late in getting to sleep. I don't know if the sleep drives it. Does the fatigue drive the sleeplessness?

INTERVIEWER: Is he hard to wake up in the mornings?

MS. MONAHAN: Not when he's doing well. Then he wakes up with a big smile.

ERNEST: And I just hop up.

INTERVIEWER: Do you need an alarm?

ERNEST: I'm groggy sometimes.

MS. MONAHAN: You know we had a joke in the family, because Mom and son both wake up really slowly. Dad is opposite. He's gotten really good about sneaking out in the morning so he doesn't wake us up.

According to this description, the mother and son share characteristics, whereas the father is different; this suggests that the team of Ernest and Mom may exclude Dad. Such forms of enmeshment are not uncommon in families that somaticize.

INTERVIEWER: Do you ever have bad dreams?

ERNEST: I don't really remember my dreams.

MS. MONAHAN: We've noticed that he can't sleep over at anybody else's house, because they go and have a great time, and the next day he can't get out of bed.

INTERVIEWER: Well, are you too tired to be athletic?

ERNEST: I love to ride my bicycle, but I hurt. I don't really like to go on recreational walks, but—

INTERVIEWER: Do you play soccer or do anything else?

ERNEST: I used to play soccer, but when I got sick, I stopped.

MS. MONAHAN: One of the things—this is not a criticism, sweetheart—Ernest is not a smooth runner; he's always been a clumper. It's like he's got three left feet down there and they interfere with each other, so he's not really well coordinated.

Once again, the mother denigrates Ernest's abilities; is she trying to keep him from partaking in the wider world?

ERNEST: It's *two* left feet.

MS. MONAHAN: And he didn't have the coordination to ride a bicycle until he was 8; it was last year, 9, I guess. But you're superb when it comes to video games and computer games and—

INTERVIEWER: Fine motor skills.

MS. MONAHAN: He's writing—he's going to be writing our home page for our business. We go to my office on the weekends if he wants to do that.

INTERVIEWER: You're at the college?

MS. MONAHAN: Yeah.

INTERVIEWER: In what department?

Ms. Monahan: Biology. So the main reason that I wanted to get counseling for Ernest is—how should I put it? He's extremely talented; he's a highly intelligent child with a fabulous future. He has the capability to be anything, to do anything in this life he wants.

Interviewer: There's a "but" coming here.

Ms. Monahan: And my goal in life is to make sure that he's educated and prepared. That's why my goal is to keep him going in school, to make sure he's got fun and exciting things in school. I've had absolutely *no* backup on my diagnosis of chronic fatigue syndrome. In all the reading I've done, he fits every single profile. Not a single physician that I've talked to has said, "Yes, chronic fatigue syndrome."

Interviewer: It's hard to diagnose in children. It's hard to diagnose in anybody.

Ms. Monahan finally begins to talk about why she has sought a mental health interview when her view so strongly supports a physical illness and no psychological problems have been described. She has never stated that Ernest has a possible somatoform disorder. The trap is that if she has failed in achieving her aspirations, and is expecting to achieve her goals vicariously through Ernest's efforts, she will again be disappointed. The interviewer remains supportive but avoids concurring with the mother.

Ms. Monahan: Well, the thing that made me most angry was, we went to see the pediatric infectious disease CM specialist. I blocked her name because she made me so mad. She spent 3½ hours with this child on a cold table, buck naked, with a sheet around him. And she looked at me at the end of all of this and said, "There's no biological reason for his condition. I think he's been abused."

Interviewer: Abused?

Ms. Monahan: Abused! Scared the living hell out of me. I was crying and Ernest was crying. We went home; we had a cup of hot chocolate; and I said, "OK, honey. Has anybody ever touched you, or beaten you, or done anything?" And we talked about this for 2 or 3 days, and I am absolutely confident in my heart of hearts and a mother's suspicious mind—never has he ever had any problems of this nature. It just fried me. This woman kissed off his entire physical condition by saying, "No biological cause." I want to find a physician who will work with us and take a look at the profile. I've been a patient little mom. I'm done being patient. I want somebody who's going to work with us.

The mother has now completed (and restated) her case: "Agree with me, or I will go elsewhere." The interviewer remains supportive, but does not necessarily accept the diagnosis of the mother, who also predicts lifetime morbidity.

[After some more discussion of Ernest's recent health, the Interviewer moves to other parts of the evaluation.]

INTERVIEWER: How was your pregnancy?

MS. MONAHAN: Superb. I—

INTERVIEWER: It was an easy 9 months and a full-term delivery?

MS. MONAHAN: Yep, right to the day. I knew when I got pregnant because it was a planned pregnancy. I was a single mom—a single woman and I wanted a child, so a good friend of mine donated the sperm, and so I know exactly when I became pregnant. And I had a great pregnancy.

The mother casually mentions her artificial insemination and her planning to be a single mother—facts of which Ernest appears already aware. The interviewer leaves this for a later meeting.

INTERVIEWER: Are you married now?

MS. MONAHAN: Yeah. I got married when Ernest was 4, to a college sweetheart. He and I got back together again, the flames were still there, and we got married.

INTERVIEWER: And he's adopted Ernest?

MS. MONAHAN: Yep. April 11 is our family day.

INTERVIEWER: Do you have other children?

MS. MONAHAN: No.

INTERVIEWER: Not a smoker?

MS. MONAHAN: Nope, I didn't smoke or drink. I haven't smoked since I was 21. I don't drink, don't do drugs.

INTERVIEWER: How did you get to this town—did you grow up here?

MS. MONAHAN: No, I came here to go to the university.

INTERVIEWER: Do you have an advanced degree?

MS. MONAHAN: No, I have a BS degree in biological science. I would have loved to go to medical school or to graduate school, but I ran out of money.

INTERVIEWER: Where did you grow up?

Ms. Monahan: South of here. My father was a scientist.

Interviewer: Is he alive?

Ms. Monahan: Yes, medically retired. I believe that I've had chronic fatigue syndrome since 1980. I've also always had PMS. I developed a very bad case of pneumonia in 1980. Immediately thereafter I had terrific trouble with fatigue and concentration. I just recently read an article about a genetic susceptibility in chronic fatigue syndrome. And I thought, "Oh, goody, great birthday present." But that leads me to think that this could very well be caused by me. [To Ernest] Sorry, guy!

Interviewer: Do you get pains too?

Ms. Monahan: It's interesting. For the last 4 years, I've had a terrible increase in symptoms, but I'm very, very private. I'm excellent at hiding my symptoms.

Interviewer: So you don't miss work.

Ms. Monahan: I miss 1 or 2 days a month, because I'm home shivering wrapped in a blanket because I can't move. I've just changed doctors again, because I was getting discouraged at the lack of progress. For 20 years, I've been patted on the head and sent to psychiatrists. I've been drugged and counseled, and, and—

Interviewer: And now you're bringing Ernest to a psychiatrist.

Ms. Monahan: Because I'm at my wits' end. I'm not getting any support.

Interviewer: But he's doing well. I don't understand.

Ms. Monahan: He's not doing well. Monday and Tuesday he was sick as a dog, in bed, weak from pain.

Interviewer: But you know what it is. It happens to you too.

With somatic symptoms that interfere with her life, Ms. Monahan is even more like Ernest than she has previously acknowledged. Her disclosure suggests a positive therapeutic alliance with the interviewer, who observes that both she and Ernest are coping well.

Ms. Monahan: But is there anybody that can help us? I just know that I'm not getting any information now.

Interviewer: The point of this evaluation is to get to know something about everybody in the family, and I don't understand enough yet to start answering your questions.

Ms. Monahan: OK.

As the theme broadens to "Who is the patient?", the informant's frustration turns toward the interviewer. However, she accepts this forthright explanation.

Interviewer: Is your husband's health good?

Ms. Monahan: He's a horse. He has his problem areas. He has terrible knees, because he was injured in Vietnam when a piece of a helicopter door flew back on one. The other knee took a piece of a motorcycle through it.

Interviewer: You've been married 6 years, so this was all before your time.

Ms. Monahan: Previous history, yeah.

Interviewer: But you said he was a college sweetheart?

Ms. Monahan: We met while we were in college. Then he went into the Army— medics. He was slogging around in the jungles for 33 months; he came back much more aware of his capabilities and limits. And he doesn't have any lingering nightmares or anything.

Interviewer: Did he come back and finish college?

Ms. Monahan: No.

Interviewer: What does he do?

Ms. Monahan: We are starting a software company. He's working full time on this, and I'm the primary support of the family.

Interviewer: Where'd he learn that?

Ms. Monahan: The Army. And he also taught physics and electronics.

The stepfather has high aspirations and achievement, but no college degree. It is now evident that both parents have never achieved their academic goals. Is this the developmental path that Ernest is to follow? It is difficult for Ernest to succeed in an area in which both parents appear not to have reached their expectations.

Interviewer: So everyone in this family is very bright.

Ms. Monahan: Yeah.

Interviewer: Can we just take a few minutes and go back another generation? You said that your father's alive and still healthy? How old is he, roughly?

Ms. Monahan: My dad is 71, and my mom is 66. My dad was an active alcoholic for a number of years while I was growing up. And I was the truthsayer of the family. I would scold my dad and say, "You're drinking too much. You need to see a doctor." I still have a very honest relationship with him.

INTERVIEWER: How many kids were there?

MS. MONAHAN: Four.

INTERVIEWER: Were you the oldest?

Another phrasing ("How far along were you in the birth order?") would be more open-ended, but this casual phrasing gets the job done.

MS. MONAHAN: Third. Three girls and a boy. The boy's the oldest.

INTERVIEWER: What's he doing?

MS. MONAHAN: He's a professor of engineering.

INTERVIEWER: And your sister?

MS. MONAHAN: I have an older sister who is a stockbroker. Strange person—she beds both the seller and the buyer to make a better deal.

INTERVIEWER: She brokers the best deal for both parties?

MS. MONAHAN: She takes them to bed as part of what she's doing in sales. She's done this for years.

INTERVIEWER: I don't understand.

MS. MONAHAN: I don't either. She's been married six times, was recently divorced because she was sleeping around. The lady has a lot of problems. My younger sister is very much the same way—compulsive liar and extremely self-destructive. She smokes like a chimney, weighs 320 pounds. Psychologically, and I think physically, she abuses her children. Ernest has seen her, what, twice?

A lot of family psychopathology is emerging. It seems to have struck everybody else in the family.

ERNEST: She yells a lot.

MS. MONAHAN: She's very unhappy, a very miserable person.

ERNEST: She has a bad temper.

INTERVIEWER: Really?

MS. MONAHAN: My brother is a nice man. He's not mean, he doesn't lie, but he takes the absolute path of least resistance in all things.

[After some more discussion of details of Ms. Monahan's family of origin, the interviewer announces that they will have to stop for that session. There ensue a few minutes of wrapping up and arranging to see Ernest's father during the next session the following week.]

In the course of this evaluation, decisions need to be made about what further evaluation is necessary, whom it will involve, and when it should take place. Will treatment be necessary? Of what sort? With whom? With what professional(s)? What are its goals? How many sessions, over what period of time, are likely to be needed?

| The Written Report

Written reports constitute the standard medium for communicating the findings of mental health investigations to other practitioners, to insurance companies, to relatives, and sometimes even to patients themselves. A report offers a clinician the opportunity to organize all the material about a patient into a logical narrative that concisely presents all of the evidence gathered thus far and supports the most likely diagnosis. Although many formats are possible for the written report, years of experience and tradition stand behind the format we use here. We illustrate each portion of the written report with portions taken from all available material about Casey, whose interview has been presented in Chapter 8.

IDENTIFYING DATA

A brief sentence or two of identifying data provides the description the reader needs to form a mental image of the patient. Include sex, race, occupation, religion, marital status (for adults), and any other such information that may seem relevant. Previous experience with mental health treatment is often included, as is some statement about the quality of information provided by the informants (especially useful if reliability seems low).

> This is the second mental health inpatient evaluation of Casey P., a 14-year-old ninth-grader referred by Dr. Z., his outpatient therapist. Casey and his mother are the principal informants. They were seen independently first and then for a brief session together. Mrs. P. is considered a good observer and reliable; Casey was minimally cooperative, but seemed to be reliable in what information he did provide.

THE CHIEF COMPLAINT

In the case of an older adolescent, the chief complaint is the patient's stated reason for entering treatment. For a child or a younger teenager, it will usually be the statement of the principal informant. In either case, it will usually be recorded as a direct quotation, though a statement that is complex, long, or vague is often better summarized. A double recording of chief complaints from both patient and parent may sometimes be useful in demonstrating their different perspectives on the problem.

Of course, this scheme represents only one of myriad ways to formulate an assessment. It depends almost entirely on DSM-IV's approach to diagnosis, which is *categorical* (i.e., it divides disorders into groups based on discrete signs and symptoms that are ascertained in the course of the evaluation). Other diagnostic systems measure degrees of variability on one or more axes; patients are therefore not compartmentalized, but rather are measured on various dimensions. DSM-IV allows for some dimensional ratings—on Axis V (when it asks for a number that corresponds to a general assessment of overall functioning), and in the severity ratings of mood disorders and some other Axis I disorders. However, some diagnosticians prefer to describe behavioral and emotional characteristics as points on continua, rather than assigning any patient—child, adolescent, or adult—to a compartment.

> Casey's mother states, "He's just changed since last year. I want him to be OK."
> Casey reports, "I just wanna get out of here."

HISTORY OF THE PRESENT ILLNESS

The principal focus of any report, the history of the present illness is a chronological account of the reason or reasons the patient has been brought to treatment. Often it begins with a statement such as "The patient was well until age 7, when he suffered the first [episode of . . .]." In the case of a disorder such as Mental Retardation or cerebral palsy that has been present since birth, however, the story might begin with a recounting of the mother's health during pregnancy or of any problems during delivery or the postnatal period.

Many life histories, even those of young children, contain multiple threads that must be disentangled. Sometimes this means presenting one strand at a time—for example, one paragraph devoted to behavior problems, another to learning disabilities. Alternatively, less relevant material may be reserved to later portions of the report. Regardless of approach, the history of the present illness should set forth all the pertinent positive data that help to support the best diagnosis, as well as any pertinent negative data that would help refute less likely or incorrect diagnoses. All of this should be presented as succinctly as possible in jargon-free language, beginning with first symptoms and flowing smoothly to the precipitant(s) for the present evaluation.

Ever since he was a toddler, Casey has had behavioral problems. Overly active from a very early age, he was distractible and had poor attention span in school. Throughout his childhood, he was defiant towards his parents and had repeated temper tantrums; since the age of 11, he has run away from home overnight on at least four occasions. Upon return, he would never tell where he had stayed, but at least once he was treated by the family physician for a sexually transmitted disease.

His mother thought that at one time there seemed to be a cyclic quality to his moods and behavior, with Casey behaving much better in the springtime. In the past year, however, there has been no discernible pattern, and his behavior has become progressively worse. His downward mood swings last only a few days and include feelings of depression, some difficulty sleeping (initial and interval insomnia), but no stated suicidal ideas.

As a first-grader, Casey was treated for hyperactivity. Old school records indicate that he frequently talked out in class, answered questions "almost before they were asked," interrupted teachers and other children, and would wander from his seat. Even his mother noted that he fidgeted and had trouble playing quietly. Nonetheless, because he is bright and has received help with homework from his engineer father, he has never failed a grade and is currently in the ninth grade at C— High. He responded well to Dexedrine, which he took from ages 6 through 13, stopping about a year ago when it seemed to lose its effectiveness. By that time, his overactivity in class had abated to the point that further treatment with medication did not seem warranted.

Casey has recently taken Zoloft (150 mg/day) and lithium (900 mg/day). Besides Dexedrine, he has previously tried Wellbutrin, Norpramin, Tofranil, Catapres, Mellaril, Tegretol, Depakote, and Ritalin. The last two of these reportedly increased his degree of violence, and the others either sedated him excessively or produced no benefit. He has had two seizures described as grand mal in nature, once in the second grade and once in the seventh grade. A seizure workup has reportedly found nonspecific, nonlocalizing slowing on his EEG; an MRI was negative. In the past 6 or 8 months his behavioral problems have escalated. First he cut school; now he curses his teachers. He was recently arrested on burglary charges and placed on probation. On at least two occasions he has physically assaulted and threatened to kill his father. The present hospitalization was precipitated when he responded to what he felt were unreasonable amounts of homework by spitting on his teacher and threatening his principal.

PERSONAL, FAMILIAL, AND SOCIAL BACKGROUND

In a paragraph or so, relate details of the patient's birth, developmental milestones, schooling (including disciplinary as well as academic problems), physical health, friends and social life, hobbies and interests, and (when appropriate) dating and sexual history. Other information that is increasingly a factor in young patients' lives includes details of adoption, parental separations or divorces, and living arrangements such as shared custody and visitation schedules. Use of substances (drugs, alcohol, tobacco), to the extent that any of this material has already been covered in the history of the present illness, may be omitted here.

> Casey's mother was 37 when he was born, in D—, Delaware. She is European American; his father is African American. She completed 1 year of college, then quit to support herself. He is a college graduate who is now employed as an electronics engineer. They were married when they were in their early 20s and intentionally delayed having children until they felt financially able to do so. Throughout the pregnancy, Mrs. P.'s emotional health was good. At birth Casey weighed 7 pounds, 4 ounces and was 21 inches long. He remained in the hospital for several days due to mild jaundice, but did not require a transfusion. His developmental milestones occurred at the expected ages. He sat by 6 months, walked by 15 months, and began to speak words at 16 months. His fine motor skills appeared clumsy—he frequently dropped objects and tripped. He entered day care at about 6 weeks and continued there until age 3, when Mrs. P. quit work. His sister was born when Casey was 2; 3 years later the family moved West and has lived in California ever since.
>
> Casey began to use alcohol when he was 12 and has had some difficulties with it since. However, he has never had symptoms of Alcohol Dependence. Although he has occasionally smoked cigarettes during the past year, he has had no symptoms of Nicotine Dependence.
>
> Although Casey can be induced to cooperate in a one-on-one situation, in a group setting he can be difficult to manage, showing off and demonstrating negative leadership talents. He often tests limits and is quick to alienate peers with rude, deliberately provocative comments.

FAMILY HISTORY

Mental disorders in both close and more distant family members, through biological or environmental means (or both), may have influenced the patient's development. Any noteworthy characteristics of personality or temperament in members of the patient's nuclear family should also be described.

> About 4 years ago Mrs. P. had a several-month period of depression, for which she received Prozac. Casey's father has always been mentally stable. There is no family history of substance use other than that of Casey's maternal grandfather, who was a heavy drinker until about 25 years ago, when he joined Alcoholics Anonymous.

MEDICAL HISTORY

The content of a medical history seems pretty obvious: history of immunizations, childhood diseases, major illnesses, operations, hospitalizations, medications, and allergies. Where appropriate, a medical review of systems will include any positive responses to questions about past or current problems concerning any of the organ systems of the body.

> Other than the apparent seizure disorder, Casey's physical health has been good. He has had no operations or nonmental hospitalizations. He takes only the medications mentioned above and has had no allergies. He has had careful pediatric care and is current in his immunizations. Physical examination revealed no abnormalities.

MENTAL STATUS EXAMINATION

For adults, adolescents, and many children, the report of the mental status examination will include appearance, speech and language, motor activity, sensory capacities, affect and mood, thinking, intelligence, attention, orientation, and relationship with the examiner. Of course, the emphasis will vary, depending on the age and developmental stage of a patient. For adolescents, the information will vary little from that for adults; for preverbal children, the differences will be marked. For the majority of children, Table 1.1 will provide a satisfactory outline, whereas the material in Table 3.1 provides a guide to behaviors expected at different developmental stages.

> Casey is a slightly built but well-nourished boy of mixed racial ancestry who appears small for his stated age of 14. He was dressed casually in baggy jeans, a sweatshirt with the hood pulled up, and flashy, name-brand basketball shoes. Initially his psychomotor activity was mildly depressed, though it quickened as the session progressed.

At times he showed some irritability, but his predominant mood was mild to moderate depression with a somewhat constricted range of affect. His mood was appropriate to his content of thought at all times. He was tearful several times during the initial interview and during subsequent interviews.

Although Casey's rate of speech was normal, the volume and tone were subdued; only occasionally did he offer spontaneous comments. Speech was relevant and coherent. Content of thought largely concerned his desire to be released from the hospital and feelings that he had been unfairly blamed for his recent problems with his teachers and parents.

Casey was fully oriented to person, place, and time. Despite the fact that he had some difficulty recalling all three of a short list of words after 5 minutes, his memory was felt to be unimpaired, because he responded to cognitive testing with little effort. He could spell *world* backward, but was concrete in his interpretation of proverbs.

He had little insight as to how difficult it was for other people to tolerate his behavior, though he did appear to understand at a basic level that his own behavior was responsible for this hospitalization. His recent history reveals extremely poor judgment, though he said he "hoped" he would behave differently, given another chance.

FORMULATION

The case formulation attempts to synthesize from interviews, school reports, and reports of previous mental care all that a clinician has learned about a patient—symptoms, medical history, current living situation and environment, family history, mental status examination, and any other aspects that may help predict the future. Although various formats have been used, we recommend one that is simple yet covers all the important aspects of the child's history and presentation.[1] Above all, the formulation should be brief. We briefly present the relevant sections, then present an example based on Casey's history.

Sections of the Formulation

1. **Brief restatement of the material.** Here are stated a few bits of identifying data and a précis of core material about the symptoms and course of the illness, along with the most important mental status material.

[1]Some clinicians also attempt to formulate the dynamics pertaining to a given clinical problem.

2. **Differential diagnosis.** This lists the possible diagnoses for the patient that should be considered prior to the beginning of treatment. Although all diagnoses (even those that are only remotely likely) should be included, obviously some will be more likely than others. At the top of the list will appear those diagnoses that, because they may be dangerous (e.g., cognitive disorders) or more readily treatable (e.g., mood disorders), are most urgently in need of treatment or elimination from consideration. A detailed formulation will include arguments for and against each Axis I and Axis II diagnosis on the list. Be sure to include any diagnoses suggesting that the difficulty may lie not with the identified patient, but with the family or within the patient's greater social milieu.

3. **Best diagnosis.** This is the diagnosis that, regardless of its place on the differential list, is considered most likely for the given patient.

4. **Contributing factors.** Here is described how the various hereditary and environmental factors promote the development of the patient's main problems. Depending on the availability of material, this section may be quite short, perhaps only a sentence. Statements as to significant strengths and the use of coping (defense) mechanisms can be included here.

5. **Additional information needed.** What further records, interviews, or tests might confirm the diagnosis?

6. **Treatment plan.** An outline of treatment should include biological, psychological, and social methods (the time-honored mental health biopsychosocial approach).

7. **Prognosis.** Based to the extent possible on systematic follow-up and randomized, controlled treatment studies of similar patients, this last section should state the likely outcome for this particular patient.

Formulation for Casey P.

[The bracketed numbers would not ordinarily appear in a written formulation; we include them as a road map.]

[1] Casey is a 14 year-old boy of mixed parentage who was hyperactive throughout his earlier childhood and has persistently defied and argued with adults, blamed others, and easily lost his temper. In the past few months he has used alcohol and tobacco, though no prob-

lems characteristic of Substance Dependence have resulted. He has been in physical conflict with his father, a teacher, and peers. He was recently arrested on burglary charges and admits to at least one episode of joy riding. Although his EEG has been reported as mildly abnormal and he has had two seizures, he has had no recent seizures.

[2] Differential diagnosis:

> Mood Disorder Due to Seizure Disorder, with Depressive Features
> Alcohol-Induced Mood Disorder
> Rule out Major Depressive Disorder
> Possible Bipolar II Disorder
> Depressive Disorder Not Otherwise Specified
> Attention-Deficit/Hyperactivity Disorder (by history)
> Alcohol Abuse
> Oppositional Defiant Disorder
> Rule Out Conduct Disorder

[3] The most likely diagnosis is Oppositional Defiant Disorder in a child who clearly had Attention-Deficit/Hyperactivity Disorder when he was younger. Despite several symptoms of depression by history, no definite mood disorder diagnosis can be made now.

[4] Contributing factors include a depressive disorder (unspecified) in his mother and a history of Alcohol Abuse in a grandfather. There have been no obvious precipitating factors. A significant personal strength is above-average intelligence.

[5] Further information should be sought from Casey's father, who has contributed only indirectly to the data base; further exploration with Casey is needed about his sexual experience; additional neurological evaluation is indicated for his abnormal EEG.

[6] Treatment will focus on (a) further attempts at treating depression and preventing seizures with medication; (b) individual brief psychotherapy to help Casey identify the origins of his anger toward adults and explore other behavioral responses; and (c) discussion with teachers to determine whether his school placement is optimal, even after several moves.

[7] Prognosis could be quite good if a biological basis for his mood symptoms can be found and treated. However, if his current downward spiral from Attention-Deficit/Hyperactivity Disorder through Oppositional

Defiant Disorder continues through Conduct Disorder and beyond, the possibility of Antisocial Personality Disorder is worrisome.

A preliminary five-axis diagnosis for Casey P. is as follows (a similar diagnostic summary will be provided for each of the vignettes we present in Part II):

Axis I	313.81	Oppositional Defiant Disorder
	314.01	Attention-Deficit/Hyperactivity Disorder, Predominantly Hyperactive–Impulsive Type, In Partial Remission
	311	Depressive Disorder Not Otherwise Specified
Axis II	799.9	Diagnosis deferred
Axis III	780.39	Seizure disorder not otherwise specified
Axis IV		None
Axis V	GAF = 55	(upon admission)
	GAF = 65	(at discharge)

PART II

DSM-IV Diagnoses Applicable to Children and Adolescents

| Disorders Usually First
Diagnosed in Infancy,
Childhood, or Adolescence

Quick Guide to Disorders Usually First Diagnosed in Infancy, Childhood, or Adolescence

In this Quick Guide, we have somewhat changed DSM-IV's order of listing to facilitate comparison of disorders. In the text, each of these disorders is fully discussed in its actual DSM-IV order. (The page number following each item in the Quick Guide indicates the point at which the text discussion of it begins.) The diagnosis of each Not Otherwise Specified category (see sidebar following Quick Guide) should be made only when the current data do not justify a more specific diagnosis.

Limited Intellectual Functioning

Mental Retardation. Beginning before the age of 18, Mental Retardation involves low intelligence and resulting difficulties requiring special help for an individual in coping with life. Note that Mental Retardation is the only disorder of infancy, childhood, or adolescence coded on Axis II. The code number is assigned according to its severity: Mild, Moderate, Severe, Profound, or Unspecified (p. 175).

Borderline Intellectual Functioning. This V-code (the V-codes are discussed separately in Chapter 27) is used for persons in the IQ range of 71–84 who don't have the problems in coping with life associated with Mental Retardation (p. 444).

Pervasive Developmental Disorders

Children with pervasive developmental disorders fail to develop normally in a number of areas, including the ability to interact socially, to communicate verbally and nonverbally, and to be imaginative. Many will also have Mental Retardation; when this is the case, it should be coded on Axis II.

Autistic Disorder. A child has impaired social interactions and communication, and develops stereotyped behaviors and interests (p. 200).

Asperger's Disorder. This condition is similar to Autistic Disorder, except that language is not delayed or impaired (p. 210).

Rett's Disorder. After 6 months of apparently normal development, a child develops abnormally, as shown by slow head growth, delayed language, poorly coordinated gait, loss of purposeful hand movements, and social isolation (p. 206).

Childhood Disintegrative Disorder. Following 2 years of normal development, a child loses skills previously acquired (p. 208).

Pervasive Developmental Disorder Not Otherwise Specified. This category is used for such conditions as atypical autism (p. 213).

Learning Disorders

As the label suggests, children with learning disorders have far more difficulty than normal in learning specific academic skills. Although these disorders will be suspected on the basis of classroom reports, each of these diagnoses is made on the basis of a standardized, individualized test. (Disorder of Written Expression can also be diagnosed from a nonstandard functional assessment.)

Reading Disorder. A child's reading skills develop far more slowly than those of peers (p. 184).

Mathematics Disorder. Math skills are markedly poorer than expected for a child's age (p. 186).

Disorder of Written Expression. Writing skills are slow to develop (p. 187).

Academic Problem. This V-code is used when scholastic problems are the focus of treatment (p. 445).

Learning Disorder Not Otherwise Specified. Use this category for learning disorders that do not meet the criteria for any of the disorders above (p. 187).

Communication Disorders

Expressive Language Disorder. A child may have a limited vocabulary or trouble producing grammatically correct sentences (p. 191).

Mixed Receptive–Expressive Language Disorder. A child has problems as noted just above, plus difficulty understanding words or sentences (p. 194).

Phonological Disorder. Speech develops slowly for a child's age or dialect (p. 195).

Stuttering. There is frequent disruption in the normal fluency of speech (p. 196).

Selective Mutism. A child elects not to talk, other than to the immediate family (p. 250).

Communication Disorder Not Otherwise Specified. Use this category for problems of communication that do not meet the criteria for the disorders listed above (p. 198).

Movement and Tic Disorders

Developmental Coordination Disorder. A child is slow to develop motor coordination and is *not* necessarily mentally retarded (p. 188).

Transient Tic Disorder. Tics occur for no longer than 1 year (p. 234).

Chronic Motor or Vocal Tic Disorder. Either motor or vocal tics occur, but not both (p. 234).

Tourette's Disorder. Multiple vocal and motor tics occur frequently throughout the day (p. 234).

Stereotypic Movement Disorder. Children repeatedly rock, bang their heads, bite themselves, or pick at their own skin or body orifices (p. 258).

Tic Disorder Not Otherwise Specified. Use this category for tics that do not meet the criteria for Tourette's Disorder or the other tic disorders (p. 239).

Disorders of Intake and Elimination

Pica. The child eats material that is not food (p. 229).

Rumination Disorder. There is persistent regurgitation and chewing of food already eaten (p. 231).

Feeding Disorder of Infancy or Early Childhood. A child's failure to eat enough leads to weight loss or a failure to gain weight. A problem with interaction with the primary caregiver causes this behavior (p. 231).

Enuresis. At 5 years of age or later, a child repeatedly voids urine (voluntarily or involuntarily) into bedding or clothing (p. 243).

Encopresis. At 4 years of age or later, a child repeatedly passes feces into clothing or somewhere else inappropriate (p. 241).

Other Eating Disorders. See Chapter 22 for information about children or adolescents who refuse to eat until they become ill (Anorexia Nervosa), or who repeatedly overeat but purge themselves to maintain an appropriate weight (Bulimia Nervosa).

Attention-Deficit and Disruptive Behavior Disorders

Attention-Deficit/Hyperactivity Disorder. In this common condition—usually (and in text hereafter) abbreviated as ADHD—individuals are hyperactive, impulsive, or inattentive, and often all three (p. 215).

Attention-Deficit/Hyperactivity Disorder Not Otherwise Specified. Use this category for symptoms of hyperactivity, impulsiveness, or inattention that do not fulfill the criteria for ADHD (p. 219).

Conduct Disorder. A child or adolescent repeatedly violates rules or the rights of others (p. 219).

Oppositional Defiant Disorder. Multiple examples of negativistic behavior persist for at least 6 months (p. 224).

Child or Adolescent Antisocial Behavior. This V-code can be used when antisocial behavior cannot be ascribed to a mental disorder, such as Oppositional Defiant Disorder, Conduct Disorder, or ADHD (p. 444).

Disruptive Behavior Disorder Not Otherwise Specified. Use this category for disturbances of conduct or oppositional behaviors that do not meet the criteria for Conduct Disorder or Oppositional Defiant Disorder (p. 227).

Disorders of Relationship

Separation Anxiety Disorder. A patient becomes anxious when away from parents or home (p. 246).

Reactive Attachment Disorder of Infancy or Early Childhood. Beginning before age 5, a child either fails to interact with others or socializes indiscriminately (p. 253).

Parent–Child Relational Problem. This V-code is used when there is no mental disorder, but a child and parent have problems getting along (p. 439).

Sibling Relational Problem. This V-code is used for difficulties between siblings (p. 439).

Problems Related to Abuse or Neglect. A single V-code number is used to cover the three categories of difficulties that arise from neglect or from physical or sexual abuse of children (p. 442).

Other

Disorder of Infancy, Childhood, or Adolescence Not Otherwise Specified. This is a catch-all category for mental disorders beginning in early life that do not meet the criteria for *any* disorder described above (p. 260).

MENTAL RETARDATION

DSM-IV does not list Mental Retardation with the cognitive disorders, though the two categories share attributes (both are brain disorders that create problems in daily life). Mental Retardation refers, as most people know, to low intelligence (as determined by a standard intelligence test) that begins before the age of 18. But low IQ alone will not qualify a patient for this diagnosis: There must also be present a variety of problems in performing the activities of everyday life such as working, communicating with others, and providing self-care (see the criteria in Table 11.1). The patient's success in coping can be modified by the effects of education, training, motivation, personality, and support from family members and other important friends and caregivers.

The Not Otherwise Specified diagnoses have been a DSM staple since 1980. They should be used only when DSM-IV criteria for more specific diagnoses cannot be made within the same diagnostic category (e.g., depressive disorders, psychotic disorders). Although the text of DSM-IV suggests other situations when such a diagnosis might be appropriate—for example, when data collection has been fragmentary—we caution against setting uncertain or vague diagnoses down in other than a differential list. We worry that too-casual use of the Not Otherwise Specified categories can provide a misleading sense of closure to a diagnostic puzzle that ought to occupy the clinician's attention until all the missing pieces have been collected. See the Introduction (p. 10) for suggestions about other ways of indicating diagnostic uncertainty.

TABLE 11.1. Criteria for Mental Retardation

- The patient's intellectual functioning is markedly below average (IQ of 70 or less on a standard, individually administered test).
- In two or more of the following areas, the patient has more trouble functioning than would be expected for age and cultural group:
  - ✓ Communication
  - ✓ Self-care
  - ✓ Home life
  - ✓ Interpersonal and social skills
  - ✓ Using community resources
  - ✓ Self-direction
  - ✓ Academic functioning
  - ✓ Work
  - ✓ Free time
  - ✓ Health
  - ✓ Safety
- The condition starts before age 18.

Code based on approximate IQ range:

317	Mild Mental Retardation (IQ 50–55 to 70)
318.0	Moderate Mental Retardation (IQ 35–40 to 50–55)
318.1	Severe Mental Retardation (IQ 20–25 to 35–40)
318.2	Profound Mental Retardation (IQ less than 20–25)
319	Mental Retardation, Severity Unspecified (the patient cannot be tested, but significant retardation seems highly likely)

Coding Note: Mental Retardation is coded on Axis II.

Although an IQ of 70 is usually considered the upper limit of Mild Mental Retardation, some individuals who score a few points below this mark may care for themselves competently. Unless they are functionally impaired in two or more areas, such persons should not be given a Mental Retardation diagnosis. On the other hand, a functionally impaired individual whose IQ ranks in the low 70s *can* receive this diagnosis. If measured IQ were the sole criterion for Mental Retardation, the number of diagnosed individuals would approximately double, to 2–3% of the general population.

Aside from functional cognitive impairment, mentally retarded children may have additional problematic behaviors, including aggression, dependence, impulsiveness, passivity, self-injury, stubbornness, and poor tolerance for frustration. Low attention span and hyperactivity have also frequently been noted, as have mood-related symptoms such as depression and low self-esteem. Indeed, Axis I mental disorders affect from one-third to two-thirds of mentally retarded individuals. It is not clear whether these behavioral and emotional symptoms are primary consequences of the Mental Retardation syndrome or are due to an interaction between cognitive development and environmental stressors—for example, problems resulting from attempts to measure up to unmeetable expectations of family members or friends.

Approximately 1% of the general population is affected by Mental Retardation; for reasons that are still debated, males predominate by a ratio of about 3:2. About 85% of these individuals have Mild Mental Retardation, which implies that they can attain at least sixth-grade academic skills. Although schoolwork comes more slowly to them, such individuals can profit from tutoring. They can learn to read for

The number of additional mental and physical conditions that may be comorbid in a patient with Mental Retardation is staggering. Take, for example, a patient with Williams syndrome, a rare condition inherited on an autosomal recessive basis (it is caused by microdeletion of a segment of the long arm of chromosome 7 that includes the elastin gene). Physical syndromes can include severe intolerance to sound, poor binocular vision, "elfin" face (fullness around the eyes, protuberant upper and lower jaws, thick lips), mild deficiency of growth, congenital heart disease (aortic stenosis), abnormal gait, dental problems, and chronic or recurrent urinary symptoms. Sudden death has occurred in some cases. The mental symptoms and disorders include hyperactivity with attention deficit, sleep disturbances, daytime wetting, feeding problems during infancy that may present as failure to thrive, and incoordination. How many of these syndromes and conditions, when their criteria are fully met, should be included on Axis I or Axis III? Should personality features of these children—described as affectionate, charming, gentle, open, and talkative—be included on Axis II?

pleasure, can use computers, and can develop friendships and intimate relationships. With family and other social support, many hold jobs, living more or less independently in the community.

When still young, individuals with Moderate Mental Retardation (IQ of about 45–55), who comprise about 10% of the retarded population, usually learn to speak well enough to communicate their basic needs effectively; some will be able to hold simple conversations. Although they can learn social, job-related, and self-care skills and can work in sheltered workshops, they probably will never live independently.

Those with Severe Mental Retardation (IQ of about 20–40) comprise 5% of all mentally retarded children. They may learn to talk, perform simple jobs with appropriate supervision, and perhaps even read a few words. The most severely affected individuals of all, those with Profound Mental Retardation constitute 1–2% of all mentally retarded persons.

In the overwhelming majority of those with Mental Retardation, there is no specific known etiology. An individual's Mental Retardation can have more than one cause (see Table 11.2).

TABLE 11.2. Common Causes of Mental Retardation

Suspected etiological conditions	% of total	Examples
Early pregnancy	30	Down's syndrome, maternal infections, maternal substance use (fetal alcohol syndrome)
Later pregnancy and perinatal period	10	Anoxia, birth trauma, fetal malnutrition, prematurity
Environmental and mental disorders	20	Cultural deprivation, early-onset Schizophrenia
Hereditary conditions	5	Fragile X syndrome, tuberous sclerosis, Tay–Sachs disease
Acquired physical conditions	5	Anoxia (e.g., near-drowning), infections, lead poisoning, trauma
Unknown	30	

Mel

Mel was 10 years old when he was brought to the mental health clinic for evaluation. The foster mother in the home where he had been living for the past 4 months voiced the chief complaint that he had exhibited himself to other children at school.

Mel's biological mother was just 18 when he was born; he and his twin brother were her fourth and fifth babies. Although she received prenatal care, she was probably using cocaine during much of her pregnancy. Mel and his brother each weighed just under 5 pounds at birth; however, it was Mel whose jaundice required light therapy for a week before he could be discharged from the hospital. Three months later he was back, suffering from seizures that for a time were treated with phenobarbital.

Until he was a year old, Mel lived with his mother; after that, she paid more attention to her crack habit than to Mel and his siblings. According to records, at 7 months Mel still could not remain in a seated position when placed there and didn't respond to sounds the way his twin did. During that first year of life, he had three hospitalizations, once when he stopped breathing and twice for seizures. When the time came for his third hospital discharge, he went to the first of many foster homes.

The foster mother with whom Mel lived the longest—from the time he was 6 until just before he turned 8—had noted how slowly he learned even the rudiments of self-care, such as tying his shoes and brushing his teeth. At the child guidance clinic, he received a Wechsler Intelligence Scale for Children—

Revised (WISC-R) Full-Scale IQ of 71, with identical Verbal and Performance scores. When he started first grade at the age of 6 years, 8 months, he was initially mainstreamed but quickly fell behind his younger classmates. Thereafter, he attended special education classes.

Throughout school, Mel's special education teachers regarded his progress as adequate, if unspectacular, for his developmental level. Although he was sometimes restless, Mel would mostly sit quietly in his seat unless disturbed. His attention span was normal, especially for the activities he enjoyed—drawing spaceships and coloring. He sometimes lashed out verbally or physically if required to engage in less desirable activities. His progress cards noted that he generally spoke distinctly, but that his language skills lagged behind his age level by at least 2 years.

Mel's current teacher reported that he was easily led. On the playground and after school, he was often seen associating with Terry, a boy 2 years younger who attended a regular class. Terry was described as "sneaky and hyperactive." On several occasions he persuaded Mel to implement some of his own plans, such as taking sandwiches from another child's lunch box. Once he even got Mel to steal money from a teacher's desk drawer, but Mel cried about it afterward. The current evaluation was precipitated when Terry persuaded other children to applaud each time Mel removed an article of clothing, which he did, right down to the skin. He later repeated the performance at his foster home.

When evaluated in the clinic, Mel looked a lot like other 10-year-olds. His posture, gait, and psychomotor activity were completely normal. His grooming was passable, but his glasses had slipped far down on his nose and he didn't bother to adjust them; his runny nose also needed more attention than he gave it. However, he was attentive throughout the course of the interview. He spoke mainly in response to questions and tended to answer in one- or two-word statements. When he did speak at greater length, he didn't really have much to say. His sentence structure betrayed no illogicalities or incoherence of thought.

Although Mel said that he felt "OK," his affect appeared somewhat sad during portions of the interview. However, after the session he was observed interacting with another child in the hallway with an affect that appeared to be "about normal." He denied wanting to hurt himself or other people, or feeling that anyone was trying to harm or otherwise interfere with him.

Mel had considerable difficulty understanding the concept of hallucinations, which, after several minutes of repeated explanations (and often giggling responses), he finally denied. His insight was evaluated as "limited": When first asked about any possible connection between taking his clothes off and the current interview, he appeared to see none. When asked the same question later on, he admitted that there might be a connection, adding, "Geez, I've told you a hundred times!" Because of his recent history, his judgment was regarded as poor.

Evaluation of Mel

Mel's tested IQ was 71, just above the arbitrary line dividing individuals with Mental Retardation from those with a borderline normal IQ. Remember that the test used must be individually administered; group IQ tests are less accurate. Even a test administered by a skilled psychometrician will only be accurate within about 5 IQ points, yielding a potential range for Mel of 66 to 76. However, unless young patients have difficulty functioning in at least two of the life areas mentioned in the criteria, they should not receive a Mental Retardation diagnosis.

Mel's academic difficulties were noted early in his school career. Although the clinician noted that his speech was impoverished, which could be taken as evidence of poor communication skills, many children will respond to a strange interviewer with apparent poverty of speech. In Mel's case, however, the observation was consonant with reports from his teachers. (DSM-IV recommends using multiple sources to verify information about areas of malfunctioning.) There was ample evidence of problems with school and communication, not to mention the social problems caused when he removed his clothing in public. In all, at least three life areas had been affected by his intellectual impairment, adequately sustaining the diagnosis of Mental Retardation. Had life areas not been affected, a V-code designation of **Borderline Intellectual Functioning** would be appropriate. His intellectual impairment had been noted from infancy, ruling out any of the **dementias** as a possible alternative diagnosis. Pervasive developmental disorders such as **Autistic Disorder** necessitate difficulty in relating socially to others, although many such children will also be diagnosable as having Mental Retardation. Those with **learning disorders** may appear slow in certain areas but will function normally in many others.

Mentally retarded persons can have nearly any other diagnosis found in DSM-IV. In fact, the prevalence of such conditions as **mood disorders and psychotic disorders** may be several times as great as in individuals with normal intelligence. **Seizure disorders** (as Axis III diagnoses) will also be found in around one-fourth of mentally retarded individuals. **Stereotypic Movement Disorder** should be diagnosed if body rocking, head banging, or other repetitive behavior is so severe that it would require treatment, regardless of intelligence level.

The actual IQ score tells us what level of Mental Retardation should be diagnosed. The physical condition responsible (e.g., Down's syndrome), if known, should be recorded on Axis III. In Mel's case, the five-axis diagnosis would be as follows:

Axis I	V71.09	No diagnosis
Axis II	317	Mild Mental Retardation
Axis III		None
Axis IV		None
Axis V	GAF = 51	(current)

Assessing Mental Retardation

General Suggestions

Perhaps one of the greatest challenges in interviewing mentally retarded children (and adults) is to pitch the questions at just the right level—neither so complex as to confuse nor so simple as to insult. Here is an excellent reason to begin with an open-ended invitation to speak freely and at length: This will give you time to judge how to tread that fine line. Generally, simplicity is the best rule; brief sentences with short words and concrete concepts will be better understood. Avoid preambles and lengthy or complicated explanations that may divert attention from the focus of inquiry. Don't hesitate to repeat a question that goes unanswered, and give examples if they appear needed.

However, with increasing degrees of Mental Retardation, open-ended questions are less and less likely to be productive. Although yes–no questions have the virtue of being simple, they may encourage inaccurate information because retarded persons tend to favor "yes" responses; multiple-choice questions are often better for this reason. Also, be careful not to use positive reinforcement excessively—this can also yield answers biased toward what the patient believes you want to hear.

Keep in mind several points about interviewing patients with Mental Retardation:

- Some individuals "look retarded" (e.g., those with Down's syndrome), but most do not.
- Don't avoid discussing physical handicaps as you review the problems a retarded child or adolescent faces.
- Higher-functioning patients may have a sense of humor and will enjoy a joke, as long as they do not perceive it to be at their expense.
- Younger or more severely retarded patients will require questions that are more concrete, more tightly structured, and more simply phrased. Especially if an answer you obtain seems irrelevant, obscure, or bizarre, make sure the patient has understood the question by requesting a repetition of the question itself.
- Some children and adolescents with Mental Retardation may have a rich fantasy life that renders them vulnerable to an inappropriate diagnosis of psychosis. It is vitally important to evaluate carefully material that is reported by caregivers as "hallucinations" (it might be fantasy) or "delusions" (mentally retarded children and adolescents are often suspicious of the new or unknown).
- Self-esteem, which is often low in the mentally retarded, needs careful and repeated evaluation. Although these patients can become depressed, poor self-image is more nearly universal.
- An initial evaluation will in all likelihood take longer than one for a nonretarded patient, and because a retarded individual's attention span is short, evaluation may require several sessions.
- Finally, many causes of Mental Retardation (e.g., fragile X syndrome, phenylketonuria, tuberous sclerosis) can be detected by means of laboratory studies, whose use is beyond the scope of this volume.

Developmental Factors

The tools appropriate to determine the developmental quotient (DQ) and IQ will vary, depending on the patient's chronological age. The WISC-R is appropriate for children aged 6–16 years. Measurement of infants' DQ is more problematic. The Denver Developmental Scale is often used by pediatricians. The Bayley Scales of Infant Development can be used to assess children aged 1–42 months. Except for the Denver Developmental Scale, all of these instruments are usually administered by specially trained developmental or clinical psychologists. Of course, children with severe or profound Mental Retardation and those who have associated characteristic physical features (such as Down's syndrome) are likely to be diagnosed at an earlier age. Look for information about these scales in Appendix 1.

LEARNING DISORDERS

In the United States, as in most of the world, a learning disorder is a specific problem in acquiring information that is out of proportion to a child's native intelligence and cannot be explained by factors such as culture, other mental disorder, or economic status. These exclusions are important, for they help to define a set of problems in which there is a discrepancy between the child's actual academic achievement and theoretical ability to learn.

Each of the learning disorders (other than Learning Disorder Not Otherwise Specified)—Reading Disorder, Mathematics Disorder, and Disorder of Written Expression—requires evidence obtained from an individually administered, standardized test before a diagnosis can be made. (See Table 11.3 for the criteria for these three disorders.) Of course, to be valid, any such instrument must be culturally appropriate and sensitive. Like so many DSM-IV disorders, learning disorders cannot be diagnosed unless they have consequences for scholastic, work, or social life. Many Americans—perhaps 5%—would qualify for a lifetime diagnosis of a learning disorder. About 40% of children formally diagnosed with learning disorder drop out of school without completing high school, as compared with the national average of about 6%.

The magnitude of a learning disorder's behavioral and social consequences

---

TABLE 11.3. Criteria for Three Learning Disorders

315.00 Reading Disorder; 315.1 Mathematics Disorder; 315.2 Disorder of Written Expression

- As measured by a standardized test that is given individually, the patient's [ability to read (accuracy or comprehension)] [mathematical ability] [writing ability] is substantially less than you would expect, considering the patient's age, intelligence, and education. (Only in the case of Disorder of Written Expression may diagnosis be based on a functional assessment of the patient's overall performance.)
- This deficiency materially impedes academic achievement or daily living.
- If there is also a sensory defect, the deficiency is worse than you would expect with it.

Coding Note: On Axis III, code any associated sensory deficit or general medical condition (such as a neurological disorder).

When you are diagnosing learning disorders, it is important what country you are in. For reasons best known to them, British mental health professionals have recently begun applying the term *learning disorder* to mean Mental Retardation. The results are likely to be nightmares for MEDLINE indexers and years of confusion for anyone wanting to review the literature on the subject.

is directly related to the severity of the impairment and to the educational remediation and social support available. Associated childhood behavioral disorders include Conduct Disorder, Oppositional Defiant Disorder, and ADHD. Also associated with the learning disorders are Phonological Disorder and Expressive Language Disorder, the latter only when it is of the developmental, not the acquired type (see p. 191). In fact, some authorities believe that communication disorders and learning disorders belong on a continuum, rather than being separate entities. DSM-IV does not take this approach, however.

315.00 Reading Disorder

Also known as *dyslexia,* Reading Disorder is the best studied of the several specific learning disorders. It occurs when a child (or adult, should it persist) cannot read at the level expected for age and intelligence. Reading Disorder can actually take any of three forms: difficulty with either comprehension or speed when reading silently, or with accuracy when reading aloud. (The criteria, however, mention only comprehension and accuracy.) Normally distributed throughout the population, it affects about 4% of school-age children. Most of those who have been studied are boys, but in populations carefully defined by research criteria, the male-to-female ratio is closer to unity. This suggests that boys are only more likely to be referred; perhaps other factors, such as activity level, make them stand out in parents' or teachers' minds as needing evaluation.

Reading Disorder has been attributed to a variety of environmental and familial causes. Lead poisoning and fetal alcohol syndrome have both been implicated, but they can only account for a small percentage of cases. Because early stimulation is so important to childhood development, socially disadvantaged individuals are especially at risk. Phonological skills are important to the development of reading ability, and Phonological Disorder is often found in the families of patients with dyslexia. In fact, some studies suggest that up to 30% of Reading Disorder cases may be accounted for by genetic inheritance.

As with so many other childhood disorders, the prognosis for those with Reading Disorder depends on a number of factors. Foremost among them is the severity of the disorder: Reading at two standard deviations below the mean carries an especially poor prognosis. Other factors that suggest a poor prognosis are parents who are poorly educated and a child's lower overall intellectual capabilities (though not absolute IQ—we know of one Down's syndrome child with an IQ of barely 70 who learned to read sentences phonetically by age 3½). In one study of children treated at age 7, 40% were reading normally at age 14. Prognosis in this group was not related to gender, the presence of phonological problems, or ADHD.

Tad

Tad Lincoln, the youngest son of Abraham Lincoln, provides an example of how several childhood disorders may be found in a single individual. Tad (his real name was Thomas, but his father thought that his squirming as an infant resembled the motions of a tadpole) probably had what today would be called ADHD. At that time, his always spirited, often frenetic behavior earned him a variety of epithets, including "spoiled brat" and "the madam's wildcat."

As one biographer put it, "Tad's mind teemed with plans and his body never rested." Even his doting mother, Mary Todd Lincoln, who herself almost certainly had a somatoform disorder, referred to him as "my troublesome Sunshine." White House staff of the era related tales of Tad's energetic mischief. He ate the strawberries the cook had cultivated out of season for a state dinner; he kicked a chess board balanced across the knees of his father and a visiting judge; he whittled the White House furniture; he drove goats through the East Room, riding a kitchen chair behind them. He fired a gun from an upstairs window and waved a Confederate flag when his father was reviewing Union troops.

Besides his conduct and activity level, Tad had other developmental problems. He had difficulty with pronunciation, for example: Following his father's assassination, 12-year-old Tad said "Papa's tot," meaning that his father had been shot. Another story from about the same time described Tad's efforts to read. His mother showed him a picture of a primate with the word *ape* printed below it. "Monkey," pronounced Tad.

Not long after his father died, Tad was reportedly behaving better. "I am not a President's son now," he was quoted as saying. "I won't have many presents anymore. Well, I will try and be a good boy . . . " He began his schooling in earnest and drew abreast his agemates in both learning and ambition by age 18, when he died of tuberculosis.

Evaluation of Tad

Was Tad's delay in learning to read better explained by the fact that he abhorred books and study, or was the cause–effect relationship the reverse? Tad's subsequent history argues against physical causes such as **impaired vision or hearing**, and other Axis I or II disorders such as a **pervasive developmental disorder** or **Mental Retardation**. All of these conditions constitute the differential diagnosis of any learning disorder. One can argue that word substitution (*monkey* for *ape*) is evidence for dyslexia. And what about Tad's difficulty with pronunciation? Of course, a diagnosis of **Phonological Disorder** requires a much larger sample of speech than has come down to us by report, as well as evidence that the difficulties with speech production made an independent contribution to Tad's relationships at home, at work, or with studies. At least one observer claimed that Tad had a cleft palate, which is one of the structural defects commonly associated with Phonological Disorder. **Cultural factors** should sometimes be considered, as in cases where there is inadequate exposure to the native language.

In the opinion of contemporary observers and some biographers, Tad's developmental delay and naughty behavior stemmed from pampering and laziness. A modern diagnosis of ADHD (found in up to 20% of children with a learning disorder) would require additional symptoms of overactivity, impulsiveness, distractibility, and inattentiveness in a variety of school and social situations.

Without benefit of modern-day observation and testing, Tad's diagnosis remains uncertain. Because we believe that clinicians should not diagnose children they have not had the opportunity to examine, we will give no five-axis diagnosis for Tad Lincoln.

315.1 Mathematics Disorder

Far less is known about Mathematics Disorder than about Reading Disorder. It may be found in about 1% of schoolchildren, and (obviously) does not appear until children are expected to learn to do mathematics—as early as kindergarten, but in most cases by the beginning of second grade. These children may have difficulty performing mathematical operations, ranging from the elementary to the complex: counting, recognizing mathematical symbols, learning math facts (such as multiplication tables), performing simple addition or other operations, comprehending mathematical terms, and understanding story problems.

315.2 Disorder of Written Expression

Even less is known about Disorder of Written Expression than about either of the previous two. Children with this disorder make mistakes in grammar, spelling, punctuation, and paragraph organization, and may have indecipherable handwriting. (But don't make the diagnosis if the *only* problem is spelling or penmanship.) The diagnosis is generally not appropriate if a patient is poorly coordinated, as in Developmental Coordination Disorder.

315.9 Learning Disorder Not Otherwise Specified

Problems of learning that don't meet criteria for any of the more specific learning disorders can be coded as Learning Disorder Not Otherwise Specified. DSM-IV gives the example of a combination of reading, mathematical, and writing problems that only *together* impede academic ability.

Assessing Learning Disorders

General Suggestions

Each of the learning disorders (aside from the minor qualification for Disorder of Written Expression) requires standardized, individually administered tests for diagnosis. Of course, before an evaluation ever gets this far, in nearly every case there will be a history that points the way to the correct diagnosis. For that reason, an interview of a patient with, say, Reading Disorder might best be spent looking for accompanying disorders, such as another learning disorder, a communication disorder, or ADHD.

An effective screen for dyslexia is often to have a child read an age-appropriate selection while you observe for the cardinal three features: slow reading, inaccurate reading, and poor comprehension of what has just been read.

Developmental Factors

Obviously, the learning disorders are unlikely to be diagnosed until a child reaches school age. Then diagnosis requires that the area of learning be measured as "substantially below" expectation for the child's intelligence. This requires testing that takes into consideration the child's chronological age—in a word, IQ.

MOTOR SKILLS DISORDER

315.4 Developmental Coordination Disorder

Developmental Coordination Disorder (abbreviated DCD for convenience in this section only) has been a focus of controversy ever since it first appeared in DSM-III-R in 1987. Can it be differentiated from neurological conditions such as dyspraxia? Is it only a fancy way of saying, "This is a clumsy child"? Does it deserve to be called a mental disorder, any more than any physical condition that produces social, educational, or occupational disability does? Whatever the eventual answers to these questions, the current notion of such a child—one whose motor coordination is seriously below expectation for intelligence and age (see Table 11.4 for the full criteria)—may fit up to 6% of children aged 5–10 years. Very young children may have delayed milestones, whereas older children may have difficulty with sports or handwork skill that involve fine motor coordination.

The cause of DCD is unknown and does not appear to be anything so simple as a problem with vision. With some studies showing as many as five different patterns of dysfunction, the ultimate "cause" will probably turn out to be a heterogeneous array, including physiological, genetic, neurological, and other contributions. At that point, a name change may be in order.

Tripper

Tripper (his family's nickname for him) was referred for evaluation at the age of 9 with the sole complaint that he was poorly coordinated for his age—

TABLE 11.4. Criteria for Developmental Coordination Disorder

- Motor coordination in daily activities is substantially poorer than you would expect, considering the patient's age and intelligence. This may be shown by dropping things, general clumsiness, poor handwriting, or problems with sports, or by pronounced delays in developmental motor milestones such as sitting, crawling, or walking.
- This incoordination materially impedes academic achievement or daily living.
- It is not due to a general medical condition, such as cerebral palsy or muscular dystrophy.
- Criteria for a pervasive developmental disorder are not fulfilled.
- If there is Mental Retardation, the incoordination is worse than you would expect with these problems.

Coding Note: On Axis III, code any sensory deficit or general medical condition (such as a neurological disorder).

"preternaturally clumsy," in the words of his father, a professor of early English literature. As a child, Tripper's father had himself been "locally famous" for poor coordination. "I could stumble on a bare wood floor," he told the interviewing clinician. But by the time he was 16, he had improved enough to play on his school's junior varsity tennis team.

It didn't look as though Tripper would excel at organized sports any time soon. "I couldn't even make the walking team," he said morosely. "Everyone laughs at me and says I'm the clumsiest guy in the galaxy." When he played at all, he was always chosen last for team sports; for the past couple of years, he had spent lunch and recess in the classroom, reading. He did well in classes such as math and English, but his handwriting was nearly illegible. At a time when he should be developing some fluency, his letters slanted and careened into one another, even when he painstakingly drew each character, lifting his pencil several times in the course of a single word. Homework "took forever," and his badly smeared pages often ended up crumpled in a wastebasket.

The product of a full-term, normal delivery, Tripper had no allergies or unusual diseases. He sat up at 7 months and took his first steps at 13 months. He spoke words and sentences at the developmentally expected ages. His mother remembered that he had required much longer than his siblings to learn to manipulate a spoon, however.

On neurological examination, Tripper attended to the tasks well and appeared normal except when asked to perform motor tasks, such as copying a diamond. "This is going to be tough," he said, then drew a shaky, five-sided figure. His WISC-R Verbal IQ was 123, but his Performance IQ was only 79. On the Beery Developmental Test of Visual Motor Integration, he scored a borderline 77; however, when the motor component was ignored, his Visual Spatial Integration score was a normal 105.

Evaluation of Tripper

Although Tripper's developmental milestones (sitting, walking) occurred within the normal range, he fully met the criteria for DCD, by virtue of being particularly clumsy and demonstrating it on standardized testing (not required for diagnosis). His sociability and schoolwork both suffered from it. He did not have Mental Retardation (which can co-occur with DCD, so long as the motor difficulties exceed what one would expect, given the extent of the **Mental Retardation**.

His ability to attend to tasks suggested that he did not have ADHD, in which children often have accidents or bump into things because their attention is on other matters. Children with **pervasive developmental disorders** (especially Asperger's Disorder) are sometimes clumsy, but this diagnosis was rendered vanishingly unlikely by Tripper's ability to relate to the examiner. The normal physical exam rendered **neurological causes** of dyspraxia unlikely. If his handwriting had been accompanied by mistakes in grammar, spelling, punctuation, and paragraph organization, **Disorder of Written Expression** would be an appropriate additional diagnosis. (Other learning disorders may also accompany a diagnosis of DCD and should be sought.) Tripper's full diagnosis would be as follows:

Axis I	315.4	Developmental Coordination Disorder
Axis II	V71.09	No diagnosis
Axis III		None
Axis IV		None
Axis V	GAF = 75	(current)

Assessing Developmental Coordination Disorder

General Suggestions

Unlike the communication and learning disorders, DCD does not require standardized tests for diagnosis. Rather, you need to be familiar enough with norms for physical ability in children of all ages to recognize deviations. (A toddler learning to walk is naturally wobbly; a 4-year-old who wobbles may have DCD.) Table 3.1 provides approximate ages for some of these milestones. If it seems difficult to draw these children into discussion of their symptoms, focus first on areas where they excel; this may bolster their self-esteem enough to enable them to talk about the areas of deficiency. It is also important to learn what the norms are for an individual child's playmates and classmates. Ask, "What is your class doing in gym? How do you spend recess?"

Obtain a firsthand demonstration of physical abilities by asking the child to hop on one foot, climb stairs, tie a shoe, catch and throw a ball; to copy symbols such as a diamond, a triangle, and intersecting polygons; to rotate the hand rapidly back and forth at the wrists; and to touch a finger first to the child's own nose, then to your finger. Instead of asking the child to perform these tasks directly, it is often helpful to play the game "Simon Says." Then you can also test the child's ability to concentrate and follow instructions while assessing coordination. Begin with easy tasks and make them progressively more complicated. Join in and have fun. Make testing enjoyable.

Developmental Factors

Of course, because symptoms change with age, assessment depends heavily on the appropriateness of the task in relation to a child's chronological age. Many children seem to outgrow their immaturity spontaneously; yet, by the age of 15, nearly half of those in one study diagnosed as having DCD when they were 5 were still demonstrably different from an age-matched comparison group. Note that assessment may depend as much on history (delayed developmental milestones) as on a cross-sectional evaluation of the child in an office setting.

COMMUNICATION DISORDERS

The disorders described in this section impair a child's ability to communicate with others. Despite the fact that they occur frequently, several of these disorders have not been well studied. Except for Stuttering (which, though much less common, is well known because it is so obvious), communication disorders are not commonly known and may often go unrecognized.

315.31 Expressive Language Disorder

Despite normal intelligence and the ability to understand what is said to them, children with Expressive Language Disorder (abbreviated ELD in this section) have trouble communicating verbally. The difficulty can show up in a variety of ways. They learn to speak late, and they speak little for their age. When they do speak, they use short sentences and simple grammar. They may have trouble learning new words, use words incorrectly, omit important parts of sentences, and/or invent their own word order. As they grow older, they may fail to develop the varieties of grammatical structure (e.g., the use of different verb forms) and sentence type (e.g., the use of commands) that characterize the speech of their agemates. Table 11.5 presents the criteria for both ELD and Mixed Receptive–Expressive Language Disorder (see below).

ELD can be either developmental or acquired. Developmental ELD has no known cause, though it tends to run in families and may have a genetic component. It may be suspected in early infancy, when babbling fails to occur, and it affects 3–5% of young children. The acquired type usually results from brain trauma or a disease such as chronic middle-ear infection. It can begin suddenly, at any age, and is much less common than the developmental type.

In its mildest forms, ELD may remain unidentified, even after a child has been referred to a mental health clinic for another reason. In one study, up to 25% of children referred for disruptive behavior were diagnosed as having previously unsuspected ELD. It has been more commonly reported in multi-problem families, but this may reflect the fact that such children are more often evaluated in mental health clinics. Up to half of children with developmental ELD grow out of it (sometimes within 6 months), but the outcome of the acquired type depends on its cause, severity, and the age of the child. ELD is associated with negativism and behavior disorders.

TABLE 11.5. Criteria for Expressive Language Disorder and Mixed Receptive–Expressive Language Disorder

315.31 Expressive Language Disorder	315.31 Mixed Receptive–Expressive Language Disorder
• On standardized measures, the patient's expressive language development scores are materially lower than scores for both nonverbal intellectual capacity and receptive language development. Clinically, the patient may have severely limited vocabulary, make errors of tense, recall words poorly, or produce sentences that are shorter or less complex than is developmentally appropriate.	• On standardized tests that are given individually, the patient's receptive and expressive language development scores are materially lower than those for nonverbal intellectual capacity. Clinically, the patient may have the same problems as with Expressive Language Disorder, as well as problems understanding sentences, words, or specific classes of words (such as spatial terms).
• It does not fulfill criteria for Mixed Receptive–Expressive Language Disorder or a pervasive developmental disorder.	• It does not fulfill criteria for a pervasive developmental disorder.

- The problem hinders educational or occupational achievement or social communication.
- If the patient also has Mental Retardation, environmental deprivation, or a speech–motor or sensory deficit, the problems with language are worse than you would expect with these problems.

Coding Note: On Axis III, code any neurological condition or a speech–motor or sensory deficit.

Susan

On an Internet chat group, Mrs. Barrett discussed the development of her daughter, Susan:

> "I just finished searching for 'Expressive Language Disorder,' and it brought me to this Web site. I think my 26-month-old daughter has this problem—at least, that's what the pediatrician said. She seems to understand everything we say, even tries to do little chores like her older brother. But she hardly speaks any words. She tries so hard to communicate with us, uses a lot of hand gestures to let us know what she wants or means. It's really heartbreaking! At first we thought it might be her hearing, but the audiometry was normal. We know she has a problem—her two older brothers both spoke early. Any advice?"

Communication disorders constitute, broadly, two sorts of problems—problems with language and with speech. The American Speech–Language–Hearing Association categorizes them as follows:

Language Disorder: Impaired comprehension or use of spoken or written language (or other symbolic systems). The disability can be in the form of language (including its system of sounds, the structure of words, and syntax—the rules that govern the formation of sentences); the context of language (semantics); or the function of language (how it is used to convey meaning).

Speech Disorder: Impaired articulation of speech, its fluency, or voice.

In a subsequent telephone interview, Mrs. Barrett expanded on Susan's symptoms. Although her sentences were largely limited to one or two words ("I got," "You bed"), by pointing she could identify subtle shades of color (indigo, azure, aqua). But when asked, "What color is this?" she would just laugh and point to it. She also lisped quite badly, even to the extent of pronouncing her own name "Thuthan." She habitually mispronounced many words ("bullah" for *butter* and "ikeem" for *ice cream*).

"She's a dear, sweet, usually happy child," her mother concluded. "She adores TV, especially if there is a program about babies. She loves to curl up on my lap; she'll pull on my sleeve and hum a little, which means she wants me to sing to her. But she can't talk. She just can't talk."

Another parent responded to this plea with the information that many school districts had testing programs for children as young as 2. This was the case where the Barretts lived. Susan's Verbal IQ on the WISC-R and the Carrow Elicited Language Inventory were both at least two standard deviations below expectations, but her Performance IQ was in the bright normal range.

Evaluation of Susan

Of course, the confirmation of this diagnosis would require standardized measurement of IQ and receptive language, both of which had been administered to Susan. But the diagnosis could be strongly suspected just from her mother's description of excellent speech comprehension, ruling out the less common **Mixed Receptive–Expressive Language Disorder**. The fact that Susan related well emotionally to her family rendered a **pervasive developmental disorder** highly unlikely, though abnormal communication skills figure prominently in the criteria for **Autistic Disorder**. (Seeking physical comfort from family members would not be found in an autistic child.) Although Susan was too young for anything to interfere with her educational or occupational achievement, her language problem was an undeniable social impairment. Other problems that can be mistaken for Expressive Language Disorder include **impaired hearing**, which was already ruled out in Susan's case with audiometry studies, and **environmental deprivation**, for which there wasn't a shred of evidence.

Like many other children with (and without) ELD, Susan also had difficulty with pronunciation. Her mother noted that she dropped certain sounds (the sibilant in *ice cream*) and substituted consonants (*l* for *t* in *butter*, for example). Her lisp even extended to the pronunciation of her own name. In defining the diagnosis of Phonological Disorder (see Table 11.6, later), many of the same conditions must be identified (or ruled out) as for ELD.

Susan had no known physical cause for either of her two Axis I disorders, which would both be considered developmental. Otherwise, any causative physical condition would be coded on Axis III. Susan's complete diagnosis would be the following:

Axis I	315.31	Expressive Language Disorder
	315.39	Phonological Disorder
Axis II	V71.09	No diagnosis
Axis III		None
Axis IV		None
Axis V	GAF = 65	(current)

315.31 Mixed Receptive–Expressive Language Disorder

Besides all the symptoms of ELD, children with Mixed Receptive–Expressive Language Disorder (abbreviated MRELD in this discussion) also have difficulty with receptive language. In plain talk, this means it is hard for them to understand what is said to them. Children with milder degrees of receptive language disability may have problems with only certain types of words (such as nouns or verbs) or with complex sentence structures. Severely affected children may be able to comprehend only the simplest words or sentence structures. These children may appear inattentive; sometimes they respond inappropriately during a conversation. Because language reception is by definition passive, deficits in this area will not often be apparent to the casual observer. Usually parents recognize that something is wrong by a child's fourth year.

Like ELD, MRELD can be either acquired or developmental. It occurs somewhat less frequently than ELD, affecting perhaps 3% of school-age children. Prognosis, somewhat worse than for patients with ELD, depends on etiology and severity: The more severe the deficit, the more likely it is that a child will have a concomitant learning disorder. Because the ability to produce language relies so thoroughly on the ability to understand it, a pure receptive language disorder is a theoretical construct that is not encountered clinically.

315.39 Phonological Disorder

Children with Phonological Disorder make errors in the production of speech (see Table 11.6 for the full criteria). They may omit certain sounds completely or substitute one sound for another (lisping is a common example). Consonants are most often affected. In milder cases, the effect may be only cute or quaint; more severely affected individuals may be difficult to understand or even unintelligible. Obvious physical causes include hearing impairment, cerebral palsy, cleft palate, and Mental Retardation, but in most cases the actual cause is unknown.

Clinically important Phonological Disorder (in DSM-III-R it was called Developmental Articulation Disorder) is diagnosable in 2–3% of preschool children. Spontaneous improvement often occurs, so that by the late teens the prevalence has declined to about 1 in 200. Phonological Disorder runs in families and is often associated with ELD or MRELD. Other mental and emotional disorders that

One cause of acquired language deficit is found in a rare neurological disorder called Landau–Kleffner syndrome. In this condition, the child's development is normal until about age 4, when progressive loss of the ability both to understand and to produce spoken language occurs. The inability is so profound as to be called "acquired aphasia" by some writers. It is accompanied by seizure disorders or abnormal EEG. The pattern of normal development during the first few years of life has also led some clinicians to confuse this syndrome with Pervasive Developmental Disorder Not Otherwise Specified.

TABLE 11.6. Criteria for Phonological Disorder

- The patient doesn't use speech sounds that are expected for age and dialect. Examples: substituting consonant sounds for one another; omitting final consonants.
- The problem hinders educational or occupational achievement or social communication.
- If the patient also has Mental Retardation, environmental deprivation, or a speech–motor or sensory deficit, the problems with language are worse than you would expect with these problems.

Coding Note: On Axis III, code any neurological condition or a speech–motor or sensory deficit.

---

often accompany Phonological Disorder include anxiety disorders and ADHD. For a clinical vignette and evaluation, see the case of Susan, presented above to illustrate ELD.

307.0 Stuttering

The stutterer's speech pattern is marked by an often agonizing loss of fluency and rhythm that is instantly identifiable by every layperson. (See Table 11.7 for the full criteria for Stuttering.) Less familiar may be some of the stutterer's sensations when grappling with the burdens of sound production. These individuals often experience a sense of momentary loss of control, and may take extreme measures to avoid difficult sounds or situations (such as using a tele-

TABLE 11.7. Criteria for Stuttering

- The patient lacks the fluency and time patterning of speech appropriate for age. At least one of the following occurs frequently:
  ✓ Repetitions of sounds and syllables
  ✓ Sound prolongations
  ✓ Interjections
  ✓ Broken words (a pause within a word)
  ✓ Blocking that is audible or silent
  ✓ Circumlocutions (substitutions to avoid words hard to pronounce)
  ✓ Words spoken with excessive physical tension
  ✓ Repetitions of monosyllabic whole words (such as "a-a-a-a-a dog bit me . . . ")
- The problem hinders educational or occupational achievement or social communication.
- If the patient also has a sensory or speech–motor deficit, the problems with language are worse than you would expect with these problems.

Coding Note: On Axis III, code any neurological condition or a sensory or speech–motor deficit.

phone) that exacerbate their misery. They typically feel anxiety or frustration; many report considerable physical tension. Even a child of 4 may be seen clenching fists, blinking, raising an upper lip, or jerking the head.

Stuttering is especially likely with consonants; initial sounds of words; the first word of a sentence; and words that are accented, long, or infrequently used. It may be provoked by telling jokes, saying one's own name, talking to strangers, or speaking to an authority figure or someone who is perceived as critical. Stutterers often achieve fluency when singing or swearing, or speaking to the steady beat of a metronome.

Stuttering typically begins in early childhood; it may com-

A tangential note on *cluttering* is in order here. In cluttering, abnormalities of both rate and rhythm of speech create dysfluency, impairing intelligibility. Whereas stutterers repeat only a single sound, clutterers may repeat syllables, words, or even short phrases, often backtracking and substituting words or ideas in speech that comes too rapidly, before their thoughts are adequately organized.

> Stutterer: "I've got to g-g-g-g-go to the store to buy some muh-muh-muh-muh-milk."
> Clutterer: "I've got to go-go-go to the st-, to the, uh, sto-sto, to the market to buy, uh, to get some, um, some m-m-m-, some ice cream."

Pure cluttering is rare; it is seen in perhaps only 5% of patients with disorders of fluency. However, many stutterers also clutter at times. Barely mentioned in DSM-III, cluttering shared Stuttering's code number in DSM-III-R, wherein it enjoyed a full-page write-up. Now, in DSM-IV, cluttering has disappeared completely as a diagnosable entity. Its demise can be traced to a paucity of research and lack of advocates, along with the belief of some that cluttering is really a problem of expression, not speech.

mence as early as the age of 2, but starts at about age 5 on average. Of course, it is quite usual for tiny children to have nonfluencies of speech, so early Stuttering is often ignored. Onset may be either gradual or sudden; the latter may be correlated with greater severity. As in so many other childhood mental disorders, there is a high male-to-female ratio—in this case, about 3:1.

Depending on age and a host of other factors, a normal person may speak up to 220 words per minute and will be dysfluent on 2% of words; a stutterer speaks roughly 25% slower and will be dysfluent about 5 times as often. As many as 3% of young children stutter; the percentage is higher for brain-damaged or mentally retarded children. Although opinions vary, the prevalence rate of Stuttering in adults is on the order of 0.1%, of whom about 80% are male.

The causes of these physical symptoms have not been fully worked out. Although tension worsens stuttering (public speaking is a notorious example), it does not account for the tendency to stutter. In fact, apart from other communication disorders and ADHD, stutterers may have fewer emotional ills than you would find in the general population. Stuttering runs in families, though not as the result of imitation; there is some evidence of heritability, and even the tendency to chronicity or spontaneous recovering (which occurs in nearly half of stutterers) may be genetically determined.

Because of its frequency and the common awareness of symptoms, no vignette has been provided for this disorder.

307.9 Communication Disorder Not Otherwise Specified

Use Communication Disorder Not Otherwise Specified for patients whose disorders of communication don't fit the criteria for any more specific disorder. DSM-IV gives examples of abnormalities in the pitch, loudness, quality, tone or resonance of the voice.

Assessing Communication Disorders

General Suggestions

Because these disorders manifest themselves as childhood speech problems, you would think that casual conversation would suffice for their identification. But two of them, ELD and MRELD, require the results of special testing for diagnosis. Furthermore, any of them can be mild to the point of being missed in the brief responses a child may make to an interviewer who relies on closed-ended questions.

Encouraging a child to talk uninterruptedly for prolonged periods may be the best way to obtain samples of speech that will demonstrate problems with rate, repetition, lack of prosody, dropped sounds, and other possible deficits of speech perception and speech production. Asking the patient to tell a story or recount an event is one way to accomplish this objective—for example, "Tell me how you get to school in the morning," or "Can you finish this story? Once upon a time, in a land far away, there lived a . . . " Patients with ELD may speak in one- or two-word sentences; leave sentences incomplete; and have trouble coming up with the right words in describing their experiences, feelings, and needs. Those with MRELD may respond inappropriately or appear not to understand. They may seem not to pay attention, ask many questions before comprehending, or appear to forget easily what they have been told.

An audio recording of the evaluation (obtained with parental permission) can facilitate speech analysis after the child has left the office; a video recording may help discern signs of tension (blinks, fist clenching, and grimaces) that often accompany Stuttering. Follow up responses that seem inappropriate by asking the child, "What did I just ask?" Also watch for shyness, aloofness, or withdrawal, any of which may indicate a communication disorder.

Apart from listening to the child produce language, assess the following:

- Use of symbols—for example, does the child let a paper cup represent a house, or a stick stand for a car?
- Ability to comprehend language—can the child follow a command that is given without the use of gestures?

Developmental Factors

As with so many other childhood disorders, early identification of communication disorders often occurs in severely affected patients. In the case of developmental ELD, a mild case may not be noticed until a patient's teens—the age at which language normally begins to develop the rich complexity characteristic of adult speech. However, even mild cases of MRELD usually become evident by the grade school years. Rarely, very young children with MRELD may have so much difficulty comprehending speech that they appear deaf when spoken to; older children may appear more confused.

In older children, a deficit in vocabulary may only affect certain word types—nouns, for example, or personal pronouns. However, younger children affected to a similar degree may commit vocabulary errors for all sorts of words.

Older children and those with less severe Phonological Disorder will have trouble with the more difficult consonant sounds, such as *s, z, sh,* and *ch*. Younger children may also have problems with the easier consonants that are learned earlier—*b, m, t, d, n, h,*—and are especially likely to omit sounds, such as at the beginnings and ends of words. Stuttering usually begins in early childhood, between the ages of 2 and 7; onset after the age of 10 is rare. Because stutterers often avoid words that they know will cause them trouble, asking older children to read from a text may help in identifying Stuttering.

PERVASIVE DEVELOPMENTAL DISORDERS

The essence of a pervasive developmental disorder (abbreviated PDD in this section) is delay: Development is slow, and sometimes never comes, in multiple areas of a child's life. Children with PDDs suffer from delayed or incomplete development in their ability to socialize, to communicate, and to control their motor movements. IQ scores range from bright to moderately retarded levels.

Although the degree of disability varies widely, the effect upon the lives of most patients and their families is profound and permanent. Table 11.8 compares some of the important features of the four major PDD syndromes.

299.00 Autistic Disorder

Children with Autistic Disorder appear quite normal; only rarely do they bear the physical stigmata of handicap or retardation. Though some are cross and contrary, parents more often describe them as easy to rear. Motor milestones

TABLE 11.8. Characteristics of Pervasive Developmental Disorders

	Autistic Disorder	Asperger's Disorder	Rett's Disorder	Childhood Disintegrative Disorder
Age at onset	Before 3 years	Recognized later than Autistic Disorder	Normal to 5–12 months	Normal to 2 years
M:F ratio	4–5:1	8–10:1	F only	M > F?
Prevalence	2–10 per 10,000	10–25 per 10,000	1 per 15,000 female live births	Rare; 10% that of Autistic Disorder
Mental Retardation	Moderate	IQ often normal	Severe or profound	Usually severe
Social impairment	Marked	Qualitative	Loss of previously acquired skills	Loss of previously acquired skills
Communication problems	Marked impairment	No significant delay	Severe impairment	Loss of previously acquired skills
Stereotypies	Marked motor	Yes	Hand-washing movements	Yes
Seizures	In 25%	Not prominent	May be present	May be present
Motor incoordination		"Clumsy"	Gait/trunk	Yes

are usually reached on time; they sleep and eat well and, when left alone, rarely fuss or cry.

In the second 6 months of life, parents become concerned about socialization. The infant does not make eye-to-eye contact, smile, or nuzzle into a parent's neck and chest when being held; instead, the infant may arch away and prefer to stare into space. During early visits to the pediatrician, parents are frequently told, "Everything will be OK—your baby will outgrow your concern." Pediatricians show their concern only when language is late in appearing, most often after 3 years of age. By then, a full range of symptoms is probably evident (see Table 11.9 for the full criteria):

The PDDs were included on Axis II until DSM-IV moved them to Axis I, where they joined nearly all other clinical disorders except Mental Retardation and the personality disorders. DSM-IV also specified criteria for Rett's Disorder, Asperger's Disorder, and Childhood Disintegrative Disorder, whereas in DSM-III-R these three would have been classified as PDD Not Otherwise Specified. (Thus the PDDs are the group of DSM-IV disorders that has been most augmented since DSM-III-R.) In part, this has been done to make DSM-IV congruent with the *International Classification of Diseases,* 10th revision (ICD-10). Be aware, however, that the science of these disorders is still young and developing, and there is considerable controversy as to the distinction between, for example, Asperger's Disorder and high-functioning Autistic Disorder. Some writers have worried about the premature creation of false distinctions in what some regard as a continuum of pervasive developmental disability.

- Lack of social interests and responsiveness, including failure to cuddle, point to objects, play with other children, and meet the gaze of another when there is a shared interest in something. Toddlers may not extend their arms in anticipation of being picked up, or may not demonstrate the normal bonding (such as following a parent from room to room). Normal fear of strangers or anxiety at separation from parents may be absent.
- Impaired use of language, ranging from peculiar speech patterns to absence of speech (in nearly half) to failure to use even nonverbal communication, such as head nods or facial expressions appropriate to mood or situation. Those who do speak may be unable to comprehend humor; communication may suffer because autistic children do not understand that words can have multiple or abstract meanings. Their speech may lack the normal lilt (*prosody*) that makes it musical. They may talk to themselves or hold forth at great length on subjects that interest no one else; others may be unable to begin or sustain normal conversation.

TABLE 11.9. Criteria for Autistic Disorder

- The patient fulfills a total of at least six criteria from the following three bulleted lists, distributed as indicated:
  - Impaired social interaction (at least two):
    - ✓ Markedly deficient regulation of social interaction through multiple nonverbal behaviors, such as eye contact, facial expression, body posture, and gestures
    - ✓ Lack of peer relationships that are appropriate to developmental level
    - ✓ Absence of seeking to share achievements, interests, or pleasure with others
    - ✓ Absence of social or emotional reciprocity
  - Impaired communication (at least one):
    - ✓ Delayed or absent development of spoken language, for which the patient doesn't try to compensate with gestures
    - ✓ In patients who can speak, inadequate attempts to begin or sustain a conversation
    - ✓ Language that is idiosyncratic or repetitive and stereotyped
    - ✓ Appropriate to developmental stage, absence of social imitative play or spontaneous, varied, make-believe play
  - Activities, behavior, and interests that are repetitive, restricted, and stereotyped (at least one):
    - ✓ Abnormal (in focus or intensity) preoccupation with interests that are restricted and stereotyped (such as spinning things)
    - ✓ Rigid performance of routines or rituals that don't appear to have a function
    - ✓ Repetitive, stereotyped, motor mannerisms (such as hand flapping)
    - ✓ Persistent fascination with parts of objects
- Before age 3, the patient shows delayed or abnormal functioning in one or more of these areas:
  - ✓ Social interaction
  - ✓ Language used in social communication
  - ✓ Imaginative or symbolic play
- These symptoms are not better explained by Childhood Disintegrative Disorder or Rett's Disorder.

- Although most have concomitant Mental Retardation, about one-fourth register an IQ of greater than 70. Seizure disorders are especially likely to develop in those autistic individuals who are also mentally retarded.
- Motor behaviors that may include stereotypies, posturing, and other ritualistic or compulsive actions (twirling, rocking, hand flapping, head banging, maintenance of posture oddly reminiscent of catatonic behavior). Play may be repetitive and nonsymbolic; toys are objects to suck or twirl. Although younger autistic children are often hyperactive, as teenagers they tend to slow down and may even become less active than normal adolescents. Autistic youngsters prefer sameness and will resist change in their environments. Their sleep may be abnormal, including initial insomnia and a reduced need for sleep; some patients may experience a complete reversal of the night–day sleep–wake pattern.

In general, social development takes place much more slowly than normal; developmental phases may occur out of the expected sequence. Some children are exquisitely sensitive to sensory input: They hate bright lights or loud sounds, and even the prickly feel of certain types of cloth or other surfaces may bother them horribly. Sometimes present are so-called *cognitive splinter skills,* including abilities in computation, music, or rote memory that far exceed a normal person's capabilities (*savantism*).

Although the prevalence of Autistic Disorder is low in the general population, it approaches 20% in children with severe Mental Retardation. The disorder affects all socioeconomic and cultural groups. Boys strongly outnumber girls, but an autistic girl is likely to be more severely affected.

The etiology is unknown, but most experts believe that genetic vulnerability and biological failures in neuronal development during gestation are responsible. Family pedigree and twin studies suggest genetic loading. Several medical illnesses are associated with Autistic Disorder: congenital rubella, phenylketonuria, tuberous sclerosis, and a history of perinatal distress. Seizures develop in up to one-fourth of these patients, especially as they approach adulthood. Minor abnormalities (e.g., high-arched palate) are often discovered on physical examination. Ventricular enlargement has been reported in 25% of cases, and high serotonin levels in platelets in 30% (an abnormality also noted in many children who have Mental Retardation without autistic features).

Jonathan

Because his mother's concerns about Jonathan's peculiar behavior had been dismissed as trivial by their family physician, he was almost 5 when she first brought him to the clinic. Now many aspects of his behavior worried her. In public places he had gradually become unmanageable. In school he would not follow directions and refused structure; when confronted, he boisterously disrupted those about him. Yet, when left alone, he watched TV by the hour and didn't seem to care what show was on. He had no friends and did not seem to want any; for long stretches he played alone in his room, preferring objects that he could twirl. Sometimes he would spin himself, as if he enjoyed becoming dizzy. If these routines were interrupted, he could become angry. Then he might hit, kick, or bite the person who interfered with his rituals.

Jonathan was an attractive, blond-haired, blue-eyed youngster—neatly dressed and groomed—who appeared his stated age. When he and his mother entered the playroom, he did not acknowledge the presence of the examiner, whom he seemed to gaze right through with a nearly blank, somehow distressingly pleasant expression on his immobile face.

Jonathan went directly to a toy car on the table and began sniffing it. Next he ran it back and forth across his chest, while swaying and humming quietly to himself. He refused to speak with the examiner and avoided all eye contact. Yet his hearing was not impaired; he looked up whenever there was a noise outside the playroom. While his mother related his history, he occupied himself by rubbing the car along his leg. Occasionally he returned to his mother and, without speaking, took her hand and guided it toward an object out of his reach. At one point during the interview, Jonathan noticed the light switch and began turning it on and off. Later, he flapped his arms repeatedly while walking on his toes around the room, and could not be persuaded to stop. During much of the interview he showed little change in facial expression. Even as he screeched loudly while his mother led him away from the light switch, his mouth was fixed in a smile, rather than an expression appropriate to pain, anger, or defiance. Results of the Peabody Picture Vocabulary Test suggested an IQ of 75.

When the examiner sat on the floor and began parallel play with a toy car, Jonathan sat nearby and copied the behavior. To the question "What's your name?" Jonathan replied, using exactly the same intonation, "What's your name?" When the examiner tried (with the mother's permission) to hug him, Jonathan froze and arched back. ("He's reacted like that since before he was a year old," his mother commented.) At one point when his mother left the room, Jonathan hardly seemed to notice her absence, and he ignored her when she returned. At the end of the session, at first he resisted leaving. Then suddenly, without saying goodbye, he darted from the playroom, his mother in rapid pursuit.

Evaluation of Jonathan

The criteria for Autistic Disorder are among the more complicated DSM-IV has to offer in child and adolescent mental health. Partly this is because they need to reflect the way this disorder pervades all areas of the patient's (and family's) life. Here is a description of how Jonathan fulfilled these criteria.

From an early age, his social interactions were abnormal. Two such deficiencies are required by the criteria. His symptoms included multiple impairments of nonverbal behavior (refusal to cuddle, avoidance of eye contact, blank or inappropriate facial expressions) and lack of peer relationships and social reciprocity. Though only one impairment of communication is required, he communicated poorly in several ways: stereotyped speech (echolalia as he exactly repeated the examiner's questions), lack of symbolic play, and inability to carry on a conversation with the examiner. Stereotyped behavior or interests was shown in arm flapping and an intense interest in twirling things, including himself.

In the playroom, Jonathan exhibited many behavioral symptoms of Autistic Disorder. He did not engage the examiner and seemed to use his mother as a part-object (guiding her hand) rather than as a whole person. He played in isolation, using a toy car as an object for self-stimulation rather than as the symbolic representation of a vehicle. He resisted physical comfort from the examiner and did not acknowledge his mother's disappearance from the room. He demonstrated a number of stereotypies and rituals, including hand flapping, toe walking, sniffing of objects, and repeatedly flicking the light switch. As required by the criteria, two other PDDs could be excluded: **Childhood Disintegrative Disorder** because Jonathan's development was not normal prior to his second birthday, and **Rett's Disorder** on the basis that he did not demonstrate the characteristic hand-rubbing behavior and was not a girl.

Besides other PDDs, several Axis I disorders would need to be considered in the differential diagnosis. Note that Autistic Disorder doesn't protect against the development of **Schizophrenia**, which occasionally occurs during the first few years of life; their (rare) co-occurrence can lead to diagnostic chaos. Some symptoms of autistic youngsters can look like prodromal or residual symptoms of Schizophrenia—isolation, disorganized behavior, blunted affect, peculiar beliefs or interests. However, patients with Schizophrenia almost always appear normal for the first 12 or more years of life, and certainly during the first 3–4 years. For the two diagnoses to be made in a single individual, DSM-IV requires the presence of prominent delusions *and* hallucinations for 1 month—perhaps less, if treatment is rapidly successful. In Jonathan's case, this differential diagnosis was easy: Although he had a notable lack of affect and odd motor behavior, he had no delusions or hallucinations.

Although the ability to use language is compromised in **Stereotypic Movement Disorder**, these children are free of the social and language abnormalities that characterize Autistic Disorder. A similar argument can rule out the **communication disorders**. Although Jonathan had significant language delays in both verbal and nonverbal (pragmatics) domains, DSM-IV explicitly states that a child with any PDD cannot also receive a diagnosis of **Expressive**

Language Disorder. His parents were supportive and sensitive to his needs, which effectively eliminated **severe psychosocial deprivation**.

Finally, the possibility of concomitant **Mental Retardation** must be considered. Even though Jonathan's *measured* IQ was 75 (borderline range), the limits of error could place his *actual* IQ in the high 60s. DSM-IV notes, however, that an additional diagnosis is usually made only in the case of Severe or Profound Mental Retardation. Jonathan's five-axis diagnosis would thus be as follows:

Axis I	299.00	Autistic Disorder
Axis II	V71.09	No diagnosis
Axis III		None
Axis IV		None
Axis V	GAF = 35	(current)

299.80 Rett's Disorder

Rett's Disorder was first described in 1966, but it did not achieve worldwide recognition until the first English-language publication appeared in 1983. Although the criteria (see Table 11.10) do not specify gender, the condition has so far been identified only in girls, thereby fueling speculation that it originates from a locus somewhere on the X chromosome. Rett's Disorder differs from Autistic Disorder in that, after a normal pregnancy and delivery, a child develops normally for the first few months. Only then do problems begin.

To accommodate the rapidly growing brain, head circumference in a nor-

---

TABLE 11.10. Criteria for Rett's Disorder

- All of the following suggest normal early development:
  - Prenatal and perinatal development
  - Psychomotor development, for at least 5 months
  - Head circumference at birth
- After this apparently normal beginning, *all* of these occur:
  - Head growth slows abnormally between 5 and 48 months.
  - Between 5 and 30 months, the child loses already acquired purposeful hand movements and develops stereotyped hand movements, such as hand washing or hand wringing.
  - Early in the course, the child loses interest in the social environment. (However, social interaction often develops later.)
  - Gait or movements of trunk are poorly coordinated.
  - Severe psychomotor retardation and severe impairment of expressive and receptive language are seen.

mal infant expands rapidly during the first 6 months of life and less so thereafter: On average, a baby's head measures 34 cm at birth, 43 cm at 6 months, and 46 cm at 1 year. After an initial few months of normal growth, a child with Rett's Disorder grows far less rapidly than would be expected for the child's chronological age. As in Childhood Disintegrative Disorder, there is a loss of already acquired purposeful movements of the hands and the onset of stereotyped hand-washing movements. Other motor manifestations include tooth grinding and trouble with chewing, breathing difficulties (hyperventilation, air swallowing, or apnea), and a stiff-legged gait in patients who can walk at all. These children lose already acquired language abilities and show little or no interest in objects or other people; three-fourths or more have seizures.

After initial deterioration, stabilization may occur; cognitive and social abilities may even improve slightly. With adolescence, motor disability (loss of the ability to walk), scoliosis, and rigidity may once again set in. The Mental Retardation that often attends this disorder is often Severe or Profound, with loss of social and language skills. Rett's Disorder affects 1 girl in 10,000, and usually becomes apparent during the second year of life. With capacity for self-care often completely lost, the effects upon child and family are devastating.

Alicia

The diagnosis of Rett's Disorder was made when 12-year-old Alicia was discovered in a county-sponsored home for retarded children. She had lived there ever since she was 2 years old, when her parents had decided that they could no longer care for her.

According to the meager records, Alicia's progress had been unremarkable for about the first 16 months. She could speak words and short sentences; she had begun to walk at 12 months. Then, some time prior to her second birthday, she had gradually stopped speaking and had withdrawn from ordinary social contact. The seizures that later developed were poorly controlled with medication, leading to institutionalization. Medical records from her infancy revealed a head size of 33 cm at birth, 40.5 cm at 6 months, and 42 cm at 18 months. The pediatrician noted the nearly static head size and diagnosed "secondary microcephaly."

Now Alicia spoke no words, but often verbalized grunts or cooing sounds. When angry, she might scream loudly and repeatedly. She could walk, but with a wide-based gait that seemed to compensate partly for a poor sense of balance. During the time she spent with the consulting clinician, she almost constantly rubbed the backs of her hands together. Although she made some eye contact during the interview and was obviously able to hear, she appeared to understand little of what was said to her and followed none of the requests made of her.

Evaluation of Alicia

On the basis of a single assessment at age 12, anyone who did not have access to her medical records would be unlikely to identify Alicia as having a diagnosis other than **Mental Retardation**. It was the history in her medical chart that allowed the correct diagnosis to be made—specifically, the decelerated growth in head size (which militated against a diagnosis of **Childhood Disintegrative Disorder**), loss of hand control and motor coordination (gait), and near absence of speech. The severity of speech and intellectual capabilities ruled out **Asperger's Disorder**. Her early history of normal development until about 16 months suggested that **Autistic Disorder** was not the correct diagnosis.

Axis I	299.80	Rett's Disorder
Axis II	318.2	Profound Mental Retardation
Axis III	None	
Axis IV	None	Lives in institution
Axis V	GAF = 11	(current)

299.10 Childhood Disintegrative Disorder

An older child (or adult) with Childhood Disintegrative Disorder (abbreviated CDD in this discussion) greatly resembles one with Autistic Disorder. That is, the typical CDD patient exhibits deficits in social interaction, little interest in the environment, and poor communication skills; and may even be unable to provide self-care, including toileting. Where the two conditions differ is in their early development. (See Table 11.11 for the full criteria for CDD.) Whereas autistic children typically show symptoms during the first 2 years of life, a patient with CDD develops normally for the first 2 to 4 years. After an onset that can be abrupt or gradual, there begins a 6- to 9-month decline in which the child loses abilities already gained, resulting in a cross-sectional picture that cannot be differentiated from Autistic Disorder: motor restlessness, incontinence, loss of language and self-feeding abilities, deterioration in interpersonal relationships,

TABLE 11.11. Criteria for Childhood Disintegrative Disorder

- At least until age 2, the child develops normally, as shown by having age-appropriate adaptive behavior, play, social relationships, and nonverbal and verbal communication.
- Before age 10, the child experiences clinically important loss of previously learned skills in the following areas (two or more required):
  ✓ Language (expressive or receptive)
  ✓ Adaptive behavior or social skills
  ✓ Bladder or bowel control
  ✓ Play
  ✓ Motor skills
- The child functions abnormally in two or more of the following ways:
  ✓ Social interaction is characterized by impaired nonverbal behaviors, peer relationships, or emotional or social reciprocity.
  ✓ Communication is characterized by delayed or absent spoken language, inability to converse, language use that is repetitive or stereotyped, or absence of varied make-believe play.
  ✓ Activities, behavior, and interests are repetitive, restricted, and stereotyped. This includes motor mannerisms and stereotypies.
- These symptoms are not better explained by Schizophrenia or another specific pervasive developmental disorder.

and interest in the environment. Thereafter, the course is variable. Some children stabilize; others continue the gradual decline. Seizures often develop. A few patients actually improve, but this is rare.

Although the etiology of CDD is not known, autopsy studies reveal abnormalities of brain neurons. The rarest of all PDD conditions, CDD affects only about 1 child in 100,000. Boys are more likely than girls to be affected.

Andrew

The product of a full-term, normal delivery, Andrew was the third child and first son in an intact family. He spoke his first words at 11 months and sentences at 20 months. He sat at 6 months, walked while holding on to furniture at 11 months, and walked independently at 13 months. Not long after his second birthday, however, his mother noticed that he had begun having difficulty holding a spoon to feed himself.

Over the next several months, Andrew gradually lost the ability to manipulate objects with his hands. His mother soon noted that he would rub his hands against each other, as if he were doing a poorly controlled job of washing them. Whereas he had been speaking short sentences, he gradually stopped speaking at all except for a single syllable ("kah"), which he used as an all-purpose expression of distress, contentment, and (to a limited extent) inquiry. On his fourth birthday, he showed no interest in his presents or cake. By this time, he had lost control of his bowels and bladder.

Evaluation of Andrew

With his severe loss of language, interest in activities, and social skills, Andrew ultimately resembled a child with **Autistic Disorder**, but this would be beginning with the end. It was his early history, when he appeared to be developing normally, that set Andrew apart. Of course, other PDDs would need to be ruled out. The manifestations of **Asperger's Disorder** are less extreme; **Rett's Disorder** has been reported only in girls, and in Andrew's case there was no evidence of decelerated growth in head size. No **general medical condition** was reported that could cause a dementia, another possible entry in the differential diagnosis. Although Andrew was markedly mentally retarded, his other deficits prevented adequate assessment of IQ. Therefore, his Axis II diagnosis had to be stated in somewhat uncertain terms. His full diagnosis would be the following:

Axis I	299.10	Childhood Disintegrative Disorder
Axis II	319	Mental Retardation, Severity Unspecified
Axis III		None
Axis IV		None
Axis V	GAF = 11	(current)

299.80 Asperger's Disorder

Although Asperger's Disorder was first described far earlier (1908) than Autistic Disorder and affects more patients, until the last few years it has been less well known. This is related partly to Autistic Disorder's obvious, devastating psychopathology, and partly to the ease with which patients with Asperger's Disorder may be misdiagnosed as having other Axis I or Axis II diagnoses.

Their areas of apparent normality and high functioning differentiate Asperger's Disorder patients from those with other PDDs (see Table 11.12 for the full criteria). Not only may early growth and development appear completely unremarkable, but in many cases intelligence remains normal throughout life (some individuals suffer from Mild Mental Retardation). Although they usually like the company and conversation of other people, individuals affected by Asperger's Disorder lack a sense of "social intelligence," making them appear insensitive to the feelings of others. As a result, they often become

TABLE 11.12. Criteria for Asperger's Disorder

- At least two demonstrations of impaired social interaction. The patient:
  - ✓ Shows a marked inability to regulate social interaction through multiple nonverbal behaviors, such as body posture and gestures, eye contact, and facial expression.
  - ✓ Doesn't develop peer relationships that are appropriate to developmental level.
  - ✓ Doesn't seek to share achievements, interests, or pleasure with others.
  - ✓ Lacks social or emotional reciprocity.
- At least one demonstration of activities, behavior, and interests that are repetitive, restricted, and stereotyped:
  - ✓ Abnormal (in focus or intensity) preoccupation with interests that are restricted and stereotyped (such as spinning things)
  - ✓ Rigid performance of routines or rituals that don't appear to have a function
  - ✓ Repetitive, stereotyped motor mannerisms (such as hand flapping)
  - ✓ Persistent fascination with parts of objects
- The symptoms cause clinically important impairment in social, occupational, or personal functioning.
- There is no clinically important general language delay (the child can speak words by age 2, phrases by age 3).
- There is no clinically important delay in developing cognition, age-appropriate self-help skills, adaptive behavior (except social interaction), and normal curiosity about the environment.
- The patient doesn't fulfill criteria for Schizophrenia or another specific pervasive developmental disorder.

---

solitary, perhaps desiring friends but lacking the skills necessary for normal social communication. Young adults with Asperger's Disorder may produce words and sentences that seem perfectly normal when written on paper, but their speech is marked by repetition, mild circumstantiality, and absence of the normal prosody and body language that accompany speech in normal persons. Although less physically impaired than is typical of those with other PDD syndromes, these individuals are often notably clumsy as children.

Asperger's Disorder is a new diagnosis in DSM-IV, and its meaning and value are thus still somewhat uncertain. Some authorities claim that it is not a discrete disorder, but a less severe variant of Autistic Disorder. Others, finding the clinical picture similar to that of Schizotypal Personality Disorder, wonder about a possible relationship between the two.

Arthur

When Arthur was born, his mother expressed relief. Her first baby, a premature boy, had died when he was only 2 weeks old. But pink, chubby Arthur had been the picture of health, as his milestones attested. He spoke words at 14 months and sentences at 18 months. He was toilet-trained when he was 28 months old.

Although he stood alone at 10 months and walked at 1 year, he fell down a good deal and walked with a rolling gait; his mother called him her "little sailor."

After only a few weeks of nursery school, the teacher requested a conference with Arthur's parents. She thought that Arthur enjoyed the company of other children, but that his approach to them—screaming or punching to get their attention—was self-defeating. She also noted that whenever she tried to talk to him, he would gaze away from her. When he spoke, his voice had a certain steady quality to it she couldn't quite define—"like he was singing, only just on one note."

Nevertheless, with above-average intelligence (Full Scale WISC-R IQ = 116), Arthur made good progress throughout school. He was referred for evaluation when he was in the sixth grade, only because he seemed have no friends outside his own family. Instead, he had two consuming interests: telephone systems and his CD collection. Arthur had memorized huge quantities of information about the history, construction, maintenance, and even financing of telephone systems. Parts of numerous old telephones were strewn about his room, and in the basement he had assembled a manual switchboard with plugs that actually worked. His CD collection was highly specialized—nothing but original-cast musicals. According to his mother, if anyone disturbed the precise order in which he had arranged his collection, he would fly into a rage. Even then, his voice showed little modulation.

During the interview, Arthur spoke clearly but monotonously about telephone line repair, ignoring the examiner's attempts to change the subject.

Evaluation of Arthur

Had Arthur been referred for evaluation a few years later, someone not alerted by his early history might have considered him for an Axis II diagnosis, such as **Schizoid Personality Disorder**. However, that diagnosis generally becomes apparent later in life and impairs social interaction less seriously. With no history of early loss of functioning, other PDDs such as **CDD** and **Rett's Disorder** could be ruled out. The absence of any marked delay in development of speech ruled out **Autistic Disorder**, though the line of demarcation may not be as clear-cut in every case. Although Arthur's highly circumscribed interests superficially resembled the obsessions of **Obsessive–Compulsive Disorder**, the latter does not usually restrict a child's interests so severely as was the case with Arthur. Obsessive–Compulsive Disorder does often begin in childhood, however. Arthur's five-axis diagnosis would be as follows:

Axis I	299.80	Asperger's Disorder
Axis II	V71.09	No diagnosis
Axis III		None
Axis IV		None
Axis V	GAF = 45	(current)

299.80 Pervasive Developmental Disorder Not Otherwise Specified

Prior to DSM-IV, children with Asperger's Disorder had to be categorized as having PDD Not Otherwise Specified. Even now, with several new categories, many children (perhaps the majority of those with any PDD diagnosis) must be given this diagnosis—for example, those who don't meet criteria for Autistic Disorder because of late age of onset or symptoms that are too few or atypical.

Assessing Pervasive Developmental Disorders

General Suggestions

Perhaps more than any other diagnostic group, the PDDs will tax your ability to evaluate a differential diagnosis. This is because aspects of these disorders overlap so many others; you may need to rule out neurological disorders, many other Axis I disorders, and (when a patient has reached young adulthood) Schizotypal or Schizoid Personality Disorder. PDD children may be clumsy or have other voluntary motor problems, so you must pay careful attention to gross and fine motor coordination—a child may even be diagnosable as having concomitant Developmental Coordination Disorder.

Some PDD children don't speak; those who do may use language inappropriately. They may ask personal questions. (An appropriate response to a personal question is often some variation of "I can't tell you that, but I can let you look to see what's in this toy box.") As with other young patients, following a child's own favorite interests or pastimes and demonstrating willingness to enter into the child's activities may help you to form some relationship with the child. As with mentally retarded children, the default answer for PDD children to questions they don't completely understand is "yes."

It is critical in diagnosing PDD to note the facility with which a child interacts verbally and affectively with you. A given child may appear indifferent, refuse physical contact, or even fail to make eye contact. You may find it helpful to rock or sway, mirroring (but being careful not to mock) the child's own behavior. After a time, the child may be willing to follow your motions, thus establishing an emotional connection at some level and helping you to assess how far the child is willing/able to relate to others, even on an entirely nonverbal level.

About three-fourths of PDD children are also cognitively impaired; Performance IQ is usually better than Verbal IQ. Like mentally retarded children, PDD patients can have such widely varying abilities that it is dangerous to hold preconceived notions about any one patient's capabilities. Such a child can challenge your interactional skills and experience as an interviewer, perhaps more than one with any other severe handicap. Several sessions may be needed to complete an evaluation.

Developmental Factors

Differences in age of onset are obvious from the criteria for various PDDs. Rett's Disorder patients develop normally for the first 6–18 months of life; for CDD youngsters, deterioration may commence only after 3–4 years. Recognition of children with Asperger's Disorder may occur even later, as expected degrees of socialization fail to develop. But the diagnosis of Autistic Disorder may be suspected in children as young as 1 year by their stiff resistance to cuddling, failure to raise their arms to be lifted, irregular social smile, and resistance to new experiences (especially new foods). In the second year, their social aloofness may become apparent in their lack of shared attention, failure to point, or failure to hold the gaze of an adult. Later, the lack of spoken language will become apparent.

ATTENTION-DEFICIT AND DISRUPTIVE BEHAVIOR DISORDERS

Although any child will misbehave from time to time, a substantial minority of children have behavior problems that go far beyond the occasional stolen candy bar, schoolyard fist fight, or classroom outburst. The disorders in this section comprise a spectrum of disruptive behaviors that exist along the dual continua of age and severity. Some difficult children grow through successive stages of aggressive behavior → Oppositional Defiant Disorder → Conduct Disorder → Antisocial Personality Disorder; far more, of course, do not. Some research seems to demonstrate that those who do progress from one stage to the next have more family history of psychopathology and use more psychoactive substances. However, the line of demarcation between Conduct Disorder and Antisocial Personality Disorder is entirely arbitrary, and no one is entirely sure that *any* of these stages is a distinct entity. ADHD, though not strictly in the line of succession with these other disorders, is often associated with them.

Although the current definitions may not discriminate disorders with a uniform etiology or prognosis, they do allow clinicians to describe a cluster of disorders that accounts for a major portion of any child mental health practitioner's practice. Specific causes for these disorders are not known, but both genetic and environmental influences are suspected. These conditions may flourish in the aftermath of a bitter divorce or harsh or restrictive parenting; Oppositional Defiant Disorder is reported more commonly in families with low socioeconomic status. Parents and other relatives may have other conduct-related disorders, depressive disorders, Substance Abuse, and Antisocial Personality Disorder. ADHD and Somatization Disorder are often found among relatives of children with ADHD.

314.0x Attention-Deficit/Hyperactivity Disorder

Through multiple changes in criteria and even more changes of name, ADHD remains one of the most common mental health diagnoses of childhood. Found in 3–5% of school-age children, it affects two or three times more boys than it does girls. (It is less commonly diagnosed in Europe, where they think that North Americans sometimes mislabel children who "only" have a disorder of conduct.)

Symptoms usually begin before a child goes to school, and the criteria (see Table 11.13) require some symptoms before age 7, but the diagnosis is not usually made for several years after the beginning of school. Mothers sometimes report that their ADHD children cried more than their other babies, or that they were colicky, irritable, or wakeful. Some even remark that these children kicked more before they were born.

Although some children may show only symptoms of hyperactivity–impulsiveness, the vast majority also (or exclusively) have symptoms of inattention. Because of disruptiveness, poor-quality schoolwork, impulsive comments, and clumsiness, these children are often unpopular with peers and adults alike. Dysthymic Disorder or anxiety disorders may be comorbid in 25–30% of children with ADHD. The symptoms of ADHD usually lessen in adolescence, but studies suggest that many such children eventually abuse drugs and alcohol.

TABLE 11.13. Criteria for Attention-Deficit/Hyperactivity Disorder

- The patient has *either* inattention or hyperactivity–impulsiveness (or both), persisting for at least 6 months to a degree that is maladaptive and immature, as shown by the following:

  ✓ **Inattention.** At least six of the following nine items *often* apply:
    ✓ Fails to pay close attention to details or makes careless errors in schoolwork, work, or other activities
    ✓ Has trouble keeping attention on tasks or play
    ✓ Doesn't appear to listen when being told something
    ✓ Neither follows through on instructions nor completes chores, schoolwork, or jobs (not because of oppositional behavior or failure to understand)
    ✓ Has trouble organizing activities and tasks
    ✓ Dislikes or avoids tasks that involve sustained mental effort (homework, schoolwork)
    ✓ Loses materials needed for activities (assignments, books, pencils, tools, toys)
    ✓ Is easily distracted by extraneous stimuli
    ✓ Is forgetful

  ✓ **Hyperactivity–Impulsiveness.** At least six of the following nine items *often* apply:
    Hyperactivity
    ✓ Squirms in seat or fidgets
    ✓ Inappropriately leaves seat
    ✓ Inappropriately runs or climbs (in adolescents or adults, this may be only a subjective feeling of restlessness)
    ✓ Has trouble quietly playing or engaging in leisure activity
    ✓ Appears driven or "on the go"
    ✓ Talks excessively

    Impulsiveness
    ✓ Answers questions before they have been completely asked
    ✓ Has trouble awaiting turn
    ✓ Interrupts or intrudes on others

- At least some symptoms begin before age 7.
- Symptoms must be present in at least two types of situations, such as school, work, home.
- The disorder impairs school, work, or social functioning.
- The symptoms do not occur solely during a pervasive developmental disorder or any psychotic disorder, including Schizophrenia.
- The symptoms are not explained better by another mental disorder, such as a mood, anxiety, dissociative, or personality disorder.

Coding Notes: Specify "In Partial Remission" for patients (especially adults or adolescents) whose current symptoms do not fulfill the criteria.

Code number is based on the symptoms during the past 6 months:

  314.00 Attention-Deficit/Hyperactivity Disorder, Predominantly Inattentive Type: The patient has recently met the criteria for inattention but not for hyperactivity–impulsiveness.
  314.01 Attention-Deficit/Hyperactivity Disorder, Predominantly Hyperactive–Impulsive Type: The patient has recently met the criteria for hyperactivity–impulsiveness but not for inattention.
  314.01 Attention–Deficit/Hyperactivity Disorder, Combined Type: The patient has recently met the criteria for both inattention *and* hyperactivity-impulsiveness. (Most ADHD children have symptoms of the Combined Type.)

Randy

Her experience with his two placid brothers left his mother ill prepared for 8-year-old Randy. "He never did learn to walk—when he was 10 months old, he started to run. He's been running ever since," she told the interviewer.

"Even before he went to school, I knew he was different. His brothers could sit and color or build with blocks by the hour, but Randy would only last a few minutes. And every evening I'd have to remind him to feed the dog. But he was very quick to learn even complicated things, if you could just get his interest."

In the first grade Randy did quite well. It was a small "demonstration" class, and there was a student teacher who redirected his obvious, persistent overactivity enough to keep him out of trouble. But this year the class size had grown, and complaining notes from his new teacher accompanied Randy home in a steady stream. One read in part: " . . . and he answers questions I've asked other children. He often interrupts me, even before I've finished asking. It doesn't help that he's often right." He often talked during "quiet period" and *never* stayed in his seat longer than 5 minutes, unless the teacher stood directly over him. Then he would wriggle, squirm, tap his fingers, or make popping sounds with his mouth until no one near him could concentrate any better than Randy could.

His mother had noted many of the same problem behaviors at home. He wouldn't finish his homework unless she or his father stood over him; he would be distracted by his brothers, the TV, the cat, or a spider spinning a web in the corner. The work he completed was hurried and "filled with mistakes that he shouldn't have made, he's so bright."

"His father was like that when he was a kid—he's a research chemist now, but he still has trouble concentrating. But Randy must have gotten his disposition from my side of the family; he's pretty happy-go-lucky and positive. Even his brothers like him, though they sometimes complain that he's always butting in."

During the first interview, Randy sat at the art table and cheerfully drew a crayon picture of a child drawing a picture with crayons. He was a freckle-faced redhead who admitted that sometimes he didn't behave very well. "I can't seem to help it," he said, then added brightly, "Maybe I'll learn how next year." He said that his teacher didn't seem to like him much. "Miss Rucker says I'm careless and lose my things, like my pencil and my books. And when she lifted up my desk top and showed the class how it looked inside, the kids all laughed."

Later, commenting on Randy's quiet behavior during the interview, his mother said, "He was that way when we took him to the pediatrician, too. It's like trying to get your TV fixed—it always works fine in the shop."

Evaluation of Randy

ADHD can be diagnosed with as few as six symptoms, but then those must all occur in either the inattention or the hyperactivity–impulsiveness group. Randy had symptoms in both of these groups. In the inattention group, he often made careless mistakes, did not sustain attention, seemed not to listen, didn't complete chores, lost school supplies, and was easily distractible. In the hyperactivity–impulsiveness group, he squirmed, roamed the classroom, was excessively on the go, talked far too much, and answered questions for the other children in the classroom. Even his brothers found him intrusive.

Some of Randy's symptoms had been present from youngest childhood, and the problems that resulted from his behavior were evident both at school and home. But from the Axis I exclusions listed in the criteria, DSM-IV seems to regard ADHD as something of a diagnosis of late (though not last) choice. Therefore, could any other disorder explain Randy's symptoms? In **pervasive developmental disorders**, such as **Autistic Disorder**, children do not communicate as well as Randy. **Mental Retardation** could be ruled out by the fact that his development was entirely normal; also, he learned quickly, once his attention was captured. Patients with **depressive disorders** may be agitated or have a poor attention span; although Randy's demeanor was cheerful, more information needed to be obtained from his parents about depressive symptoms, as well as symptoms of **anxiety disorders**. Of course, there was no evidence whatsoever for a **psychotic disorder** such as **Schizophrenia**. Many patients with **Tourette's Disorder** are also hyperactive; the vignette includes no details about **motor or vocal tics**, and his parents would have to be asked about these. Although the criteria advise ruling out **personality disorders**, such a diagnosis would be hard to sustain in a child so young.

Children reared in a **chaotic social environment** can be hyperactive or inattentive; as far as our information goes, Randy's home was stable and supportive. There is no evidence from the vignette of willful misbehavior that would suggest other **behavior disorders**, such as **Oppositional Defiant Disorder** or **Conduct Disorder**, both of which often accompany ADHD. In fact,

Randy seemed to feel bad that he could not control himself. **Learning disorders** can also be comorbid with ADHD and the disruptive behavior disorders, and should be considered in the differential of any child who acts out in school.

Because Randy exhibited symptoms in each of the hyperactivity–impulsiveness and inattention groups, his subtype diagnosis would be Combined Type. In fact, this is the most common subtype. Randy's diagnosis (pending a further interview with his parents) would be as follows:

A couple of generations ago, the hallmark of ADHD was fidgety behavior, which determined one of its names: Hyperactive Child Syndrome. These children were described as "motorically driven," always running, and as having trouble sitting quietly. In the last decade or two, problems maintaining attention became the focus for this disorder, now somewhat clumsily renamed Attention-Deficit/Hyperactivity Disorder (no wonder the abbreviation "ADHD" has found currency!). Recent work suggests yet another theory: namely, that it develops as a failure of brain mechanisms responsible for self-control and the inhibition of impulses. The brain areas involved may be the caudate nucleus and the globus pallidus, both of which are portions of the basal ganglia. Although the theory has not yet been adequately tested, it is at least possible that DSM-V or DSM-VI will give yet another name to this puzzling, widely prevalent condition.

Axis I	314.01	Attention-Deficit/Hyperactivity Disorder, Combined Type
Axis II	V71.09	No diagnosis
Axis III		None
Axis IV		None
Axis V	GAF = 65	(current)

314.9 Attention-Deficit/Hyperactivity Disorder Not Otherwise Specified

Children who are hyperactive or who have problems maintaining attention but who do not fulfill the criteria for ADHD may be coded as having ADHD Not Otherwise Specified.

312.8 Conduct Disorder

To one degree or other, the behavior of children with Conduct Disorder is persistently antisocial. The behavior can occur in any of four different categories, with the specific symptoms arranged so that symptoms in only one category will suffice for diagnosis (see Table 11.14). Note that most of these symptoms, whether they occur in a juvenile or an adult, can lead to arrest or other legal consequences. In fact, for an adult to be diagnosed as having Antisocial Personality Disorder, the exact criteria listed under the first bullet in Table 11.14 must have been present prior to the age of 15 (for truancy and staying out at night, 13).

From the age of 2–3, boys are more aggressive than girls. Children who are

In 1970, Eli Robins and Samuel Guze specified five criteria for validating mental health diagnoses. Their seminal work is often quoted today. To what extent does the category of Conduct Disorder fulfill their criteria?

1. Clinical description of a disorder is the first step in diagnosis. In 14 years, the DSM has changed criteria sets for Conduct Disorder three times. With each iteration, the diagnosable subtypes have changed completely. Although the inclusion criteria have retained some consistency from one edition of DSM to the next, their severity ranges from staying out late at night through breaking and entering to rape and use of a weapon.
2. Laboratory findings should support the classification. Unhappily, no consistent lab or radiographic findings have been found for Conduct Disorder.
3. Delimitation from other disorders should be facilitated by exclusion criteria. In regard to Conduct Disorder, DSM-IV does not state criteria for ruling out other diagnoses; in fact, comorbidity is the rule.
4. Follow-up studies should confirm a homogeneous outcome. Children who have been diagnosed as having Conduct Disorder can have a broad range of adult Axis I and II diagnoses, including no mental disorder at all. Even the most severely conduct-disordered child has no more than a 50% likelihood of developing Antisocial Personality Disorder.
5. Family studies should demonstrate the increased prevalence of the same disorder in close relatives. The relatives of children affected by Conduct Disorder often have alcoholism, Antisocial Personality Disorder, or Somatization Disorder, but so far, it has not been conclusively demonstrated that these represent forms of the same disorder.

Our understanding of Conduct Disorder appears to be in its infancy, with a range of psychopathology that is too broad, is too often confounded with other disorders, has insufficient support from family and genetic studies, and has no support at all from the lab. The outcome of Conduct Disorder is too inconsistent to support the validity of its use. Many authors seem hardly able to write about the diagnosis without disparaging it.

Children diagnosed with Conduct Disorder are at risk for a variety of personality disorders, and these criteria actually form a part of the requirements for the adult diagnosis of Antisocial Personality Disorder. The question must therefore be raised: Is Conduct Disorder more properly considered an Axis I or an Axis II disorder? Perhaps it is neither; perhaps it is a hybrid of symptoms that bridge two worlds. Further research, and not a little additional thought, may be needed to sort out these perplexing relationships.

TABLE 11.14. Criteria for Conduct Disorder

- For 12 months or more, the patient has repeatedly violated rules, age-appropriate societal norms, or the rights of others. This is shown by 3 or more of the following 15 symptoms, at least 1 of which has occurred in the previous 6 months:

  Aggression against people or animals
  ✓ Engages in frequent bullying or threatening
  ✓ Often starts physical fights
  ✓ Has used a weapon that could cause serious injury (gun, knife, club, broken glass)
  ✓ Has exhibited physical cruelty to people
  ✓ Has exhibited physical cruelty to animals
  ✓ Has committed theft with confrontation (armed robbery, extortion, mugging, purse snatching)
  ✓ Has forced sex upon someone

  Property destruction
  ✓ Has deliberately set fires to cause serious damage
  ✓ Has deliberately destroyed the property of others (except for fire setting)

  Lying or theft
  ✓ Has broken into a building, car, or house belonging to someone else
  ✓ Frequently lies or breaks promises for gain or to avoid obligations ("conning")
  ✓ Has stolen valuables without confrontation (burglary, forgery, shoplifting)

  Serious rule violation
  ✓ Beginning before age 13, frequently stays out at night against parents' wishes
  ✓ Has run away from parents overnight twice or more (once if for an extended period)
  ✓ Beginning before age 13, frequently engages in truancy

- These symptoms cause clinically important job, school, or social impairment.
- If 18 years or older, the patient does not meet criteria for Antisocial Personality Disorder.

Based on age of onset, specify:
    Childhood-Onset Type: At least one problem with conduct before age 10
    Adolescent-Onset Type: No problems with conduct before age 10

Specify severity:
    Mild (both are required): There are few problems with conduct beyond those needed to make the diagnosis, *and* all of these problems cause little harm to other people.
    Moderate: Number and effect of conduct problems are between Mild and Severe.
    Severe (either or both): There are many more conduct symptoms than are needed to make the diagnosis, *or* the conduct symptoms cause other people considerable harm.

highly aggressive by age 7 or 8 tend to remain so later in life and are three times more likely than other children to have police records as adults. The prevalence of Conduct Disorder in boys is high, ranging from 6% to 16%, depending upon the study; the rate for girls is perhaps half as high.

It is the age of onset, specified in the subtype diagnosis, that is important to the prediction of outcome. The Childhood-Onset Type (onset under the age of 10) is more often associated with marked aggression and poor outcome (up to 50% of patients with this subtype go on to receive an adult diagnosis of Antisocial Personality Disorder). Childhood-Onset patients are also far more likely to be male than female. In patients who don't become symptomatic until adolescence (more or less), the sex ratio is less extreme, and the disorder is less likely to result in the adult diagnosis of Antisocial Personality Disorder.

Jim

The interview with 10-year-old Jim was conducted in juvenile hall, which had been his home for the past 2 weeks. He had taken his penny collection to school for Hobby Day. At lunchtime it went into one of his socks, with which he then bludgeoned a second-grader who had refused to give up the jelly sandwich Jim wanted. The incident was by no means Jim's first attempt at extortion.

"He's been threatening other kids for a couple of years," his mother had said before the interview. "We had him down to the child guidance clinic. They said he had a behavior disorder. They're telling me!"

Jim had been a cranky, negative sort of baby, and his temperament hadn't improved by the time he had learned to talk. "His first complete sentence was 'I didn't do it,' " his mother remarked. He'd argue any point, even when he was caught red-handed doing something. Beginning in kindergarten, he'd blame the fights he started on his victim. When the other child objected, Jim would sometimes get even by sneaking around to that child's home to destroy a piece of play equipment. He was an angry child who by the age of 8 had cut the tires of more than one bicycle; once he had shredded the awning of a neighbor's sandbox with a pair of scissors he had stolen from a rack at Safeway.

Repeated shoplifting had prompted his first evaluation 2 years earlier. Twice that same year he had entered neighbors' homes and stolen small items, which he had then tried to sell on the school playground. School reports noted that he was bright and could have been a good student. But repeated truancy and starting fights had now earned him expulsion from three different schools.

"He comes by it naturally," his mother explained. "His father's served time in Lompoc twice for armed robbery. I guess you'd say he's a career criminal." She saw a bright spot in Jim's detention: "This is the first time in months I've known where he was at night."

Jim was a sandy-haired, chunky boy, large for his age, who swaggered across the playroom floor in a pair of overalls that had one strap undone. He disdained the various play materials that were offered him; he settled down on a wooden chair with a steady gaze and an air of complete control. For several minutes, he replied to questions with one- or two-word answers. When he finally spoke spontaneously, it was to ask how soon he would be released. He was told that it depended on the results of the evaluation, because he had struck and severely injured the younger child.

Jim gazed steadily at the interviewer. "It wasn't me—I never did nothin' wrong. Besides, the little snot prob'ly had it coming."

Evaluation of Jim

Of the many behavioral criteria for the diagnosis of Conduct Disorder, DSM-IV requires the presence of only three for the mildest cases. Jim had many more than three symptoms, including bullying, starting fights, using a weapon, property destruction, breaking and entering, lying, truancy, and staying out at night. Some of these behaviors had occurred just recently, and collectively they had greatly affected both Jim and his mother. Although lack of empathy is ignored by the official criteria (partly because it is so hard to measure), Jim's manifest absence of empathy would be regarded by many clinicians as central to the syndrome of Conduct Disorder.

Of course, there are other possible causes of antisocial behavior. **Gross brain pathology**, such as a tumor, an infection, or a seizure disorder, is one such cause; a **psychotic disorder** can be another. The clinician who saw Jim would have to look carefully for evidence of problems with cognition, hallucinations, delusions, and other symptoms of these conditions.

Besides the symptoms embodied in the criteria, other problems can be associated with this diagnosis. Children with Conduct Disorder often begin sexual activity in early adolescence. Some are depressed (they may show evidence of a **Major Depressive Episode** or **Dysthymic Disorder**); many will **abuse substances**. **Reading Disorder** and other language (oral and written) deficits have been noted in a substantial number of these children, and **ADHD** is comorbid in nearly half. Earlier in life, before he became quite so antisocial, Jim's symptoms (arguments, blaming others, angry, spiteful) might have qualified him for the diagnosis of **Oppositional Defiant Disorder**—a common precursor to Conduct Disorder. However, DSM-IV does not permit Oppositional Defiant Disorder to be coded in the presence of Conduct Disorder, which takes precedence.

We agree that because of its grave prognosis and the relative absence of effective treatment, all other possible disorders should be given serious consideration before a diagnosis of Conduct Disorder is made. However, if any case history justifies the use of this diagnosis, Jim's would appear to be the one. Because he had many more symptoms that the minimum required, and he had seriously injured the other child with his homemade sap, his Conduct Disorder would be coded as Severe. His possible future Axis II diagnosis is discussed in Chapter 26 (p. 433); his complete diagnosis would be the following:

Axis I	312.8	Conduct Disorder, Childhood-Onset Type, Severe
Axis II	799.9	Diagnosis deferred
Axis III		None
Axis IV		Incarcerated in juvenile hall
Axis V	GAF = 41	(current)

313.81 Oppositional Defiant Disorder

As disruptive behavior disorders go, Oppositional Defiant Disorder (abbreviated ODD in this discussion) is relatively mild. It occupies an uneasy niche in the broad spectrum of childhood behavioral problems. Here is the source of controversy surrounding these children: Can their persistently defiant, hostile, and uncooperative behavior be adequately differentiated from the behavior of normal toddlers (or adolescents) and from the more severe Conduct Disorder? If it can, what is the prognosis for such individuals? Is ODD then a risk factor for later Conduct Disorder?

The facts known about ODD are sparse. It usually begins early, frequently evolving from a toddler's normal quest for independence. Sometimes implicated have been coercive parenting styles that involve strict, often harsh, and inconsistently applied discipline. These children's angry and defiant behaviors almost universally disrupt their home lives. Somewhat less often, relationships in the school and in the community are also affected. (See Table 11.15 for the full criteria.)

Before adolescence, boys are more often affected than girls; thereafter, the sexes are affected equally. Overall, about 1 in 20 children can be diagnosed with ODD. Years later, some have progressed to full-blown Conduct Disorder or worse, but perhaps 25% have no signs of the disorder on follow-up. In adults who continue to show only symptoms of ODD, it resembles a personality disorder.

Shelly

"Mom can't handle me."

For the 10 or 15 minutes after stating her chief complaint, Shelly was nearly silent. An attractive though immature 13-year-old, she sat with downcast

TABLE 11.15. Criteria for Oppositional Defiant Disorder

- For at least 6 months, the patient shows defiant, hostile, negativistic behavior; four or more of the following often apply:
  - ✓ Losing temper
  - ✓ Arguing with adults
  - ✓ Actively defying or refusing to carry out the rules or requests of adults
  - ✓ Deliberately doing things that annoy others
  - ✓ Blaming others for own mistakes or misbehavior
  - ✓ Being touchy or easily annoyed by others
  - ✓ Being angry and resentful
  - ✓ Being spiteful or vindictive
- The symptoms cause clinically important distress or impair work, school, or social functioning.
- The symptoms do not occur in the course of a Mood or Psychotic Disorder.
- The symptoms do not fulfill criteria for Conduct Disorder.
- If age 18 or older, the patient does not meet criteria for Antisocial Personality Disorder.

Coding Note: Only score a criterion in the list under the first bullet positive if that behavior occurs more often than expected for age and developmental level.

eyes, answering questions with monosyllables or "I don't know." She wore lipstick and eyeshadow, and her ears had several piercings apiece.

Colicky as a baby, Shelly had been difficult right from the start. "She never seemed to sleep," her mother had reported during an earlier interview. "She moved from the terrible twos straight through the terrible threes to the terrible fours. She was—and is—the world's pickiest eater. And she always refused to go to bed. The first word she ever learned to say was 'No.' "

Almost as soon as she spoke sentences, Shelly had begun to argue. "Now she'll argue about anything. She'll argue until she's grounded. Then she loses her temper, then her allowance, but still she won't give in. She'll just sit in her room and read by the hour."

Although she sometimes became so angry that she slammed doors, Shelly was never destructive or violent toward people. Neither was she dishonest: There had been no history of stealing, and she almost always told the truth. Although in the past few months she had often thrown away homework assignments that she could have completed easily, when questioned she would usually own up to what she had done. But the falling grades were "not her fault."

"She's never willing to take responsibility," her mother commented. "According to her, bad things happen because the teacher has pets or I'm unfair. She says she doesn't have friends because the other girls are jealous.

But even when she was in Brownies, I've seen her pick away at another girl till the whole group turned on her."

With shakes of her head, Shelly denied feeling depressed, using drugs or alcohol, and having suicidal ideas. To questions about delusions and hallucinations, she responded, "That's dumb." Only the subject of her parents' divorce produced much interaction or affect. "It really burns me. Sure, Daddy drinks. But he never, like, hit her or anything. And she was always nagging him."

She folded her arms across her chest. "I hate them both."

Evaluation of Shelly

As is typical for this disorder, Shelly's difficulties began when she was tiny; they persisted into adolescence, far longer than the minimum 6 months required. The extremes to which she would pursue an argument are classical for ODD. Other symptoms included refusing to do her homework, blaming others for her own misconduct, and deliberately annoying another girl in Brownies. She also expressed anger over her parents' divorce, but this would have to be further evaluated before it could count as a symptom of ODD, because any symptom must occur more often than would be expected for someone of the patient's age and level of development. Of course, a degree of oppositional behavior is normal at certain developmental stages (toddlerhood, adolescence), but Shelly's problematic behaviors had been present for years. (In many other children, the issue may be less clear-cut.) They also caused social and academic problems for her.

Shelly denied symptoms of a **mood disorder** or **psychotic disorder**, and the vignette includes evidence against aggressive, destructive, or antisocial behavior (she didn't fight or lie) that would suggest the more serious **Conduct Disorder** or **Antisocial Personality Disorder**. Although the foregoing are the only diagnoses the criteria specifically prohibit, clinicians should also be on the lookout in some cases for **ADHD**, which may be associated with disruptive behavior and is commonly comorbid with ODD. Another possibility may be **Mental Retardation**, which can only be comorbid with ODD if a child's oppositional symptoms are much greater than would be expected for the age and degree of retardation. The inability to understand spoken language caused by **impaired hearing** can also mimic willful disobedience. In some cases (not Shelly's), impaired progress in school may necessitate ruling out a **learning disorder**, such as **Reading Disorder** or **Mathematics Disorder**. Shelly's five-axis diagnosis would be the following:

Axis I	313.81	Oppositional Defiant Disorder
Axis II	V71.09	No diagnosis
Axis III		None
Axis IV		None
Axis V	GAF = 55	(current)

312.9 Disruptive Behavior Disorder Not Otherwise Specified

Use this code for a child who has clinically important conduct or oppositional defiant behavior that does not fulfill the criteria for Conduct Disorder or ODD.

Assessing Attention-Deficit and Disruptive Behavior Disorders

General Suggestions

Evaluating behavior that is hyperactive, inattentive, oppositional, disruptive, or otherwise difficult to control can pose a challenge to any interviewer, no matter how experienced. Though many children who are brought for evaluation of hyperactivity or oppositional behavior may fidget and squirm, significant hyperactivity is often not evident when such a child is being interviewed. New situations or environments, such as a first office visit, sometimes act to suppress activity. After serial observations over several visits, disruptive behaviors may become more apparent. Negativism may only become evident with adults a child knows well. However, even a single meeting may be enough to reveal inattention to conversation, disorganized play with dolls and toys, or inability to wait for turns when playing a game.

In no other area of child mental health is it more important to seek out and use multiple resources; the combination of parents who are unknowledgeable with children who are often unreliable is a setup for diagnostic confusion. You may find it useful to interview parent and child separately to assess, for example, just how much of the child's time is unsupervised (which may correlate with the diagnosis of Conduct Disorder).

Asking about unsanctioned behaviors is an invitation to lie. However, if you request an opinion about similar behavior if it was exhibited by a peer or fictional child, you may learn how fully the patient approves of the behavior: "One of the kids who comes in here hit his sister last week because she hid his crayons. Do you think that was OK?" Some children and adolescents may even be induced to brag about their exploits, though your reaction must not seem to sanction the behavior.

An oppositional child may justify negativistic behavior on the basis that the request was unreasonable. Note that it does not suffice for a diagnosis of ODD merely to observe in an interview that a child is touchy, angry, spiteful, annoying, and prone to blame others—the criteria require the historical evidence that such is *often* the case.

Developmental Factors

ADHD can be difficult to discriminate from inattentiveness resulting from the drive for exploration that is normal in toddlers and preschool children. In such cases, you must place even greater emphasis than usual on the histories from parents *and* teachers. (DSM-IV requires these behaviors to be reported in at least two settings.) Older children may be self-aware enough to report feeling inner restlessness.

Of course, very young children are notorious for negativistic behavior (the "terrible twos"); even defiant behavior may be quite normal in this age range. And very young children certainly cannot be expected to sustain attention for longer than a few minutes.

In DSM-IV, for the first time, Conduct Disorder is subtyped according to age of onset: Childhood-Onset versus Adolescent-Onset. For the former to be diagnosed, a child must have had at least one symptom before age 10. Note that the milder symptoms of Conduct Disorder in younger children will usually become evident first (lying, shoplifting, staying out at night, and truancy will precede robbery at gunpoint, rape, and use of a weapon).

Since the publication of Lee Robins's seminal book *Deviant Children Grown Up* (Baltimore: Williams & Wilkins, 1966), the prognostic value of early development of symptoms has been recognized. Robins found that the younger a boy was at first arrest, the greater his risk of a poor outcome. However, over half of even the most disturbed youngsters did not develop Antisocial Personality Disorder.

FEEDING AND EATING DISORDERS OF INFANCY OR EARLY CHILDHOOD

As their new name suggests, the feeding and eating disorders of infancy or early childhood are somewhat simplified from DSM-III-R, in that this group no longer includes Anorexia Nervosa and Bulimia Nervosa. Pica has been known for hundreds of years; Rumination Disorder was introduced as a diagnosis in DSM-III. But Feeding Disorder of Infancy or Early Childhood has been newly created for DSM-IV. It is intended to comprise what is called *nonorganic failure to thrive*, which is partly coextensive with Rumination Disorder and Reactive Attachment Disorder of Infancy or Early Childhood.

307.52 Pica

Derived from the word *magpie* (a bird whose scientific name is *Pica*), Pica as a term for abnormal eating behavior dates back at least four centuries—perhaps to a time when someone, watching these large black-and-white birds as they collected clay and mud for nests, assumed that that they were eating it instead. Pica (see Table 11.16 for the full criteria) has for centuries been identified with two groups: young children and pregnant women. Dirt is one of the more common substances these people ingest, but any nonnutritive substance—chalk, wall plaster, soap, burnt matches, or (in extremely rare cases) even feces—will fulfill the definition. In some patients, Pica may be a sign of iron deficiency. Others may develop any of a variety of medical complications. Children who eat paint risk lead toxicity; intestinal obstruction can result from ingestion of hair and other bulky, indigestible material.

Individuals with Autistic Disorder and/or Mental Retardation are especially prone to develop Pica, and the risk increases with the severity of these disorders. Adult women with the condition are likely to have a family history of Pica and a personal history of it when they were children. A background of neglect and low socioeconomic status is common among affected children. The behavior usually begins between the ages of 1 and 2 years, and remits with the onset of adolescence or with the correction of iron deficiency anemia.

TABLE 11.16. Criteria for Pica

- For at least 1 month, the patient persists in eating dirt or other nonnutritive substances.
- This behavior is not appropriate to the patient's developmental level.
- It is not sanctioned by the patient's culture.
- If this behavior occurs solely in the context of another mental disorder (such as Mental Retardation, a pervasive developmental disorder, or Schizophrenia), it is serious enough to require independent clinical attention.

Melanie

Melanie was 12 when her parents both died in an automobile accident and she went to live with her older sister in Philadelphia. She was a slender, awkward girl who seemed to hunger for friends, always hanging about the fringes of a group at school. So, when she was 14 and a freshman in high school, the few who knew her expressed amazement to learn that she was pregnant. "I don't think she's ever even had a period," remarked her sister, "and I've never heard anything about a boyfriend."

Even then, the pregnancy was only discovered when her sister found her one afternoon in the backyard eating potting soil. It had happened several times in the past 2 months, and it was behavior even Melanie couldn't explain. ("I don't know why I do it, I just do it.") She was whisked away to see the pediatrician, who diagnosed anemia and a 4-month pregnancy. Although she had never before eaten dirt, her sister recalled that as a toddler, Melanie would pick up chewing gum and other discarded material from the park and put it into her mouth.

Evaluation of Melanie

Eating material that had no nutritional value (at least for humans) had persisted longer than a month and was behavior foreign to Melanie's culture. She was old enough and mature enough (a freshman in high school at age 14) that her developmental stage could not explain the symptoms (such behavior would be considered developmentally appropriate in a toddler). Other diagnoses with which Pica can co-occur include **Schizophrenia** (but Melanie did not explain her behavior with delusions). There is no information that would suggest a **pervasive developmental disorder**, in which unusual eating habits may also be encountered.

Although no personality disorder diagnosis could be made, Melanie's relatively poor social relationships suggested avoidant features. The fact that Axis II features needed to be further evaluated is indicated by the V-code. For the moment, Melanie's diagnosis would be as follows:

Axis I	307.52	Pica
Axis II	V71.09	Diagnosis deferred
Axis III	V22.2	Normal pregnancy
Axis IV		Pregnancy
Axis V	GAF = 65	(current)

307.53 Rumination Disorder

During rumination, an individual regurgitates a bolus of food from the stomach and chews it again. This is a normal part of the digestive process for cattle, deer, and giraffes, which is why they are called *ruminants*. In humans, it is abnormal and can lead to physical complications. When people ruminate, they do not experience nausea. In most cases, the food is later swallowed once again to be digested, but some persons (especially infants and the mentally retarded) will spit it out instead. Then malnutrition, failure to thrive (in infants), or a reduced resistance to disease can occur. Mortality rates as high as 25% have been reported.

Mentally retarded individuals are more often affected by Rumination Disorder than are persons of normal IQ, though occasionally a case of it in a nonretarded adult has been reported. In most cases the behavior subsides spontaneously, though it can persist throughout life. One adult ruminator was reportedly Samuel Johnson, the 18th-century lexicographer, whose acquaintances noted his "cud-chewing" behavior.

Rumination Disorder (see Table 11.17 for the criteria) is uncommon, though more frequent in males than in females. It most often develops in infants, beginning after solid foods are introduced into the diet. Voluntary regurgitation may not be present initially. Often gastroesophageal reflux precipitates the onset. The act of ruminating may be associated with medical conditions such as hiatus hernia, although such a condition would rule out the diagnosis of Rumination Disorder. The cause is unknown, though social problems (abnormal parent–child interaction) may be a factor.

Because the criteria are quite descriptive, we have provided no clinical vignette.

TABLE 11.17. Criteria for Rumination Disorder

- After a period of normal functioning, for at least 1 month the patient repeatedly regurgitates and rechews food.
- This behavior is not caused by a gastrointestinal illness or other general medical condition (such as esophageal reflux).
- The behavior doesn't occur solely during Anorexia Nervosa or Bulimia Nervosa.
- If it occurs solely during Mental Retardation or a pervasive developmental disorder, it is serious enough to require independent clinical attention.

307.59 Feeding Disorder of Infancy or Early Childhood

The first word of this disorder's name was chosen carefully to reflect the fact that the problem is presumed not to be with the child's eating, but rather with a disturbance in the child's relationship to the mother (or other care-giver). As a result, child and mother cannot regulate the child's nutritional intake satisfactorily, and the child fails to gain weight. It is not all that uncommon, and the disorder might have been defined as a Parent–Child Relational Problem (see p. 439). Indeed, this was one suggestion considered by the creators of DSM-IV, whose consensus was that the consequences (potential for death) were too serious for a V-code diagnosis. (See Table 11.18 for the full criteria.)

Inadequate nutrition can render these children fussy or withdrawn. Some-times the diagnosis is made when they rapidly gain weight once hospitalized, separated from their mothers, and consistently fed by sensitive nurses. Neglect, abuse, and parental psychopathology are often described in extreme cases of failure to thrive. Nonorganic failure to thrive has now been linked with a num-ber of conditions besides Feeding Disorder, among them Rumination Disorder, Reactive Attachment Disorder, and Breathing-Related Sleep Disorder. We have probably not yet heard the last word on this group of potentially fatal condi-tions that still await adequate definition.

Derek

Deborah had been only 17 when her first son, Raymond, was born. Hours after the delivery she had left the baby with relatives, put all the clothes she could carry into a plastic satchel, and headed for San Diego, where she waited on ta-bles. Now Raymond was nearly 13 and lived with his paternal grandmother on the Oregon coast, and it had been years since Deborah had thought about ba-bies. Beyond taking iron tablets and visiting the obstetrician twice, she hadn't prepared at all for Derek.

When Deborah was at work, Derek was watched by an immigrant woman from upstairs, who spoke almost no English. "Don't talk foreign to him,"

TABLE 11.18. Criteria for Feeding Disorder of Infancy or Early Childhood

- For 1 month or more, the patient has persistently failed to eat adequately and has either not gained weight or lost weight.
- This behavior is not due to a gastrointestinal illness or other general medical condition (such as esophageal reflux).
- Neither another mental disorder (such as Rumination Disorder) nor the lack of available food better explains the symptoms.
- It begins before age 6.

Deborah had told her irritably. "I don't want him growing up with an accent." When she returned from work, she was too tired to pay him much attention. As a result, Derek spent most of his first year staring at the sides of his crib.

When Derek was nearing his first birthday, it was the sitter who, in halting words, pointed out that he still weighed only 14 pounds—in fact, for the past several months he had hardly gained weight at all. She noted that when she tried to feed him, he often cried and turned his head away or pushed back the spoon. "He jus' don' wanna eat," she had said. Those occasions when Deborah herself fed him often ended in tears for both.

When he was finally taken to the well-baby clinic, Derek was pronounced "undernourished and neglected" and was hospitalized for further evaluation.

Evaluation of Derek

Notice that the first bulleted criterion in Table 11.18 actually includes two requirements. The sitter's testimony that he failed to eat adequately fulfilled the first; the second depended on the objectivity of the scales. However, Derek's diagnosis could not be definitively stated until the appropriate laboratory and radiographic exams had ruled out other causes of failure to thrive, such as **endocrine**, **gastrointestinal**, or **neurological disorders**. Therefore, as the introduction to DSM-IV requests, the diagnosis would at first have to be stated as provisional.

Although he was kept clean, the Axis IV diagnosis was given because of the lack of adequate psychological stimulation. Had Derek not qualified for the Feeding Disorder diagnosis, his Axis I diagnosis might instead have been Neglect of Child, coded 995.5 instead of V61.21 to indicate a focus on the child as victim (see p. 442). Depending on the outcome of medical investigations, in addition to underweight, malnutrition might have to be coded on Axis III. Derek's interim diagnosis would be as follows:

Axis I	307.59	Feeding Disorder of Infancy or Early Childhood (Provisional)
Axis II	V71.09	No diagnosis
Axis III	783.4	Underweight (failure to thrive)
Axis IV		Problem with primary support group: Neglect of child
Axis V	GAF = 65	(on admission)

Assessing Feeding and Eating Disorders of Infancy or Early Childhood

General Suggestions

Although direct observation of parents and child at mealtime may reveal much about early feeding or eating disorders, most of the concrete information about Rumination Disorder and Feeding Disorder of Infancy or Early Childhood will come from the parents. To elicit behaviors associated with Pica, you can ask older children: "Do you like to taste things that other people don't eat? Do you ever eat dirt, chalk, soap, that sort of thing?" Of course, children may not be forthcoming about behaviors they perceive adults to frown on, so you might preface your questions with "Sometimes kids eat things that aren't food . . ." On the other hand, Pica may only come to light during the investigation of medical problems such as iron deficiency or malnutrition. Watch for other oral behaviors, such as nail biting and thumb sucking.

Developmental Factors

As the generic name suggests, each of these three disorders occurs early in life; Rumination Disorder and Feeding Disorder of Infancy or Early Childhood usually begin prior to a child's first birthday. Normal toddlers will put nearly anything into their mouths, so the diagnosis of Pica should not be made unless the inappropriate eating lasts longer than 1 month in a child developmentally past the toddler stage.

TIC DISORDERS

307.23 Tourette's Disorder

307.22 Chronic Motor or Vocal Tic Disorder

307.21 Transient Tic Disorder

Tics can be motor or vocal, simple or complex, transient or chronic. These three dimensions define the three main members of the tic disorder family (see Table 11.19). Simple motor tics include grimaces; eye muscle twitches; abdominal tensing; and jerks of shoulder, head, or distal extremities. Simple vocal tics may

TABLE 11.19. Criteria for Tourette's Disorder and Two Other Tic Disorders

	Tourette's Disorder	Chronic Motor or Vocal Tic Disorder	Transient Tic Disorder
Motor tics	• Multiple motor tics required for diagnosis.	• At some time, the patient has had either vocal or motor tics, *but not both* (may be single or multiple).	• Requires either *or* both vocal or motor tics (may be single or multiple).
Vocal tics	• One or more required for diagnosis.		
Duration	• For longer than 1 year, these tics have occurred many times each day, nearly every day or at intervals. During this time, the patient never goes longer than 3 months without the tics.		• For at least 4 weeks but no longer than 12 consecutive months, these tics have occurred many times each day, nearly every day.
Must rule out	—	• Tourette's Disorder	• Tourette's Disorder *and* Chronic Motor or Vocal Tic Disorder
Other criteria	• The symptoms begin before age 18. • The symptoms are not directly caused by the effects of a general medical condition (such as Huntington's disease or postviral encephalitis) or substance use (such as a central nervous system stimulant).		
Specifiers	—	—	• Specify whether: Single Episode or Recurrent

include barks, coughs, throat clearing, sniffs, and single syllables that may be muttered or called out. Complex tics are more organized patterns of speech or motor movement. Although tics are generally involuntary, patients can often suppress them for periods of time; they usually disappear during sleep. Under conditions of stress, fatigue, or illness, their frequency and intensity may increase.

Motor tics first appear during childhood, sometimes in a child as young as 2, and classically involve the upper part of the face. Vocal tics begin somewhat later. It is clear, however, that affected children present with a wide range of symptoms. On one end of the continuum is the simple, occasional eye blinking tic when a child is under stress. On the other end are the multiple motor and vocal tics so extreme that they preclude participation in the normal classroom.

Tics leave children feeling out of control of their own bodies and mental processes—an experience that is especially true of Tourette's Disorder, first described in 1895 by Georges Gilles de la Tourette. These patients have not only multiple motor tics, but also vocal tics; often (but by no means always), they eventually utter coarse language (*coprolalia*) at socially inappropriate times. It is still not clear whether there is a developmental progression from transient tics to chronic tics to Tourette's Disorder.

Tics are common among children; community surveys find them in perhaps 10% of boys and 5% of girls. Of course, these are predominantly transient motor tics, many of which never cause enough concern to warrant an evaluation. The prevalence in adults is lower, though male predominance persists. For Tourette's Disorder, the prevalence is about 5 per 10,000 in the general population, with males far more often affected than females. The perceived frequency and severity of tics in any child are complicated by the social context in which they occur. Family studies suggest that in at least 65% of cases, Tourette's Disorder is familial. What is inherited seems not to be a genotype for Tourette's Disorder but for a broadly defined spectrum of disorders that includes tics, Tourette's Disorder, and Obsessive–Compulsive Disorder. Other factors possibly associated with the development of Tourette's Disorder include stress and low birth weight.

Although there are a number of effective pharmacological treatments for Tourette's Disorder, once diagnosed it tends to persist throughout life. Some families (and classrooms) are better able than others to mitigate the shame, embarrassment, and guilt that attend the vocal outbursts. The presence of a compassionate, understanding, supportive environment greatly increases the likelihood of enhanced self-esteem and improved social relationships. The prognosis for other tic disorders is far better. Of course, by definition, transient tics disappear within a few months. Even "chronic" motor or vocal tics usually wane and disappear within a few years. Motor tics rarely persist into adulthood and beyond.

Because the symptom of tics is the same, regardless of which of these three DSM-IV disorders it occurs in, we present only one vignette.

Neal

When Neal was 5, he was referred to a day treatment program because of his hyperactivity and motor tics. Though his verbal skills seemed normal, he had difficulty listening to his kindergarten teacher, who felt that he was impulsive and had a short attention span. These difficulties were first noted at about the time of his parents' divorce. Then Neal cried a great deal, which progressed to temper tantrums and aggressive acting out in school. At the request of the teacher, the family physician started him on Ritalin. He was referred to the day treatment program largely because the Ritalin did not manage his aggression and impulsiveness.

Let's scrutinize the bare definition of a *tic*. A tic is a movement or vocalization that is all of the following:

Stereotyped. It occurs as a persistent, mechanical repetition without any apparent purpose.
Nonrhythmic. It occurs without apparent periodicity.
Rapid. An individual, simple tic lasts less than a second—in the blink of an eye, so to speak.
Repeated. It occurs over and over.
Sudden. An individual tic occurs without warning.

Neal's mother had noted no problems with hyperactivity, but had become concerned when the tics began, a few months before that first evaluation. First there was a barely perceptible blinking of his eyes, which occurred many times each day. These minor facial twitches were later coupled with a drawing down of the corners of his mouth. Over a 6-month period, these single motor tics became ever more frequent and developed into more complex patterns that involved his face, neck, arms, and hands. The treatment center staff discontinued the Ritalin when his tics became obvious, but their intensity and severity continued to increase. Sometimes Neal's tics seemed to yank him off his chair and onto the floor. All the while, the gentler facial grimacing continued as well.

When Neal was nearly 7, he began to experience vocal tics. At first, these were soft grunting sounds he would make whenever his shoulder twitched, but within a few months he was uttering barks, sniffs, and grunts that gradually became louder. Most of these verbal outbursts were unintelligible; soon, however, clearly audible, sexually explicit words crept into his output.

As the treatment team came to know him better, it was apparent that Neal was also beset with compulsive rituals. He organized his desk at school into small compartments and carefully placed his possessions into specific squares. He also counted the ceiling tiles repetitively.

On close examination, his mother was noted to have occasional facial grimaces and mild motor head-jerking tics.

Evaluation of Neal

A diagnostician who met Neal during the first few months that he had tics (motor tics only) would have been hard pressed to make any diagnosis at all. Tics are common in childhood and may cause no distress or impaired functioning.

This is why the text revision of DSM-IV (DSM-IV-TR; published in 2000), in the only criteria changes pertaining to children, discards the earlier requirement for all tic diagnoses that the symptoms cause marked distress or impair functioning in some material way. During the first year, Neal could only have qualified for a diagnosis of Transient Tic Disorder. (This diagnosis can be assigned whether motor tics, vocal tics, or both are present.) After 1 year, Chronic Motor or Vocal Tic Disorder could have been diagnosed if Neal had had only motor *or* vocal tics. By the time a year had passed, neither of the foregoing diagnoses was appropriate—one because of the time span, the other because of the two types of tics. Then the appropriate diagnosis became Tourette's Disorder.

Of course, for any of these diagnoses other **general medical conditions** must be ruled out, including neurological movement disorders such as dystonia. Abnormal movements can sometimes be found in **substance-induced toxicity**, such as with amphetamine. Neal's prescription for Ritalin may have precipitated his tics; if that were the only cause of his symptoms, no tic disorder diagnosis would be needed. Then a code describing the medication's effect could be indicated on Axis I—**Medication-Induced Movement Disorder Not Otherwise Specified** (see p. 446). Other conditions in which abnormal movements can occur include the **pervasive developmental disorders** (hand flapping and other stereotypies are prominent in the diagnostic criteria for **Autistic Disorder**, **Rett's Disorder**, **Childhood Disintegrative Disorder**, and **Asperger's Disorder**), none of which applied to Neal. Neither did he have a history or other symptoms necessary for **Schizophrenia, Catatonic Type**.

With a more complete history, a diagnosis of **ADHD**, which can also be comorbid with Tourette's Disorder and other tic disorders, might be warranted but for one fact: Neal's symptoms seemed to be present only at school, not at home. Of course, this could have been due to selective reporting on the part of his mother; however, with strict criteria and the information provided, only a diagnosis of ADHD Not Otherwise Specified would be warranted. His clinician would also need to watch for symptoms of **Obsessive–Compulsive Disorder**, with which Tourette's Disorder is

Why do only some children who receive the gene for Tourette's Disorder develop symptoms? One possibility is that a streptococcal infection may in some way sensitize their brains. A study by Harvey Singer and colleagues found higher levels of antineuronal antibodies in the putamen (an area of the brain involved in the control of movement). If nothing else, such findings demonstrate the importance of asking about a history of physical illnesses, even one as seemingly minor as a streptococcus infection.

often comorbid and which might not become obvious until much later. As matters stand, Neal's complete diagnosis would be the following:

Axis I	307.23	Tourette's Disorder
	314.9	Attention-Deficit/Hyperactivity Disorder Not Otherwise Specified
Axis II	V71.09	No diagnosis
Axis III		None
Axis IV		None
Axis V	GAF = 60	(current)

307.20 Tic Disorder Not Otherwise Specified

Use Tic Disorder Not Otherwise Specified to code tics that don't fulfill criteria for another tic disorder.

Assessing Tic Disorders

General Suggestions

Although seizures enter into the differential diagnosis of tics, an EEG is only rarely necessary. With no positive laboratory or X-ray findings, the diagnosis of tics relies primarily upon observation. And because even moderately serious tics can with effort be suppressed for a time, observation may have to extend over a longer period—hours, in some cases.

Don't forget the important role that history taking can play in diagnosis of tics. Do the tics disappear during sleep or increase with anxiety, fatigue, or stress? Some patients may require extended evaluation, involving a diary of times, places, and situations in which the tics occur.

Watch for rapid contractions in related muscle groups, producing quick blinks or grimaces of the face or twitching of other body parts (simple motor tics). Complex motor tics are slower and may appear to be performed on purpose, as in touching or smelling. Although the upper face is most often involved, the shoulder girdle and arms are sometimes affected.

Repetition is key to the identification of vocal tics. A lone, simple vocal tic can be passed off as a cough or a sneeze; repeated grunts, snorts, sniffs, or throat clearings confirm the diagnosis. Complex vocal tics include words or phrases that a patient utters or imitates from the speech of others. Vocal tics are especially likely to occur at natural pauses in speech, as at the end of a phrase or sentence.

Developmental Factors

Tics are quite common in younger children. Motor tics begin at an average age of 7 and usually precede the onset of vocal tics. In patients with Tourette's Disorder, severe symptoms such as coprolalia develop last of all.

ELIMINATION DISORDERS

Although Encopresis and Enuresis usually occur separately, they may occur together, especially in children who have been severely neglected and emotionally deprived. Both bowel and bladder training practices vary with social context and with a family's cultural background, so either disorder must be diagnosed with sensitivity to these practices and the patient's age. DSM-IV, using common standards of practice in the United States, has determined that soiling after the age of 4 years or wetting after the age of 5 years qualifies for the respective diagnosis. Criteria of frequency and of social and functional impairment are also mandated, to avoid overdiagnosing the accidents that can occasionally befall any young child. (See Table 11.20 for the full criteria for Encopresis and Enuresis.)

More often than not, these syndromes first present in the pediatric or primary care setting, where gastrointestinal and genitourinary tract abnormalities (though rare) often receive early investigation. The clinical, diagnostic, and economic value of these expensive and intrusive examinations is questionable, especially in view of the fact that a careful medical history is often sufficient to make an accurate diagnosis.

In both Encopresis and Enuresis, it is important first to establish whether the disorder is primary or secondary. A *primary* disorder is one in which symptoms have been present throughout the developmental period (toilet training was never fully successful). In *secondary* disorders, symptoms occur after at least 6 months of successful toilet training. Because these disorders present in primary care settings and because clinicians may use widely varying criteria, it has been difficult to estimate accurately the prevalence of either Encopresis or Enuresis.

TABLE 11.20. Criteria for Encopresis and Enuresis

Encopresis	307.6 Enuresis
• Accidentally or on purpose, the patient repeatedly passes feces into inappropriate places (clothing, the floor).	• Accidentally or on purpose, the patient repeatedly urinates into clothing or the bed.
• For at least 3 months, this has happened at least once per month.	• The clinical importance of this behavior is shown by *either* of the following: ✓ It occurs at least twice a week for at least 3 consecutive months, *or* ✓ It causes clinically important distress or impairs work (scholastic), social, or personal functioning
• The patient is at least 4 years old (or the developmental equivalent).	• The patient is at least 5 years old (or the developmental equivalent).
• This behavior is not caused solely by use of a substance (such as laxatives) or by a general medical condition (except through some mechanism that involves constipation).	• This behavior is not directly caused by a general medical condition (such as diabetes, seizures, spina bifida) or by the use of a substance (such as a diuretic).
Code by specific type: 787.6 Encopresis With Constipation and Overflow Incontinence 307.7 Encopresis Without Constipation and Overflow Incontinence	Specify type: Nocturnal Only Diurnal Only Nocturnal and Diurnal

Encopresis

Encopresis is usually associated with constipation. Chronic constipation, perhaps related to dietary irregularity, often leads to fissures around the anus that cause pain on defecation. To avoid this pain, children begin to withhold stools. Refusal to eat, weight loss, and dehydration all aggravate the constipation, which in turn hardens the stool and worsens the fissures. Leakage of unformed stool around the impaction in the rectum results in soiling of clothes and bed sheets. Frequent daytime changes of clothes are necessary.

Secrecy and denial are cardinal features of Encopresis that is *not* accompanied by constipation. Children hide their formed, soft, normal-size stools in unusual locations—in bureau drawers, in trash cans, under the bed. When questioned about this behavior, they often claim ignorance of how the stools got there. This form of the disorder is less common than Encopresis associated with constipation, and it is often linked with stress and other family psychopathology. Disorganization (a lack of behavioral consistency and structure) characterizes many such households. Some of these children may have been subjected to physical or sexual abuse.

With boys predominating, Encopresis affects 1.5–7% of elementary-school-age children. Soiling and chronic constipation account for 20% of complaints in pediatric gastroenterology clinics and for 10% of visits to child mental health clinics. Children who present with Encopresis should have a thorough cognitive evaluation to rule out the presence of developmental delay.

Kent

"He was murder to toilet-train," said Kent's mother. "I'd sure hate to go through all that again!"

Kent had Down's syndrome and a Full Scale IQ (WISC-R) of 68. He had been nearly 4 when he finally stopped wearing diapers. Now, at almost 6, he had started first grade in a special education class. Kent's father, a chief petty officer on a frigate in the Navy, had just deployed for a 6-month cruise in the Mediterranean—his second in the last 4 years. There had been quite a row the evening before he sailed, and Kent had cried himself to sleep. For several nights thereafter, his mother had cried herself to sleep in Kent's bed.

A week or two later, Kent had come home with dirty underpants. He had been spanked and sent to bed with only cereal for supper, but a week later, his mother found feces in one of his father's shoes. "It was at the back of our closet. I'd never have looked there but for the smell," she explained. Over the next several months, this had happened half a dozen times. Each time the feces appeared in a new location—on the front doorstep, in the sandbox of the little girl next door, behind the guest bathroom toilet. Each time, Kent denied knowing how it had happened.

The pediatrician at the naval base hospital could find nothing physically wrong. Kent's mother denied even keeping laxatives in the house. "I don't know when we'd ever need them—he sure hasn't ever been constipated."

Evaluation of Kent

Kent met the duration and frequency criteria for Encopresis. Although he was mentally retarded, he was developmentally at least the equivalent of a 4-year-old. The history reveals no evidence of any **general medical condition** or a **substance use disorder**, including laxative use, that could account for his behavior. Although Encopresis Without Constipation and Overflow Incontinence is the less common type of this disorder, Kent had had no difficulty with either constipation or overflow incontinence. There was no evidence for associated

Oppositional Defiant Disorder or **Conduct Disorder** (more commonly reported when a child is intentionally encopretic) or for **Enuresis**. Kent's five-axis diagnosis would thus be the following:

Axis I	307.7	Encopresis Without Constipation and Overflow Incontinence
Axis II	317	Mild Mental Retardation
Axis III	758.0	Down's syndrome
Axis IV		Father absent on military duty; parental discord
Axis V	GAF = 55	(current)

307.6 Enuresis

By a ratio of about 4:1, primary Enuresis (i.e., a child has never been dry) is the more common form of this disorder. It is usually limited to nighttime wetting; daytime bladder control is unaffected. By the time such a child is referred to a mental health professional, the common remedies of fluid restriction before bedtime and awakening the child at about midnight to use the toilet have usually failed; medical conditions have been ruled out; and bladder function studies have been negative. The child usually wets three to five times weekly and is too embarrassed to sleep over with friends.

In some children, enuretic episodes may be associated with Stage IV non-rapid-eye-movement sleep, which occurs especially during the first 3 hours after sleep onset. In other children, episodes occur more than once per night or randomly throughout the period of sleep. Although a child with primary Enuresis may explain the episodes by recounting dreams of urinating, awakenings immediately after episodes of bedwetting do not confirm the presence of dream reports. When dreams are elicited, they are not of nightmare quality.

Secondary Enuresis, which develops after a child has become dry, most often occurs randomly throughout the night and often appears following a traumatic event such as a hospitalization or separation from parents. Secondary Enuresis is also more likely than primary Enuresis to be associated with nightmares.

Although some enuretic children have urinary tract infections or anatomical anomalies, in the vast majority the etiology of Enuresis remains unknown. Most authorities cite genetic factors and maturational delay. Approximately 75% of enuretic children have a first-degree relative with a history of

Should Enuresis be considered a mental disorder? Although the criteria state that Enuresis can be intentional, the incidence of this must be vanishingly rare. The symptoms are physical, and the pathology is almost exclusively physiological; even its treatment is primarily provided by pediatricians, not mental health professionals. Of course, Enuresis has many emotional sequelae, but then the same can be said of obesity, which no one (certainly not DSM-IV) considers to be a mental disorder.

Enuresis. When both parents have a positive history, 77% of their children are enuretic.

Before age 6, Enuresis is equally prevalent in boys and girls. Thereafter, boys are several times more likely to present with symptoms of Enuresis, despite the fact that urinary tract infections are more common in girls.

Overall, Nocturnal Only is the most common subtype of Enuresis, though girls more often have the Diurnal Only subtype. By adolescence, the prevalence of Enuresis tails off to only about 1%.

Henry

At age 8, Henry was referred by his pediatrician because of persistent Enuresis, which occurred four or five times a week. Toilet training had been effortless, and he was dry during the day by the time he was 3 years old. His parents, unaware of any psychological problems in the family or in Henry's life, were dismayed at the mental health referral. But they were also concerned that Henry had begun to refuse to sleep at friend's houses; he was equally reluctant to have his friends spend the night with him.

Henry's developmental history and mental status examination were unremarkable. He was an accomplished bicycle rider and enthusiastic Little League baseball player. He liked his second-grade classroom teacher and enjoyed playing with his neighborhood friends. In fact, Henry was a happy, well-adjusted boy whose parents were proud of his achievements. His father and his paternal uncle had had Enuresis during their school-age years, but both had completely outgrown the problem by age 10.

After a physical exam and urinalysis found no abnormality that could explain his problem, Henry's parents were instructed to keep a sleep diary for 2 weeks. They noted Henry's bedtime, his sleep onset time, and the time of each enuretic episode. The diary revealed that Henry had wet the bed on 9 of the 14 nights of the 2-week period. On seven occasions, the episode occurred within the first 2 hours after sleep onset; twice, Henry wet later at night.

Evaluation of Henry

The only significant disorder to be considered in a differential diagnosis for Enuresis is a **general medical condition** that can explain the symptoms. In that sense, Henry was found to be completely normal (no anomalies of the genitourinary tract, no evidence of diabetes mellitus or diabetes insipidus, no urinary tract infections). The age of onset, frequency, and duration of his problems fully met the diagnostic criteria. Because his enuresis occurred only during sleep, the specifier Nocturnal Only was added. Although children with Enuresis may have other mental disorders, such as Encopresis, delayed development, or sleep disorders, Henry's history gave no reason to suspect an additional diagnosis. His complete diagnosis would be as follows:

Axis I	307.6	Enuresis, Nocturnal Only
Axis II	V71.09	No diagnosis
Axis III		None
Axis IV		None
Axis V	GAF = 81	(current)

Assessing Elimination Disorders

General Suggestions

Talking about their symptoms may be embarrassing for some children, but you will usually already have the relevant history for a diagnosis of either Encopresis or Enuresis. Focusing on the involuntary nature of the problem and the hope for improvement will often foster a positive therapeutic alliance. To help build rapport, use the child's own terms (as determined from your interview with the parents) for feces and urine. Ask whether the child has either the sensation of needing to void or of pain with defecation. Can you learn how the child perceives the parents' response—is it warmly supportive, or punitive and cold, or somewhere in between?

Colon and rectal segments that lack nerve cells (*aganglionic* segments) represent congenital megacolon (Hirschsprung's disease). During the first year of life, children with Hirschsprung's disease develop symptoms that include abdominal distention, pain, malnutrition, and Encopresis with Constipation and Overflow Incontinence. A barium enema and intestinal biopsy are required for evaluation.

Developmental Factors

As with so many other behaviors, just a few years of maturation can separate the pathological from what is developmentally appropriate. By any set of criteria one chooses, the prevalence of Enuresis is relatively high (7–33% for boys) at age 5, but it falls off by a factor of two to four by age 10. Encopresis, however, is relatively uncommon (about 1%) throughout childhood, with little reduction until the teenage years.

OTHER DISORDERS OF INFANCY, CHILDHOOD, OR ADOLESCENCE

Three of the disorders classified in the final grouping of DSM-IV's first section are characterized by the child's regulation of anxiety in relation to stressful interactions with parents. The Inhibited Type of Reactive Attachment Disorder of Infancy or Early Childhood may especially serve as an early, age-appropriate precursor of Selective Mutism, a syndrome of inhibited speech production. Both of these disorders seem related to significant childhood trauma, stress, or emotional neglect. School avoidance (or school phobia, as it used to be called) may be another manifestation of childhood trauma related to attachment and affect regulation.

309.21 Separation Anxiety Disorder

The name encapsulates the symptoms—anxiety when a child or adolescent is separated from parents or other important caregivers. Separation Anxiety Disorder (abbreviated SAD in this section) often becomes most inhibiting in school. However, reluctance to remain with babysitters at younger ages, or in day care and preschool settings, is also a common source of difficulty. A precipitating event may be identified: a minor accident, illness, or operation; a move to a new house, classroom, or school; the loss of a pet, friend, or parent. These perceived threats arouse anxiety in a youngster, who characteristically first complains, then resists separating. Physical complaints may serve as justification for remaining at home with parents. Ultimately, the youngster completely refuses separation, despite recriminations and punishment from parents and pressure from school authorities. This sequence usually progresses rapidly in younger children, but the process may be more insidious in adolescents. (Table 11.21 gives the full criteria for SAD.)

SAD is sometimes confused with truancy, but the whereabouts of a truant are usually unknown by either the parents or the school authorities, whereas children or adolescents absent secondary to SAD are most likely to be found at home or with their parents. Because young children have difficulty talking about their anxious feelings, they commonly experience SAD as somatic symptoms. Pediatricians who encounter children with headaches, recurrent abdominal pains, and muscle weakness are likely to treat these as physical disorders. Often it is a classroom teacher or school psychologist who first suggests the correct diagnosis.

Children and adolescents are particularly vulnerable to SAD at three

TABLE 11.21. Criteria for Separation Anxiety Disorder

- The patient has developmentally inappropriate, excessive anxiety about being separated from home or from parents (see Coding Note, below). Of the following symptoms, three or more persist or recur:
  ✓ Excessive distress when anticipating or experiencing separation from home or parents
  ✓ Excessive worry about loss of or harm to parents
  ✓ Excessive worry that the child will be separated from a parent by a serious event (such as being kidnapped or becoming lost)
  ✓ Fears of separation cause refusal or reluctance to go somewhere (such as school)
  ✓ Excessive fears of being alone or without parents at home or without important adults elsewhere
  ✓ Refusal or reluctance to sleep away from home or to go to sleep without being near a parent
  ✓ Recurrent nightmares about separation
  ✓ Recurrent physical symptoms (such as headache, abdominal pain, nausea, vomiting) when anticipating or experiencing separation from parents
- These symptoms last 4 weeks or more.
- They begin before age 18.
- They cause clinically important distress or impair school (work), social, or personal functioning.
- The symptoms do not occur solely during a pervasive developmental disorder or any psychotic disorder, including Schizophrenia.
- In adolescents and adults, the symptoms are not better explained by Panic Disorder With Agoraphobia.

Specify if: Early Onset (begins before age 6)

Coding Note: If patient does not live with parents, another "major attachment figure" is understood.

School phobia is a term that was once used to describe the refusal of children to attend school. Of course, it was not usually school as such that a child feared, but the consequences of being away from home or parents. *School avoidance* is a better term for a problem that can stem from a variety of causes, of which SAD is only the most frequent. Anxiety disorders, Conduct Disorder, mood disorders, substance use, and intrafamilial discord are among the other causes of school refusal.

stages: when they first begin kindergarten (5 years); at the beginning of junior high, when they shift to a more complex learning environment (11 years); and when the changes of puberty become prominent (13–14 years). Perhaps 5% of grade school children have SAD; by junior high, the number falls to around 2%. SAD may be especially prevalent in children who have serious physical illness—for example, HIV-positive boys with hemophilia, or children who require dialysis for end-stage kidney disease. Girls with SAD outnumber boys with the disorder in the general population; however, a boy with the condition is more likely to be referred for evaluation, causing the sex ratio in clinical populations to be approximately 1:1. About 3% of referrals to child mental health clinics are diagnosed with SAD. However, a larger number of children may be treated successfully in pediatric practices. Later in life, these children may be at special risk for other anxiety symptoms, such as Panic Disorder; Social Phobia may be an adult equivalent.

Eric

When he was 12 years old, Eric was referred for evaluation because he persistently feared losing his mother. When Eric was only 3, his father, a glazier working on a downtown office building, had died in a fall from a 12th-floor scaffolding. Eric's mother had gone back to work at a bank, and Eric seemed to accept day care relatively well. Yet as he was about to enter junior high, Eric's enthusiasm for school hit a snag. That summer, he had a number of dreams in which he could see his mother but could not reach her because they were separated by a wide ditch. "Maybe it was the Grand Canyon," he said. He lived just across the street from his elementary school, but the junior high was several miles from his home.

In the first week of seventh grade, Eric made several trips to the nurse's office. He repeatedly said he was worried that his mother's bank would be held up. He complained that he could not breathe, and twice his mother had to leave work and take him home. The second week he did not attend class at all because of abdominal pain. The pediatrician pronounced him healthy.

During his first mental health interview, Eric appeared verbal and cheerful. He denied symptoms of depression, anxiety, or Panic Attack. He acknowledged that his fears about his mother were probably exaggerated. "But I've only got one parent," he said. "You can't be too careful."

Evaluation of Eric

For a boy of 12, physical symptoms, persistent worry, troubled dreams, and fears about separation from a parent, common in very young children, are developmentally inappropriate; thus Eric qualified for the diagnosis of SAD. His symptoms had lasted longer than a month and he was distressed enough to be unable to attend class. Other possible diagnoses can be ruled out: He denied having **Panic Attacks**, and the circumstances of his symptoms were too constricted for a diagnosis of **Generalized Anxiety Disorder** (which, however, is often comorbid). Other disorders in which separation anxiety can be encountered include **Schizophrenia** and the **pervasive developmental disorders**, none of which could be supported by Eric's history. There was no evidence of a **mood disorder**, which co-occurs in up to half of these children.

Because Eric's symptoms began well after the age of 6, the Early Onset specifier would not apply. The absence of Eric's father would not be noted on Axis IV, because it happened long ago and seemed to be neither causing current stress nor likely to affect treatment. Eric's complete diagnosis would therefore be the following:

Axis I	309.21	Separation Anxiety Disorder
Axis II	V71.09	No diagnosis
Axis III		None
Axis IV		None
Axis V	GAF = 70	(current)

Assessing Separation Anxiety Disorder

General Suggestions

Very young children go through a stage in which they object to separation from their parents, but this does not usually last beyond the third year. Although such children may scream or have a tantrum as their parents get ready to leave, they calm down and carry on with their usual activities, once they are left in day care or with a babysitter. A child with SAD is less readily distracted, and such behavior will endure long past the stage at which it is developmentally appropriate.

Historically, look for symptoms (emotional or physical) that parallel the course of the school year—waxing when school is in session, waning on weekends or over the summer. Watch to see the degree to which a young child clings to the parent in the waiting room. Does the resistance to parting increase as the time for separation draws nearer? Is the degree of distress so severe that you cannot interview the child alone? Ask the child, "What do you fear will happen?" The answer will probably involve scenes of disaster—a parent involved in a car crash, or the kidnapping or death of the child.

Developmental Factors

Young children with SAD may react to fears of parental separation by physically clinging or trailing their parents from room to room. They are more likely to report fear of harm to a parent, whereas older children and adolescents can often describe physical symptoms or subjective feelings of distress. Older children may balk at leaving home to attend camp, sleep over with a friend, or even attend school. A teenager may express reluctance to remain home alone at an age when babysitting younger children is the norm.

313.23 Selective Mutism

Selective Mutism (Elective Mutism in DSM-III and DSM-III-R) is a disorder in which children are silent except when alone or with a small group of intimates. The condition typically begins during preschool years, after normal speech has developed. Such a child, who speaks appropriately at home among family members but becomes relatively silent when confronted by strangers, may not attract clinical attention until entering school. (Table 11.22 gives the criteria for this disorder.)

In about 20% of cases, English is a second language or a parent reports that a child has had some kind of speech delay, such as Stuttering or articulation immaturity. Otherwise, though often shy, most of these children have normal hearing and intelligence. The usual pattern is that a child speaks fluently at home, but refuses to speak at school or when brought for evaluation. When

TABLE 11.22. Criteria for Selective Mutism

- Despite speaking in other situations, the patient consistently does not speak in specific social situations where speech is expected, such as at school.
- This behavior impedes school or work achievement or social communication.
- It has lasted at least 1 month (excluding the first month of school).
- It is not caused by unfamiliarity or discomfort with the spoken language needed in the social situation.
- It is not better explained by a communication disorder (such as Stuttering).
- It does not occur solely during a pervasive developmental disorder or any psychotic disorder, such as Schizophrenia.

these children do speak, sentence structure, vocabulary, and articulation are normal.

Though at least one series of 100 patients has been reported, Selective Mutism is an uncommon disorder, with a prevalence of less than 0.1% in the general population. Girls are more often affected than boys. There is frequently a family history of Selective Mutism or Social Phobia. Although the disorder usually improves spontaneously within a period of weeks or months, the treatment process can be extremely frustrating for a therapist, whose young patient may remain completely silent during therapy sessions, even while gradually regaining normal speech when at school or with friends.

Kim

Kim was a tall, slender, tomboyish 14-year-old who stopped speaking with anyone but her mother, and then only when she was at home. The problem had begun abruptly 18 months earlier, when she was just finishing sixth grade. At about that time, her parents separated after 15 years of marriage, and her father left the family and moved to a distant city to live with a new girlfriend. Kim, her 9-year-old sister, and her mother were left behind.

Kim was born in New York City, where her grandparents had moved from Poland more than 60 years earlier. Her early growth and development were entirely normal; she had no history of Stuttering or delayed speech. Whereas

Some observers believe that Selective Mutism may not be a discrete entity, but only a symptom of social anxiety. Others suggest that it often develops as a sequel to Posttraumatic Stress Disorder. Fearfulness and anxiety consistently characterize children who have this disorder. Should it actually be classified with the anxiety disorders—as a subtype of Social Phobia, for example? Perhaps DSM-V will tell.

her previous school progress had been good, her refusal to speak had by this time brought her to the brink of failure at school and had nearly severed her peer relationships. Instead of making her repeat the seventh grade, her teacher had recommended treatment.

Although Kim had stopped talking with her friends and was completely mute in class, her speech at home with her mother and sister was perfectly normal. In fact, her mother brought a tape recording of Kim's speech at home to the initial interview. On the tape, Kim talked at some length about a dance step she had seen on MTV; twice she could be heard interrupting her sister. Although Kim refused to utter even one syllable with the examiner, she maintained good eye contact and promptly wrote out answers to questions. By this means she denied any history of depression, hallucinations, or Panic Attacks.

Evaluation of Kim

The first problem for the clinician is to rule out confounding factors (primary disorders of **language**, **learning**, or **hearing**) that can produce the appearance of Selective Mutism. None was apparent in Kim, who, as an American born to English-speaking parents, should have had no cause for discomfort with her native language. Once past these barriers, we have in Selective Mutism a one-symptom disorder for which the symptom is completely self-evident. Kim qualified for the diagnosis without a doubt.

However, several other disorders can present with mutism. **Severe Mental Retardation** and a **pervasive developmental disorder** (such as **Autistic Disorder**) could be ruled out by Kim's history of normal development and progress through elementary school. The history also states clearly that there was no evidence of another **communication disorder**. Although **Social Phobia** is often associated with Selective Mutism, Kim indicated in writing that **anxiety** did not play a major role in her difficulties. Nowhere in these written communications or in her history was there evidence of **Schizophrenia** or another **psychotic disorder**. Although children with severe **depression** may speak very little, their refusal tends to be characteristic at home as well as away. Kim's diagnosis would thus be the following:

Axis I	313.23	Selective Mutism
Axis II	V71.09	No diagnosis
Axis III		None
Axis IV		None
Axis V	GAF = 51	(current)

Assessing Selective Mutism

General Suggestions

There is something of a contradiction in the notion of interviewing anyone who won't speak. But of course, much that we seek to learn about any child comes from the history, and much else from observing nonverbal behavior. Learning that a child who utters nothing in the course of a half-hour session speaks fluently and at length at home strongly suggests Selective Mutism. Even such a child may be induced to communicate in whispers, in gestures, or by writing or drawing. Observing that a mute child appears *interested* in communicating may help sort out the differential diagnosis of one who has Mental Retardation, just as warmth or responsiveness can help discriminate the selectively mute child from one who has a pervasive developmental disorder. Carefully note any apparent anxiety; some evidence suggests that selectively mute children may suffer from an extreme variety of Social Phobia. Angry children may try to control the environment by refusing to speak, but with persistent questioning, their resolve tends to break down rapidly.

Developmental Factors

Because patients with Selective Mutism speak normally at home, it is usually not noticed until they begin school. However, some normal children are reluctant to speak when they first begin school, so make the diagnosis only if the problem does not resolve spontaneously after a month in kindergarten or first grade.

313.89 Reactive Attachment Disorder of Infancy or Early Childhood

Disorders of attachment can begin early in life. They can even be observed in infants as young as 3 months. In a severe case, by 6 months of age Reactive Attachment Disorder of Infancy or Early Childhood (abbreviated RAD in this discussion) may present as nonorganic failure to thrive. Typically, the infant's weight, length, and head circumference remain consistently at or below the 3rd percentile on standardized growth charts. To reestablish normal physical growth and psychological development, mere nourishment is not sufficient. Rather, consistent, predictable social stimulation and affective feedback are needed between an infant and a familiar, sensitive caregiver. Under these conditions, the losses are quickly regained. Less fortunate patients may die, usually of an intercurrent infection secondary to a compromised immune system.

DSM-IV specifies two major RAD subtypes (see Table 11.23 for these subtypes and the full RAD criteria). In the Inhibited Type, infants and toddlers withdraw from social contacts; when they do interact, they are shy or distant. At the prospect of separation from a parent, such a child will resist, clinging desperately or throwing tantrums. In contrast, the Disinhibited Type is characterized by promiscuity in social relationships. The infant or toddler does not exhibit age-appropriate wariness of strangers, but approaches all with equanimity and apparent lack of fear. Such a child may feign indifference to the departure of the parent. The responses in both subtypes are more obvious in the presence of strangers when the primary parent is absent. Although there

---

TABLE 11.23. Criteria for Reactive Attachment Disorder of Infancy or Early Childhood

---

- The patient's social relatedness is markedly disturbed and developmentally inappropriate. This begins before age 5 and occurs in most situations, as shown by *either* of the following:
  ✓ Inhibitions. In most social situations, the child doesn't interact in a developmentally appropriate way. This is shown by responses that are excessively inhibited, hypervigilant, or ambivalent and contradictory. For example, the child responds to caregivers with frozen watchfulness or mixed approach–avoidance and resistance to comforting.
  ✓ Disinhibitions. The child's attachments are diffuse, as shown by indiscriminate sociability and inability to form appropriate selective attachments. For example, the child is overly familiar with strangers or lacks selectivity in choosing attachment figures.
- This behavior is not explained solely by a developmental delay (such as Mental Retardation), and it does not fulfill criteria for a pervasive developmental disorder.
- Evidence of persistent pathogenic care is shown by one or more of these:
  ✓ The caregiver neglects the child's basic emotional needs for affection, comfort and stimulation.
  ✓ The caregiver neglects the child's basic physical needs.
  ✓ Stable attachments cannot form because of repeated changes of primary caregiver (such as frequent changes of foster care).
- It appears that the pathogenic care just described has caused the disturbed behavior; for example, the behavior began after the pathogenic care did.

Specify type, based on predominant clinical presentation:
  Inhibited Type: Failure to interact predominates
  Disinhibited Type: Indiscriminate sociability predominates

---

have been isolated reports of adults who qualify for this diagnosis, it remains overwhelmingly one of early childhood.

Many diagnoses include statements about what is *not* causative, but RAD is the only child diagnosis in DSM-IV that implies any etiology at all, let alone one rooted in a disturbed bonding process. Some authorities, claiming that RAD can be found in children who lack any evidence of parental neglect or absenteeism, recommend that the criteria specifying pathogenic care be deleted in future DSMs.

Various observers have voiced concerns about the concept of RAD. For one thing, the forced dichotomy of subtypes may be a bit too pat. For example, some children may simultaneously manifest symptoms of both inhibition and promiscuity; others may appear inhibited at an early age, but then become promiscuous later. Another concern is that the DSM-IV criteria require children to be seriously affected before the diagnosis can be made. Yet, as is true for other DSM-IV diagnoses, precursor or "high-risk" disturbances may foreshadow a later, full-blown disorder that early intervention could forestall. (A recent study suggests that criteria other than DSM-IV's may better identify this group of children.) It has also been noted that other DSM-IV diagnoses, especially Major Depressive Disorder and Feeding Disorder of Infancy or Early Childhood, may be equally appropriate for small children who fail to thrive.

Shawna

Almost since she could walk, Shawna had been overly friendly. When she was 3, a social services caseworker referred her to the mental health clinic. Neither the caseworker nor her mother could stop her from running up to any stranger while shopping, or, later, striking up a conversation with strangers of either sex. Once she had accompanied a newfound friend to his home for cookies. Fortunately, she had been returned to the yard of her home unmolested; however, despite a severe spanking, she remained "willing to go off with anyone."

Shawna's mother was trying to rear two daughters alone while completing her own high school education and working evenings in a variety store. The children were watched by a series of neighbor girls, one of whom had dropped out of school in the ninth grade; another might have used marijuana while on duty.

Shawna's behaviors had seemed to worsen after her sister was born. The previous summer, the two girls had lived with their maternal grandmother. The grandmother had reported a gradual reduction in Shawna's impetuous behavior after their second month together, but it recurred once the girls returned to their mother.

When she first met the interviewer, 3-year-old Shawna immediately ran up to him, arms outstretched, squealing with delight and calling, "Daddy! Daddy!" During the interview, she paid her mother hardly any attention. At first she clung to the interviewer's leg, repeatedly requesting to be picked up, asking for a shoe ride, and engaging in other familiarities. As she became increasingly provocative and difficult to manage, her mother offered to "whack her butt," but neither followed up on the threat nor made other attempts to manage her behavior. The interviewer finally suggested a walk outside to continue the interview. Away from the presence of her mother, Shawna confidently took his hand and trotted along, chattering about the dolls she had discovered in the playroom. Throughout that portion of the session, Shawna focused well on the topics at hand and used age-appropriate verbal and nonverbal communications.

Evaluation of Shawna

Shawna's behavior suggests a variety of possible diagnoses. Although it is unusual to diagnose **ADHD** at this age, it must be considered in any impulsive child. However, Shawna did appear to focus her attention when sufficiently engaged, and there was evidence of self-control in situations other than at home (e.g., when she was staying with her grandmother). Similarly, she did not show the negative behavior that would be expected in **Oppositional Defiant Disorder**, or the violation of rights or rules found in **Conduct Disorder**. Although formal testing was not attempted at this interview, her overall intellectual functioning appeared about normal for her age, so **Mental Retardation** seemed unlikely. There was nothing about her communication or socialization that would suggest a **pervasive developmental disorder**.

Rather, Shawna's too-ready acceptance of a strange male interviewer suggested a disturbance of social relatedness that is typical for RAD. Pathogenic care was evidenced by repeated changes of babysitters and her mother's prolonged absences from the home. Some of her developmentally inappropriate behavior remitted in a more stable environment (staying with her grandmother), suggesting a causal relationship between care and behavior. Her nondiscriminating sociability would require the specifier of Disinhibited Type.

Axis I	313.89	Reactive Attachment Disorder, Disinhibited Type
Axis II	V71.09	No diagnosis
Axis III		None
Axis IV		Inconsistency of parental surrogate
Axis V	GAF = 70	(current)

Assessing Reactive Attachment Disorder
of Infancy or Early Childhood

General Suggestions

In evaluating an infant or toddler with RAD, it is first necessary to establish the nature of the child's relationship to the parent(s). The attachment relationship serves to mediate the balance between security and exploration, and it may be different for mother, father, and others. Abnormal attachment interactions are likely to intensify during stress, as in new situations, when a young child often feels insecure and turns to the parent for comfort. If the parent leaves the room, the child's sense of insecurity may be reawakened. The clinical evaluation affords many opportunities to observe the response to stress, the recovery of security, and the exploration of the new setting. A careful and detailed history of such experiences during the child's development, and observations of comfort and exploration during the evaluation, constitute the basic elements of an attachment assessment.

This disorder (or, considering the rather dissimilar forms, these *two* disorders) calls for you to deal carefully yet effectively with both the patient and the parent. You may need to redirect the inhibited patient you have just peeled off your leg, taking care neither to encourage the behavior nor to reject the child, whereas a relaxed, friendly, nonintrusive attitude permits an inhibited child time to become comfortable with the interview situation and with you. Dealing with the parent may necessitate even greater caution, to preempt resistance and reduce the suspicion and hostility that may be the natural lot of parents whose behavior qualifies by DSM-IV criteria for this disorder. Of course, a friendly, open attitude is likely to carry you far. But certain interviewing techniques may help set the informant at ease:

- Begin with other topics. Never underestimate the value of a few minutes of nonthreatening information gathering to demonstrate your compassion and establish rapport.
- Suggest an excuse for unfavorable information, to relieve embarrassment—for example, "Working two jobs makes every minute with your child doubly precious."
- Emphasize the positive: "Shawna's doing very well in a number of areas."

Developmental Factors

By definition, this disorder must begin before a child's fifth birthday. As of this writing, there are still no data that would suggest greater prevalence of either subtype at any particular age.

307.3 Stereotypic Movement Disorder

Stereotypic movements or stereotypies are behaviors that an individual seems compelled to repeat over and over without any particular goal in mind. Early in life, stereotypies are common and normal; babies all rock themselves and put things into their mouths, apparently deriving comfort or information from these behaviors. But when stereotypies create problems well into later childhood, they may be said to constitute Stereotypic Movement Disorder (abbreviated SMD in this discussion). In addition to the more benign behaviors (e.g., hand flapping), these behaviors include such self-injurious acts as head banging, biting of lips or fingers, and hitting of the child's own body. Chronic tissue damage may result from hitting or biting. (See Table 11.24 for the full criteria for this disorder.)

SMD may affect as many as 3% of young children; no one knows how many adults may be affected, though it is probably uncommon except among adults with Mental Retardation. It is said that head bangers tend to be boys, whereas self-biters are more often girls. In a study of 20 adults with SMD, only 6 were males; many also had a mood or anxiety disorder. Its causes are unknown, though boredom, frustration, or stress may increase the behaviors.

Claudia

At the age of 14, Claudia continued to suck her thumb and rock. When she was 4, her parents tried behavior modification to stop her habit. For 2 weeks she gladly accepted the treat (extra dessert at supper), but reverted to thumb sucking when the bribe was no longer forthcoming. Throughout her childhood the habit persisted, though by the time she was 10 she had learned to suppress it most of the time when she was at school. At other times it would recur—when she was doing her homework, while she was falling asleep, and even sometimes when she was eating supper. As a result of the merciless ribbing she took, especially from the boys in her neighborhood, she had formed few friendships. She had never spent the night at another child's house.

TABLE 11.24. Criteria for Stereotypic Movement Disorder

- The patient's motor behavior seems driven, repetitive, and nonfunctional. Examples include biting or hitting self, body rocking, hand shaking or waving, head banging, mouthing of objects, and picking at skin or body openings.
- This behavior seriously interferes with normal activities or causes physical injury that requires medical treatment (or would, if the behavior were not interfered with).
- If the patient also has Mental Retardation, the stereotypic behavior is serious enough to be a focus of treatment.
- The behavior is not better explained by a compulsion (as in Obsessive–Compulsive Disorder), a tic (tic disorder), hair pulling (Trichotillomania), or a pervasive developmental disorder.
- It is not directly caused by a general medical condition or the effects of substance use.
- The behavior has persisted for at least 4 weeks.

Specify if With Self-Injurious Behavior. The behavior causes bodily injury that requires medical treatment (or would, if the behavior were not interfered with).

"Nobody much likes me," she said. After this speech, she popped her thumb back into her mouth and curled her index finger across the bridge of her nose as she gently rocked from the waist up, back and forth.

Claudia weighed 8 pounds, 4 ounces when she was born. According to her mother, her developmental milestones occurred at the expected times, and there had been no history of tics or hair pulling. Despite her isolated existence, she enjoyed the company of others and got along well with her two older sisters. Other than a red thumb and slightly protuberant front teeth, her physical examination was completely normal.

"I don't *have* to do it," Claudia said of her thumb sucking. "I just like it."

Evaluation of Claudia

Although thumb sucking isn't usually considered pathological, it was one of the stereotypies reported in 1 of the 20 adults mentioned previously. Body rocking is specifically mentioned by DSM-IV. Neither behavior would qualify at all had it not persisted far longer than 4 weeks and interfered with Claudia's social development. No other Axis I diagnosis would seem to explain the behavior better. There is no information that would suggest **Mental Retardation**, and she specifically denied any compulsive quality to the behavior, as would be the case with **Obsessive–Compulsive Disorder**. Her mother's report ruled out **Trichotillomania** and **tic disorders**.

Her physical examination was normal, suggesting that no **general medi-**

cal condition (or neurological disorder, such as Huntington's disease) could explain her illness and that she would not qualify for the specifier With Self-Injurious Behavior. Claudia's diagnosis would be as follows:

Axis I	307.3	Stereotypic Movement Disorder
Axis II	V71.09	No diagnosis
Axis III		None
Axis IV		None
Axis V	GAF = 65	(current)

Assessing Stereotypic Movement Disorder

General Suggestions

SMD is the only DSM-IV diagnosis (other than those made specifically during infancy) that can be made solely by observation. Even so, ask whether stress worsens the abnormal movements. Observe for evidence of chronic tissue damage (one preteen girl developed massive bumps on her forearms from repeatedly banging them on the edges of table tops). Ask about other such behaviors as compulsions, hair pulling, and tics.

Developmental Factors

These movements may peak during adolescence and then decrease in frequency. Nearly all children whose movement disorders persist beyond adolescence begin to have symptoms before age 12. Note that the vast majority of adult patients reported with SMD are mentally retarded.

313.9 Disorder of Infancy, Childhood, or Adolescence Not Otherwise Specified

Use the final category in this section of DSM-IV for any other disorder that begins before adulthood and is not better defined elsewhere.

CHAPTER 12

Cognitive Disorders

Quick Guide to the Cognitive Disorders

As in the Quick Guide to Chapter 11, the page number following each item indicates the point at which text discussion of it begins.

Delirium

A delirium is a rapidly developing, fluctuating state of reduced awareness in which a patient has trouble shifting or focusing attention, *and* the patient has at least one defect of memory, orientation, perception, or language. In young patients, the following types of delirium can be diagnosed:

Delirium Due to a General Medical Condition. Delirium can be caused by trauma to the brain, infections, epilepsy, endocrine disorders, and various other diseases throughout the body (p. 263).

Substance-Induced Delirium. Alcohol and other sedative drugs of abuse, as well as nearly every class of street drug, can cause delirium. Medications and poisons can also be implicated (p.263).

Delirium Not Otherwise Specified. This category is used when a patient's delirium does not meet the criteria for any of the types described in DSM-IV (p. 267).

Dementia

In a dementia, there must be multiple cognitive deficits that include memory loss, as well as one or more of the following: aphasia, apraxia, agnosia, and loss of executive functioning. If any impairment in the ability to focus or shift attention exists, it is not prominent. In adults, Dementia of the Alzheimer's Type and Vascular Dementia are the most common types, but of course these diagnoses are virtually unheard of in children and adolescents. One of the following diagnoses will usually be made:

Dementia Due to Other General Medical Conditions. A large number of medical conditions can cause dementia, including brain tumor, Creutzfeldt–Jakob disease (slow virus), head trauma, HIV disease, Huntington's disease, Parkinson's disease, and Pick's disease. The most common intermediate paths of dementia resulting from medical conditions are kidney and liver failure (p. 267).

Dementia Not Otherwise Specified. This diagnosis is used when a patient's dementia does not meet the criteria for any of the types described in DSM-IV (p. 269).

Substance-Induced Persisting Dementia. From 5% to 10% of dementias in adults are related to prolonged use of alcohol, inhalants, or sedatives, but these are rare in children and adolescents.

Other Causes of Cognitive Symptoms

Cognitive Disorder Not Otherwise Specified. This category is used when a patient has cognitive deficits that do not clearly suggest a delirium, a dementia, or an amnestic disorder (p. 269).

INTRODUCTION

Although a specific underlying etiological agent cannot always be identified, cognitive disorders are caused by general medical conditions or by the use of psychoactive substances. In each case, the result is a defect of brain anatomy, chemistry, or physiology that leads to problems with thinking and memory. Three groups of cognitive disorders have relevance for children and adolescents: delirium, dementia, and Cognitive Disorder Not Otherwise Specified (a single-disorder "group"). DSM-IV lists a fourth group, amnestic disorders; however, these are rarely if ever encountered in young patients. Some consider them to constitute a special type of dementia. In this chapter, we describe the first three groups; we also provide two case vignettes and discussions to illustrate selected disorders from these groups.

DELIRIUM

293.0 Delirium Due to a General Medical Condition

Substance-Induced Delirium

Delirium is the most common cognitive disorder—and, by some accounts, the most common of all mental disorders. It occurs especially in young children, who are easy prey to fever and infection. Other causes in young patients include endocrine dysfunction, drug withdrawal or toxicity, vitamin deficiency, liver or kidney disease, poisons, and the effects of surgical operations. Note that each of these causes is usually located somewhere in the body other than the brain.

Delirious patients have two main sorts of symptoms: (1) difficulty focusing, maintaining, or shifting attention, and (2) difficulty with thinking or memory. The symptoms develop rapidly, within a period of days or even hours, and are often more pronounced at night.

In the midst of a conversation or during a favorite activity, a delirious child or adolescent may lapse into the stupor of half-sleep (altered attention). Some delirious patients may think less quickly, appear vague, or have difficulty solving problems. Questions must be asked several times before they are answered. Other patients may seem hyperalert and distractible, shifting attention rapidly from one stimulus to another. (Picture a child with high fever who thrashes about in bed and keeps glancing into the corners of the room.) Still other patients, especially those whose delirium is caused by metabolic factors, may instead experience a slowing of physical movement.

The cognitive deficit can manifest itself as one or more problems with language, memory, orientation, or perception:

- The *language* of delirium is rambling; it may be pressured or incoherent. Older children and adolescents may have trouble writing. Speech that is only slurred, without being incoherent, does not indicate delirium.
- *Memory* is nearly always impaired, with recent memory affected first. Retention and recall are also disturbed; patients typically later recall little of their delirious experiences.
- Children and adolescents with delirium are often *disoriented*. In children old enough to be fully aware of dates, months, seasons, and years,

orientation to time is usually the first to go. They may fail to recognize their surroundings; they may misidentify parents or other people familiar to them. Only in extreme cases do patients lose orientation to personal identity.

- Distorted *perception* may be experienced in varying degrees of severity. In mild or early delirium, surroundings may appear less clear than usual: Boundaries are fuzzy, colors too bright, images distorted. Adolescents and older children may be able to describe some of these symptoms. As thinking becomes more seriously disordered, patients may experience *illusions*, which are misinterpretations of actual sensory stimuli. Still further advanced across this spectrum are *hallucinations*, which are false perceptions in the absence of an actual sensory stimulus. Younger children are especially likely to respond to illusions or hallucinations with fear or anxiety.

Delirium usually begins suddenly and often fluctuates during the course of the day. Usually this means that patients are more lucid during the morning and sicker at night—a characteristic known as *sundowning*. Most deliriums are relatively short-lived, lasting perhaps a week or less, and resolving once the underlying cause has been relieved.

Table 12.1 presents criteria for the specific types of delirium most likely to be diagnosed in children and adolescents: Delirium Due to a General Medical Condition and two types of Substance-Induced Delirium (Substance Intoxication Delirium and Substance Withdrawal Delirium). Note that the two types of Substance-Induced Delirium receive the same code numbers, but that the codes differ according to whether alcohol or another substance has been ingested (see Table 14.6 in Chapter 14 for the codes for these and many other substance-related disorders). The exact name of the substance ingested should be used when a diagnosis is made. Note also that Substance Intoxication (or Withdrawal) Delirium and Substance Intoxication (or Withdrawal) due to the same substance should not be diagnosed together; whenever symptoms are severe enough to warrant the delirium diagnosis, it alone should be made. Finally, note that delirium can be induced by the use of a prescribed medication, and that in such cases it is almost always due to toxicity. Such medications are categorized as "Other" substances and coded with the exact names of the medications, followed by "-Induced" (rather than "Intoxication").

TABLE 12.1. Criteria for Delirium Due to a General Medical Condition, Substance Intoxication Delirium, and Substance Withdrawal Delirium

General Medical Condition	Substance Intoxication	Substance Withdrawal

- The patient has a reduced level of consciousness and difficulty focusing, shifting, or sustaining attention.
- The patient shows a cognitive change (deficit of language, memory, orientation, perception) that a dementia cannot better explain.
- The symptoms develop rapidly (hours to days) and tend to fluctuate during the day.
- History, physical examination, or laboratory data suggest that . . .

. . . a general medical condition has caused the delirium.	. . . either ✓ the symptoms developed during Substance Intoxication, *or* ✓ they are caused by the use of a prescribed medication (see text).	. . . the symptoms developed during or shortly after Substance Withdrawal.

Max

Max was 5 when he was brought to the children's ward of the community hospital in a Midwestern university town. Max and Deborah, his 6-year-old sister, lived with their maternal grandparents, who told the clerk in the urgent care unit that Max had been well until that afternoon, when he had come in from play. At first they thought he was just tired; within an hour he appeared drunk. When he intentionally urinated in a corner of the living room, they realized that something was terribly wrong and brought him in for evaluation. Deborah admitted that while the two children were playing doctor, Max had swallowed several tablets of their grandfather's medications. The pill bottles she produced contained diazepam and amitriptyline.

During the initial examination that evening, Max seemed quite lethargic. Though he could be aroused, his gaze drifted off to the curtains at the side of his bed when staff members were trying to talk to him. For a time his mood was euphoric, and he talked about being a doctor—as if he were one already. Later that evening he seemed fearful and agitated; he moved restlessly in his bed, apparently trying to find a nickel he thought he had lost. He misidentified a nurse as his mother and called a ballpoint pen a gun. Then he volunteered, "I'm not a new skateboard—I'm a Frenchie." At different times he said he was at home and "in a prison for dogs." His agitation prevented a complete reading of the EEG obtained that evening, but "severe disorganization and slowing" were reported.

Max slept most of the following day, but within 48 hours of admission he was much improved. Now he could name the hospital, identify his grandparents and an already-favorite nurse, and correctly name everyday objects. The following day he was discharged as recovered.

Evaluation of Max

Max's level of consciousness was clearly compromised on the evening of and the day following his admission—he was often drowsy and he could not sustain his attention for longer than a few moments. Cognitive change was evident in his problems with language (much that he said was gibberish), orientation, and perception. These symptoms had developed within a few hours of ingesting medications known to be toxic (in overdose) to the central nervous system.

The most common alternative to consider in the differential diagnosis for delirium is another cognitive disorder—**dementia**, which was of course ruled out by the rapidity of onset. The presence of hallucinations might suggest a **psychotic disorder**, which could also be ruled out by the acute onset. Although other causes of delirium (**general medical conditions,** such as head trauma and infectious disease) must be considered in any child who presents as Max did, the vital information obtained from his sister made the correct etiology quite clear. Note that the criteria for Delirium Due to a General Medical Condition are very nearly identical to those for Substance Intoxication Delirium. DSM-IV points out that **Malingering** and **Factitious Disorder** should also be considered when the symptoms are less than classical for delirium and when no causative agent is obvious.

Although the drugs involved in Max's delirium would receive exactly the same code number, each would be coded separately on Axis I because each contributed to the intoxication. Living apart from both parents could complicate the care of Max and his sister, so it was coded as specifically as possible on Axis IV. Max's full diagnosis would thus be as follows:

Axis I	292.81	Diazepam Intoxication Delirium
	292.81	Amitriptyline Intoxication Delirium
Axis II	V71.09	No diagnosis
Axis III		None
Axis IV		Separated from parents, living with grandparents
Axis V	GAF = 90	(on discharge)

780.09 Delirium Not Otherwise Specified

The category of Delirium Not Otherwise Specified should be reserved only for cases that do not meet the criteria for the types of delirium described above or for any other types described in DSM-IV. DSM-IV specifically mentions delirium whose causes are not proven, and delirium caused by factors (such as sensory deprivation) other than those it lists.

DEMENTIA

Dementia Due to Other General Medical Conditions

On the face of it, childhood dementia seems a contradiction in terms. Childhood is a period of growth, but *dementia* means "decline"—think of Vascular Dementia and Dementia of the Alzheimer's Type. Of course, neither of these conditions affects children or adolescents; nor does Substance-Induced Persisting Dementia occur often enough in young patients to warrant its inclusion here. However, children and adolescents can fall prey to some dementia-inducing medical conditions, such as head trauma and HIV disease. The criteria for Dementia Due to Other General Medical Conditions are presented in Table 12.2. Such a dementia can be diagnosed any time after the age of 3 or 4, which is the youngest age at which intelligence can first be reliably measured with objective tests.

In contrast to delirium, the site of pathology in dementia is within the tissues of the brain itself. Although we usually think of dementia as permanent and often progressing inexorably, in some cases it is reversible. Such an outcome is most likely in the case of young children, whose brains are still resilient enough to recover from injuries that would permanently incapacitate an adult.

Dementia usually begins gradually. A child may lose interest in school or in recreational activities. Judgment and impulse control begin to suffer. With reduced ability to understand, analyze, and remember, patients of any age must get through the day by relying upon the skeleton of old habits—for children, often a fragile structure.

All demented patients have the following features in common:

- **Memory loss.** In milder cases this usually affects only recent memories; when dementia is more severe, remote memories also become involved. Although patients who have always functioned at a low level (such as those with Mental Retardation) are not automatically considered to be demented, a retarded child can develop dementia just like anyone else. As is well known, many patients with Down's syndrome develop Dementia of the Alzheimer's Type later in life.

- **Other cognitive deficits.** Besides memory loss, demented patients must show evidence of at least one other cognitive deficit listed here:

    Agnosia (trouble recognizing things). Even with intact sensory functioning, a patient cannot recognize or identify familiar objects, such as a ball or a piece of doll house furniture.

    Aphasia (trouble understanding or using language). Loss of language skills does not usually occur until late in the disease; then patients may become increasingly vague, circumstantial, or even mute. A cli-

---

TABLE 12.2. Criteria for Dementia Due to Other General Medical Conditions

The patient has developed deficits of thinking, as shown by *both* of the following:

- Impaired memory (can't learn new information or can't recall information previously learned)
- At least *one* of these:
    ✓ Aphasia (problems using language)
    ✓ Apraxia (trouble carrying out motor activity, despite intact motor functioning)
    ✓ Agnosia (despite intact sensory functioning, inability to recognize or identify objects presented)
    ✓ Impaired executive functioning (problems abstracting, organizing, planning, or sequencing information)
- Each symptom materially impairs work, school, social, or personal functioning.
- These symptoms don't occur *solely* during a delirium.
- A general medical condition has probably directly caused the deficits, as judged by history, laboratory data, or physical examination.

Coding Note: Besides coding the dementia on Axis I, you should also code the underlying disease on Axis III. Some of the more common responsible general medical conditions are listed below.

Type of dementia	Axis I	Axis III
Dementia Due to HIV Disease	294.9	043.1
Dementia Due to Head Trauma	294.1	854.00
Dementia Due to Parkinson's Disease	294.1	332.0
Dementia Due to Huntington's Disease	294.1	333.4
Dementia Due to Pick's Disease	290.10	331.1
Dementia Due to Creutzfeldt–Jakob Disease	290.10	046.1
Dementia Due to Other General Medical Condition	294.1	[Specific Axis III code for condition]

nician unfamiliar with a young patient's previous developmental level will have to rely on parents or others for information about language capability.

Apraxia (trouble carrying out a motor activity). Despite intact sensory, motor, and intellectual capabilities, patients with apraxia cannot perform certain acts. An example would be a child who can manipulate a pencil, recognize a design, and understand the command to draw, but still cannot copy a design.

Executive functioning (problems with planning, organizing, sequencing, or abstracting information). This is the mechanism everyone uses to organize simple acts and ideas into complex behaviors. Loss of executive functioning means difficulty in performing activities of daily living, interpreting new information, or adapting to new situations.

294.8 Dementia Not Otherwise Specified

A diagnosis of Dementia Not Otherwise Specified should be reserved only for cases of dementia that do not meet the criteria for any of the types of dementia described in DSM-IV (most often, cases for which there is not enough evidence to confirm a particular etiology).

OTHER COGNITIVE DISORDERS

Cognitive Disorder Not Otherwise Specified

Usually as a result of head injury, many children and adolescents do develop cognitive disorders that qualify as neither delirium nor dementia. Two specific syndromes, postconcussional disorder and mild neurocognitive disorder, have been suggested for inclusion in DSM-V.

Karl

When Karl was 10, he was admitted to the trauma center after falling off his bike. On a Tuesday just

Head injuries were once the most frequent cause of dementia in children, but a number of other disorders usually encountered in adults may be etiological: Wilson's disease, Huntington's disease, metachromatic leukodystrophy, normal-pressure hydrocephalus, hypothyroidism, brain tumor, and now HIV encephalopathy. At the dawn of the 21st century, HIV/AIDS may be the single most frequent cause of dementia in children and adolescents.

after supper, he had left his bike helmet hanging on his bedroom chair and gone off with three friends. His mother had had no idea where he was until the hospital called at about 8:30 that evening.

Karl's parents had been divorced for years. He and his mother lived in subsidized housing near the center of town. When he wasn't drinking, Karl's father was at sea tending the engine on a fishing boat. Every few months he would turn up, take Karl to the movies or a ball game, then argue with Karl's mother about money and disappear again.

Perhaps it was this most recent visit, which included an afternoon Giants game, that distracted Karl's attention from the road. Even long after he had recovered, his memory for that entire day was an almost total blank. The police report stated that he swerved his bicycle into the path of a slowly approaching pickup truck and was tossed several yards into some shrubbery. He awakened hours later to the pain of a splitting headache and two broken arms.

That evening, skull X-rays and a CT scan were read as normal. An EEG obtained just after he had awakened showed nonspecific slowing; at follow-up 2 weeks later, it was completely normal.

Karl was released from the hospital on the third day and returned to school the following Monday. He had always been a good student with excellent attention span, but for several months after the accident his performance suffered. Three months after his return to class, for the first time in his school career, the "doesn't pay attention in class" box was checked on his report card. His teacher's comment read, "Karl seems restless and distractible; he frequently gets out of his seat and wanders around the room, disturbing other children. He no longer seems to care about completing his assignments."

When his mother brought Karl for evaluation, she noted several changes in him. First, sometimes during the night he would awaken, get up, and roam about the house for 15 or 20 minutes before going back to bed. Second, although much of the time he seemed to be his usual self, he rapidly grew irritable and cross when thwarted. Finally, despite the fact that his father had bought him a new bike, it remained unused in storage at their apartment.

Karl was a slightly built boy who appeared a year or so younger than his stated age. There was no evidence of secondary sex characteristics, and his voice had not yet begun to change. He admitted to having headaches almost daily since the accident, though he thought that recently they might be getting a little better. He spoke clearly and distinctly, and expressed himself in coherent, linear sentences. He emphatically denied any experiences suggestive of hallucinations or delusions. Although his attention had to be recalled to the interview several times during a half-hour session, he was able to score a perfect 30 points on the Mini-Mental State Exam.

Evaluation of Karl

Karl had suffered head trauma of the sort commonly associated with very serious cognitive disorders. Why could he not be diagnosed as having either a delirium or a dementia?

Karl did have a problem sustaining attention while in school, but there was no evidence of the sort of cognitive change (problems with memory, disorientation, language, or perception) required for **delirium**. Also, the history indicated no fluctuations with time of day in his symptoms, which by the time of evaluation had lasted longer than the typical delirium. Subsequent to his accident, Karl apparently had some classroom difficulty acquiring new information, which would suggest **dementia**. But, as measured by the Mini-Mental State Exam, the degree of this impairment was not severe; moreover, he had no evidence of other cognitive problems (aphasia, apraxia, agnosia, impaired executive functioning) necessary to diagnose dementia.

The diagnosis of **Personality Change Due to Head Trauma** might eventually be warranted (head trauma certainly can precipitate personality change), but Karl had had his symptoms for only a few months, and for children this diagnosis requires at least 1 year of altered behavior. Karl's symptoms might also suggest the possibility of a **mood disorder** or **anxiety disorder**. As is true whenever a diagnosis is in doubt, both of these categories should be carefully considered; for Karl, however, the data poorly supported such a diagnosis.

Two additional cognitive disorders should be considered, **mild neurocognitive disorder** and **postconcussional disorder**. DSM-IV gives each of these specific diagnoses in lower-case type, because neither has as yet been generally accepted. (To assist with their future evaluation, research criteria for these and other diagnoses are included in Appendix B of DSM-IV.) For mild neurocognitive disorder to be diagnosed, formal testing would have to reveal some evidence of a cognitive abnormality. Besides his wandering attention, Karl would have to have some other problem, such as memory, disturbed executive functioning, perceptual–motor problems, or impaired language use. Clearly, no convincing case for this diagnosis could be made.

Postconcussional disorder would seem to be a more likely candidate. Required are a history of head trauma and problems with *either* attention or memory, plus three or more of the following: sleep problems, irritability or aggression, apathy or lack of spontaneity, headache, easy fatigability, dizziness, mood change, and personality change. Karl had the first three or four of these symptoms and so would qualify for the diagnosis. When DSM-V arrives, early in the 21st century, we may be able to use this term officially; in DSM-IV terms, however, his diagnosis would have to be as follows:

Axis I	294.9	Cognitive Disorder Not Otherwise Specified (postconcussional disorder)
Axis II	V71.09	No diagnosis
Axis III	959.01	Head injury, unspecified
Axis IV		Family disruption through divorce
Axis V	GAF = 80	(upon evaluation)

Assessing Cognitive Disorders

General Suggestions

Like most DSM-IV diagnoses, the cognitive disorders can present in a variety of ways, depending on a patient's age and developmental stage (see below). In younger children, behavioral changes may be the most obvious. Especially in delirium, diminished attention span appears as trouble concentrating. A delirious child may doze off during an interview. Alternatively, a child's difficulty in maintaining focus may show itself as marked, often irritable restlessness. In such a case, if even the parents are unable to soothe their child, delirium may be the cause. Also, picking at bedclothes suggests a cognitive disorder.

As with every DSM-IV diagnosis, a complete history is vital. Changes in cognitive ability can only be evaluated with respect to previous levels of development. For example, did a child who now has difficulty constructing sentences or remaining continent ever possess these capabilities? The answer spells the difference between a cognitive disorder and developmental delay.

Careful and repeated observation and assessment are especially important in children who have sustained a closed head injury, whether or not they have been unconscious. Metabolic imbalances or structural brain malfunction may be suggested by physical findings such as tremor, seizures, abnormal posture, or poor visual acuity. Children with cognitive disorders other than delirium may appear slow at study or in initiating play. They have trouble planning activities and are sometimes thought lazy. They may be concrete in their responses, suggesting low intelligence that belies their actual innate ability.

Frontal lobe disinhibition can produce a variety of changes in the personality of a child, who may become oppositional, outspoken, overly talkative, impulsive, careless in grooming, or given to making inappropriate personal comments. Emotions may be described as moody (labile) or irritable.

Developmental Factors

The assessment of attention and concentration is particularly difficult in young children, whose cooperation and understanding of tasks have not fully developed. A diagnosis of dementia requires a demonstration of deterioration, so it cannot be made until a child's intellect can be reliably assessed (at about the age of 4 or 5).

The themes developed in delirious hallucinations reflect the age of the patient: A young child may dream of peanut butter sandwiches or fears of abandonment. Overall, however, the age of the child is a far less important determinant of psychopathology than are the nature, location, and severity of the injury. Nonetheless, here are two general principles: (1) The effects of a closed head injury are especially severe in children under the age of 2, who are prone to subdural hematomas; and (2) adolescents, by virtue of their boisterousness, experimentation, activity level, and often faulty judgment, are especially vulnerable to car crashes and other accidental causes of closed head injury.

| Mental Disorders Due to
a General Medical Condition

DSM-IV defines a variety of disorders that occur as the result of a general medical condition. Because not all of these apply to juveniles, and even the applicable disorders are seldom encountered by child mental health professionals, we do not give their criteria in detail. But it is sometimes necessary to consider these disorders in the differential diagnosis of other, more prevalent childhood and adolescent illnesses. We have therefore provided these criteria in tabular form (see Table 13.1). We will repeatedly refer to this table throughout the remainder of this book. (Note that Delirium Due to a General Medical Condition and Dementia Due to Other General Medical Conditions, which might also have been included in Table 13.1, have been discussed in Chapter 12.)

TABLE 13.1. Criteria for Six Mental Disorders Due to a General Medical Condition

Anxiety Disorder	Mood Disorder	Sleep Disorder	Personality Change	Psychotic Disorder	Catatonic Disorder	Sexual Dysfunction
• Prominent anxiety, compulsions, obsessions, or Panic Attacks	• Persistent (1) depressed mood or marked loss of interest or pleasure in nearly all activities, or (2) elevated, expansive or irritable mood	• Sleep problem that warrants clinical attention and doesn't meet criteria for Narcolepsy or Breathing-Related Sleep Disorder	• A lasting change from patient's established personality (in young children, a striking deviation from typical development or a change lasting at least 1 year)	• Prominent delusions or hallucinations	• Catatonic symptoms (e.g., immobility, negativism, muteness, echolalia, posturing, waxy flexibility)	• Clinically important sexual dysfunction dominates the clinical picture

• The symptoms cause clinically important distress or impair work, school, social, or personal functionings. — *(Sexual Dysfunction: • Marked distress or effect on interpersonal functioning)*

• Symptoms don't occur solely during a delirium.

• No other mental disorder better explains these symptoms.

• History, physical exam, or laboratory findings suggest that a general medical condition directly causes these symptoms.

Coding Note: On Axis III, code the general medical condition responsible for each disorder. In addition, give the condition's exact name in the Axis I diagnosis.

Anxiety Disorder	Mood Disorder	Sleep Disorder	Personality Change	Psychotic Disorder	Catatonic Disorder	Sexual Dysfunction
Code 293.89. Specify: With Generalized Anxiety, With Panic Attacks, With Obsessive-Compulsive Symptoms.	Code 293.83. Specify type: With Depressive Features, With Major Depressive-Like Episode, With Manic Features, With Mixed Features.	Code by type: 780.52, Insomnia Type; 780.54, Hypersomnia Type; 780.59, Parasomnia Type; 780.59, Mixed Type.	Code 310.1. Specify type: Labile Type; Disinhibited Type; Aggressive Type; Apathetic Type; Paranoid Type; Other Type, Combined Type, Unspecified Type.	Code based on major symptom: 293.81, With Delusions; 293.82, With Hallucinations.	Code 293.89. No subtypes or specifiers.	Code by type. 625.8, Female Hypoactive Sexual Desire; 608.89, Male Hypoactive Sexual Desire; 607.84, Male Erectile Disorder; 625.0 Female Dyspareunia; 608.89, Male Dyspareunia; 625.8, Other Female Sexual Dysfunction; 608.89, Other Male Sexual Dysfunction.

| Substance-Related Disorders

Quick Guide to the Substance-Related Disorders

Mind-altering substances yield four basic types of disorders: Substance Dependence, Abuse, Intoxication, and Withdrawal. Most of these DSM-IV terms apply to nearly all of the substances discussed; exceptions are noted below. Various other substance-related disorders are also identified by DSM-IV.

Substance Use Disorders

Substance Dependence. Substance use falling into this category is use that has produced certain behavioral characteristics and clinically important distress or impaired functioning. Found in all drug classes except caffeine, Substance Dependence doesn't have to be intentional; it can develop from medicinal use, such as the treatment of chronic pain (Table 14.1).

Substance Abuse. This is a residual category (i.e., a diagnosis of last resort) for individuals whose substance use produces problems that do not reach the level of Substance Dependence. This diagnosis applies to all substances except caffeine and nicotine (Table 14.2).

Substance-Induced Disorders

Substance Intoxication. Recent substance use causes this acute clinical state, which can apply to all drugs except nicotine (Table 14.3).

Substance Withdrawal. This class-specific collection of symptoms develops when a frequent user discontinues or markedly reduces the amount used. It applies to all substances except caffeine, cannabis, PCP, the hallucinogens, and the inhalants (Table 14.4).

Other Substance-Induced Disorders. Other substance-induced disorders sometimes diagnosed in children and adolescents include Substance-Induced Psychotic Disorder, Mood Disorder, Anxiety Disorder, and Sleep Disorder. They can be experienced during intoxication, during withdrawal, or as consequences of substance misuse that endure long after the misuse and withdrawal symptoms have ended (Table 14.5).

INTRODUCTION

No one really knows the extent of child and adolescent substance misuse, for several reasons:

- *Casual usage.* Many surveys report the percentage of youths who have used a drug, or class of drugs, within a given time period. Yet only a fraction of these children and adolescents may use drugs frequently or have problems that result from usage. (Should any degree of substance use in a juvenile be considered "normal"?)
- *Use of specific drugs in particular demographic areas.* Use of "hard" drugs, such as heroin and cocaine, is traditionally heavier in inner-city areas than in suburban or rural localities. By contrast, some studies show that the more socially acceptable substances—alcohol, tobacco, and marijuana—may be used as frequently in rural as in urban areas.
- *Comorbid diagnoses.* The vast majority of children and adolescents who misuse substances have other disorders, symptoms of which may obscure the evidence of substance misuse. These diagnoses include Conduct Disorder, ADHD, and mood and anxiety disorders, any of which may be found in a third or more of youths who misuse substances. Multiple comorbid diagnoses are not uncommon.
- *Changing criteria.* For decades, classifications and diagnostic criteria have been revised every few years. In most cases the effect upon perceived prevalence must be slight, but the generic criteria for Substance Abuse were substantially changed in DSM-IV.

THE DSM-IV APPROACH TO DIAGNOSING SUBSTANCE MISUSE

Five Diagnostic Concepts

The foregoing difficulties notwithstanding, DSM-IV takes a giant step toward unifying our understanding of the substance-related disorders. It allows us to make literally hundreds of logical diagnoses according to five diagnostic concepts:

1. **Substance Dependence.** The generic criteria for Substance Dependence (see Table 14.1) identify substance-related problems that are mainly issues of control and physiological change. Because caffeine, the hallucinogens, the inhalants, and PCP don't appear to produce clini-

TABLE 14.1. Generic Criteria for Substance Dependence

- The patient's maladaptive pattern of substance use leads to clinically important distress or impairment, as shown in a single 12-month period by three or more of the following:
  ✓ Tolerance, shown by either of these:
    –Markedly increased intake of the substance is needed to achieve the same effect
    –With continued use, the same amount of the substance has markedly less effect
  ✓ Withdrawal, shown by either of these:
    –The substance's characteristic withdrawal syndrome occurs
    –The substance (or one closely related) is used to avoid or relieve withdrawal symptoms
  ✓ The amount or duration of use is often greater than intended.
  ✓ The patient repeatedly tries without success to control or reduce substance use.
  ✓ The patient spends much time using the substance, recovering from its effects, or trying to obtain it.
  ✓ The patient reduces or abandons important social, work, school, or recreational activities because of substance use.
  ✓ The patient continues to use the substance, despite knowing that it has probably caused physical or psychological problems.

Specify whether:
    With Physiological Dependence. There is evidence of tolerance or withdrawal (see above).
    Without Physiological Dependence.

Choose one or none to specify course:
    Early Full Remission (months 2 through 12)
    Early Partial Remission (months 2 through 12)
    Sustained Full Remission (months 13+)
    Sustained Partial Remission (months 13+)

Specify either or both, when appropriate:
    On Agonist Therapy (does not apply to Cannabis, Hallucinogen, Inhalant, or PCP Dependence)
    In a Controlled Environment (does not apply to Nicotine Dependence)

cally significant tolerance or withdrawal symptoms, Substance Dependence does not apply to them. Children and adolescents are far less likely than adults to receive a diagnosis of Substance Dependence.

2. **Substance Abuse.** The residual category of Substance Abuse (see Table 14.2 for generic criteria) was redefined in DSM-IV to identify patients whose substance use has not been severe enough to create Substance Dependence but has nonetheless caused problems. In contrast to Substance Dependence, Substance Abuse identifies problems that are principally social and legal. No one yet knows how much predictive value this category has for any age group.

3. **Substance Intoxication**. Anyone can become intoxicated; therefore, Substance Intoxication is the only substance-related diagnosis that can be made for a person who uses a substance only once. Each of the substance-specific criteria sets (see Table 14.3) is applied to patients whose thinking and behavior are currently being influenced by the substance in question.

4. **Substance Withdrawal.** Each of the specific criteria sets for Substance Withdrawal (see Table 14.4) is applied to patients who have used enough of a substance that reducing or discontinuing it affects their thinking or behavior.

5. **Substance-Induced Mental Disorder**. Scattered throughout DSM-IV are criteria sets that describe the effects of substances on cognition, psychosis, mood, anxiety, sex, and sleep. Table 14.5 gives criteria for most of these that apply to children and adolescents. (Substance-Induced Persisting Dementia, Substance-Induced Persisting Amnestic Disorder, and Substance-Induced Sexual Dysfunction are rarely if ever applicable

---

TABLE 14.2. Generic Criteria for Substance Abuse

- The patient's maladaptive substance use pattern causes clinically important distress or impairment, as shown in a single 12-month period by one or more of the following:
  - ✓ Because of repeated use, the patient fails to carry out major obligations at work, school, or at home.
  - ✓ The patient repeatedly uses substances even when it is physically dangerous.
  - ✓ The patient repeatedly has legal problems from substance use.
  - ✓ Despite knowing that it has caused or worsened social or interpersonal problems, the patient continues to use the substance.
- For this class of substance, the patient has never fulfilled criteria for Substance Dependence.

TABLE 14.3. Substance-Specific Criteria for Substance Intoxication

	Alcohol/ sedatives, etc.	Caffeine	Cannabis	Cocaine/amphetamines
Use	• Recent use	• Recent use > 250 mg	• Recent use	• Recent use
Maladaptive psychological/ behavioral changes	• Some required— e.g.: ✓ Inappropriate sexuality or aggression ✓ Labile mood ✓ Impaired judgment ✓ Impaired job, school, or social functioning	• Clinically important distress or impaired job, school, social, or other functioning	• Some required— e.g.: ✓ Motor performance deficits ✓ Anxiety ✓ Euphoria ✓ Impaired judgment ✓ Social withdrawal ✓ Slowed sense of time	• Some required—e.g.: ✓ Euphoria or blunted affect ✓ Hypervigilance ✓ Interpersonal sensitivity ✓ Anger, anxiety, or tension ✓ Changes in sociability ✓ Stereotyped behaviors ✓ Impaired judgment ✓ Impaired job, school, or social functioning
Other symptoms	• During or shortly after use, one or more: ✓ Slurred speech ✓ Lack of coordination ✓ Unsteady walking ✓ Nystagmus ✓ Impaired attention or memory ✓ Stupor or coma	• During or shortly after use, five or more: ✓ Restlessness ✓ Nervousness ✓ Excitement ✓ Sleeplessness ✓ Red face ✓ Increased urination ✓ Gastrointestinal upset ✓ Twitching muscles ✓ Rambling speech ✓ Rapid or irregular heart rate ✓ Tireless periods ✓ Increased psychomotor activity	• Within 2 hours of use, two or more: ✓ Red eyes ✓ Heightened appetite ✓ Dry mouth ✓ Rapid heart rate	• During or shortly after use, two or more: ✓ Speeded or slowed heart rate ✓ Dilated pupils ✓ Heightened or lowered blood pressure ✓ Chills or sweating ✓ Nausea or vomiting ✓ Weight loss ✓ Speeded or slowed psychomotor activity ✓ Muscle weakness, depressed breathing, chest pain, or irregular heartbeat ✓ Seizures, confusion, distorted voluntary movements or muscle tone, or coma
Other	• The symptoms are not caused by a general medical condition or better explained by another mental disorder.			
Specifiers	None	None	With Perceptual Disturbances	With Perceptual Disturbances

Hallucinogens	Inhalants	Opioids	PCP
• Recent use	• Recent use or exposure	• Recent use	• Recent use
• Some required—e.g.: ✓ Depression or anxiety ✓ Ideas of reference ✓ Fears of insanity ✓ Persecutory ideas ✓ Impaired judgment ✓ Impaired job, school, or social functioning	• Some required—e.g.: ✓ Apathy ✓ Assaultiveness ✓ Belligerence ✓ Impaired judgment ✓ Impaired job, school, or social functioning	• Some required—e.g.: ✓ Euphoria, then apathy ✓ Depression or anxiety ✓ Speeded or slowed psychomotor activity ✓ Impaired judgment ✓ Impaired job, school, or social functioning	• Some required—e.g.: ✓ Assaultiveness ✓ Belligerence ✓ Impulsiveness ✓ Speeded psychomotor activity ✓ Unpredictability ✓ Impaired judgment ✓ Impaired job, school, or social functioning
• During or shortly after use, perceptual changes • During or shortly after use, two or more: ✓ Dilated pupils ✓ Rapid heart rate ✓ Sweating ✓ Palpitations ✓ Blurred vision ✓ Tremors ✓ Lack of coordination	• During or shortly after use, two or more: ✓ Dizziness ✓ Nystagmus ✓ Lack of coordination ✓ Slurred speech ✓ Unsteady walking ✓ Lethargy ✓ Slowed reflexes ✓ Slowed psychomotor activity ✓ Tremors ✓ Muscle weakness ✓ Blurred or double vision ✓ Stupor or coma ✓ Euphoria	• During or shortly after use, pupils constricted (or dilated, if severe overdose) • During or shortly after use, one or more: ✓ Sleepiness or coma ✓ Slurred speech ✓ Impaired memory or attention	• Within 1 hour of use, two or more: ✓ Nystagmus ✓ Heightened blood pressure or heart rate ✓ Numbness or decreased pain response ✓ Trouble walking ✓ Trouble speaking ✓ Rigid muscles ✓ Coma or seizures ✓ Abnormally acute hearing

• The symptoms are not caused by a general medical condition or better explained by another mental disorder.

None	None	With Perceptual Disturbances	With Perceptual Disturbances

TABLE 14.4. Substance-Specific Criteria for Substance Withdrawal

	Alcohol/ sedatives, etc.	Cocaine/ amphetamines	Hallucinogens	Nicotine	Opioids
Use	• Heavy/prolonged use before cessation/ reduction	• Heavy/prolonged use before cessation/ reduction	See table footnote	• Daily use for several weeks before cessation/ reduction	• Several weeks of heavy use before cessation/ reduction, or a period of use before use of an antagonist
Symptoms	• Within hours to a few days, two or more: ✓ Sweating or rapid heartbeat ✓ Trembling of hands ✓ Sleeplessness ✓ Nausea or vomiting ✓ Brief hallucinations or illusions ✓ Speeded psychomotor activity ✓ Grand mal seizures ✓ Anxiety	• Within hours to a few days, dysphoric mood plus two or more: ✓ Fatigue ✓ Vivid bad dreams ✓ Increased or decreased sleep ✓ Heightened appetite ✓ Speeded or slowed psychomotor activity		• Within 24 hours, four or more: ✓ Dysphoria or depression ✓ Sleeplessness ✓ Anger, frustration, or irritability ✓ Anxiety ✓ Trouble concentrating ✓ Restlessness ✓ Slowed heart rate ✓ Increase in appetite or weight	• Within minutes to a few days, three or more: ✓ Dysphoria ✓ Nausea or vomiting ✓ Aching muscles ✓ Tearing or runny nose ✓ Dilated pupils, erect hairs, or sweating ✓ Diarrhea ✓ Yawning ✓ Fever ✓ Sleeplessness
Other	• The symptoms cause clinically important distress or impair social, job, or other functioning. • The symptoms are not caused by a general medical condition or better explained by another mental disorder.				
Specifiers	With Perceptual Disturbances	None	None	None	None

Note. Hallucinogen Persisting Perception Disorder (Flashbacks) is not really a withdrawal disorder, although it occurs after a person has ceased use of LSD or another hallucinogen. It consists of the reexperiencing of at least one of the symptoms of perception that occurred during Hallucinogen Intoxication (e.g., flashes of color, trails of images, afterimages, halos, perceptions of objects as larger or smaller than they actually are, geometric hallucinations, and false peripheral perception of movement). The criteria listed as "Other" in the table body also apply to this disorder.

to children and adolescents; the criteria for the two forms of Substance-Induced Delirium have been given in Table 12.1.)

Classes of Substances That Can Be Misused

DSM-IV lists a total of 11 substance categories plus "other (or unknown)" that can alter behavior, feelings, or perceptions. However, these 11 can be condensed into just six broad categories. Interpret these usage figures cautiously—the rates continually change, and accurate data are not available for some substance classes.

TABLE 14.5. Criteria for Four Other Substance-Induced Mental Disorders

Psychotic Disorder	Mood Disorder	Anxiety Disorder	Sleep Disorder
• Prominent delusions or hallucinations (except those for which patient has insight)	• Persistence of *either* or *both:* Depressed mood or notably decreased interest or pleasure in nearly all activities; and/or elevated, irritable, or expansive mood	• Prominent anxiety, compulsions, obsessions, or panic attacks	• A sleep problem serious enough to warrant clinical attention

• Another, non-substance-induced [psychotic] [mood] [anxiety] [sleep] disorder doesn't better account for symptoms.

• Symptoms don't occur solely in the context of delirium.		• Symptoms don't occur solely in the context of delirium	

• History, physical exam, or lab data suggests either that symptoms developed within 1 month of Substance Intoxication or Withdrawal, *or* that they are caused by medication use.

        • Symptoms cause clinically important distress or impair work, school, social, or personal functioning.

Specify: With Onset During Intoxication, With Onset During Withdrawal

| Code based on major symptoms (see Table 14.6): With Delusions, With Hallucinations | Specify type: With Depressive Features, With Manic Features, With Mixed Features | Specify: With Generalized Anxiety, With Panic Attacks, With Obsessive–Compulsive Symptoms, With Phobic Symptoms | Specify type: Insomnia Type, Hypersomnia Type, Parasomnia Type, Mixed Type |

- **Central nervous system depressants**. These two substance classes have identical DSM-IV criteria sets for Substance Intoxication and Withdrawal.

   Alcohol. Of course, most adolescents have tried alcohol; the percentage of all teenagers who use it frequently is in the low double digits. With less drinking experience from which to judge, even those young people who do not go on to have an alcohol problem may underestimate its effects. As a consequence, when they do drink, they drink far too much. Perhaps for this reason, adolescent Alcohol Intoxication not infrequently results in stupor or coma.

   Sedatives, hypnotics, and anxiolytics. Readily available in parents' medicine cabinets and on the street, these drugs are reportedly often misused by children and teenagers. Documentary evidence of the extent of this misuse is still lacking, however.

- **Central nervous system stimulants**. To one degree or another, each of the drugs in this category increases central nervous system activity, resulting in alertness, elevation of mood and sense of well-being, improved task performance, and decrease in hunger and in the need for sleep. Identical criteria for Substance Intoxication and Withdrawal apply to cocaine and the amphetamines.

Amphetamines. These powerful drugs, first synthesized about a hundred years ago, are reportedly popular with young people, but no one knows to what extent. Tight government controls on manufacture and distribution have probably diminished their use somewhat in the past several decades.

Cocaine. Manufactured from coca leaves, which grow in South America and other parts of the world, cocaine is perhaps the most addictive substance ever created. As one of the most widely misused psychoactive substances in the world, cocaine undoubtedly causes problems for some young people. However, there are very few data to draw on.

Caffeine. Of course, caffeine presents far less danger than amphetamines and cocaine do; in fact, learning to drink coffee is a rite of passage for the vast majority of young people. Yet, in excess, even this benign substance can cause symptoms of intoxication. Some people experience withdrawal symptoms, even though DSM-IV does not officially recognize caffeine withdrawal; perhaps DSM-V will.

- **Opioids**. Most heroin users get their start through peer pressure when they are in their teens or early 20s. Contributing factors include parental divorce, low socioeconomic status, inner-city residence, relatives who misuse alcohol, and early experimentation with other substances such as marijuana and alcohol. Still, only about 1% of late adolescents have used opiates in some form.
- **Perception-distorting drugs**. The toxic effect of each of these drugs is to produce hallucinations or some other form of altered perception. None of these drugs has any noteworthy withdrawal syndrome.

Inhalants. The inhalants include nearly anything that evaporates or can be sprayed from a can. They are cheap, easy to obtain, and (because they are absorbed from the lungs) rapidly effective. These drugs produce changes in the way users see color, size, or the shape of objects. Sometimes they cause actual hallucinations. They can also alter a user's mood, ideas, or sense of time. They are especially popular with young people—about 20% of late adolescents have used them, though mainly when they were younger.

PCP. PCP (or phencyclidine) is cheap, but its (mostly) young male users especially value the euphoria it produces. Some experience psychosis so convincing that, in the absence of adequate history, it cannot be distinguished from Schizophrenia.

LSD. LSD (an abbreviation for lysergic acid diethylamide) is emblematic of the hallucinogens, which do not usually produce hallucinations at all, but rather illusions (misinterpretations of actual sensory stimuli). In Canada, they are sometimes called *illusionogens.* At only about 10% lifetime prevalence for graduating high school seniors, LSD may be less popular now than formerly; other drugs in the class are probably more popular (an example is MDMA, one of the so-called designer drugs). The hallucinogens can affect patients in two ways: intoxication and flashbacks (which DSM-IV somewhat clumsily calls Hallucinogen Persisting Perception Disorder).

Marijuana. Finally, there is cannabis (marijuana), the illicit drug most commonly used in the United States. By graduation, nearly a third of high school students have tried it. Those who use it feel that it sharpens their perceptions. Illusions may occur, but hallucinations rarely do.

- **Nicotine**. Here's an oddity: DSM-IV includes Nicotine Withdrawal, but not Nicotine Intoxication. Of course, when nicotine is taken in great enough quantity by a naïve user, toxic symptoms are there aplenty (ask any kid who's tried one of Dad's stogies). It is also the most widely used addictive drug in the United States.

- **Other (or unknown).** Other mind-altering substances include anabolic steroids (which may be misused by athletes who want to perform better and by others to enhance physical attractiveness). Nitrous oxide (laughing gas) produces euphoria, and a variety of over-the-counter and prescription drugs (including antihistamines, antiparkinsonian drugs, and cortisone) may be used to produce other states of altered consciousness. Finally, the "unknown" category is used when a patient has obviously ingested a substance, but its exact nature cannot be determined.

Application of the Four Basic Concepts in Clinical Practice

The generic criteria for Substance Dependence (Table 14.1) and Substance Abuse (Table 14.2) are necessary for the evaluation of any patient suspected of misuse of alcohol or other substances. They can be used with Tables 14.3 and 14.4, which summarize the criteria for Substance Intoxication and Withdrawal (respectively) specific to various drug classes listed above, and with Table 14.6, which summarizes and gives codes for the mental disorders that can be associated with each class of substance in children and adolescents. Below, we use a single case vignette to illustrate the application of the four basic DSM-IV concepts (Substance Dependence, Abuse, Intoxication, and Withdrawal) in clinical practice.

Rodney

"It was so hard to start, I had no idea it would be harder to stop." Rodney was almost 17, but he looked a lot younger. Lying on his back in a hospital bed, his left arm in a sling and his right leg strung up by pulleys. He didn't recall much about the accident that had put him there. It involved quite a few brandy Alexanders and too little instruction about hanging onto the passenger bar of the Honda motorcycle driven by his roommate. His only injuries were skeletal, and he was clear-headed enough to realize that he badly needed a cigarette.

Rodney was probably the smartest kid ever born in his part of Texas. By the time he was 12, he was already attending high school classes, had won several statewide scholastic contests, and had appeared twice on a popular TV quiz show. When he was 14, his parents reluctantly let him accept a full-tuition scholarship to a small but prestigious liberal arts college several hundred miles from home.

"Of course, I was the smallest one there—except for one guy with some sort of an endocrine disorder," said Rodney. "I didn't really think about it at the time, but I'm sure I started smoking and drinking to compensate for my size." After he had stopped feeling nauseated and dizzy every time he lighted up, one of his classmates had taught him to blow one small smoke ring right through the center of another, larger one.

By the time Rodney had been in college 6 months, he was smoking a pack and a half a day. When studying for exams (unless he got the highest grade in the class, he invariably felt that he wasn't "measuring up"), he found himself sometimes lighting one cigarette from another, going through several packs in a day this way—far more than he had meant to. The following year, in a mandatory health class, he read the Surgeon General's report on smoking and saw a video about lung cancer ("in living—no, *dying*—color"). He swore he'd never smoke again, but his resolve lasted exactly 48 hours. For two nights he couldn't sleep, and he noticed that he became restless, depressed, and "so irritable my roommate begged me to light up again." Over the next year he had tried twice more to quit. Once he attended Smoke Enders; when that failed, he asked the student health service for nicotine patches. "They wouldn't give them to me without parental consent—I'm going to be a senior in 4 months!"

Rodney's parents both worked in the small-town feed and seed store they owned. Both were hard-working churchgoers who had never touched a drop of alcohol. Growing up in the same small community, both had been appalled at what alcohol had done to their own fathers. Several times in the last few months, when he was so badly hung over he couldn't attend classes, Rodney had vaguely wondered whether he was about to follow in his grandfathers' unsteady footsteps.

The only bright spot, he observed wryly as he shifted uncomfortably in the hospital bed, was that "when I fell off the Honda, I was so drunk I didn't feel a thing." At first it was assumed that he had a concussion, but the blood alcohol level of 0.25 suggested simple intoxication. He had awakened 12 hours later with pins through his femur and a terrific hangover. Now, 2 days later, his vital signs were stable and normal—except for a pulse rate of only 56.

"I don't suppose you could smuggle in some nicotine gum?" Rodney asked.

Evaluation of Rodney

The central organizing principle behind the DSM-IV criteria for any class of substances is Substance Dependence, which is where we'll start in this necessarily long discussion. First, let's consider Rodney's smoking.

The generic criteria for Substance Dependence (Table 14.1) focus on behaviors that suggest problems with either physiology or control. Rodney's smoking involved several of the latter, each of which, as the criteria require, had occurred during the preceding 12 months. He had sometimes spent a great deal of time using nicotine (chain-smoking), and he sometimes smoked more than he intended. He no longer experienced the nausea and dizziness typical of novice smokers; this, according to DSM-IV, was evidence of tolerance. Later, he had spent much time trying to stop.

TABLE 14.6. Codes for Substance-Related Disorders Applicable to Children and Adolescents

	Delirium[a]	Persisting Dementia	Persisting Amnestic	Psychotic Disorder[b]	Mood Disorders	Anxiety Disorder
Alcohol	291.0 I/W	291.2	291.1	291.5/.3 I/W	291.8 I/W	291.8 I/W
Amphetamines	292.81 I			292.11/.12 I	292.84 I/W	292.89 I
Caffeine						292.89 I
Cannabis	292.81 I			292.11/.12 I		292.89 I
Cocaine	292.81 I			292.11/.12 I	292.84 I/W	292.89 I/W
Hallucinogens	292.81 I			292.11/.12[c] I	292.84 I	292.89 I
Inhalants	292.81 I	292.82		292.11/12 I	292.84 I	292.89 I
Nicotine						
Opioids	292.81 I			292.11/.12 I	292.84 I	
PCP	292.81 I			292.11/.12 I	292.84 I	292.89 I
Sedatives, hypnotics, anxiolytics	292.81 I/W	292.82	292.83	292.11/.12 I/W	292.84 I/W	292.89 W

Note. Adapted with permission from the *Diagnostic and Statistical Manual of Mental Disorders* (4th ed., p. 177). Copyright 1994 American Psychiatric Association.

Abbreviations in table body: I, With Onset During Intoxication; W, With Onset During Withdrawal; PD, With Perceptual Disturbances.

[a]Although a delirium is called Substance Intoxication Delirium or Substance Withdrawal Delirium, according to whether it occurs during intoxication or withdrawal, the code numbers are the same.

[b]For the psychotic disorders, the first set of numbers after the decimal point indicates the code for With Delusions; the second set of numbers indicates the code for With Hallucinations.

[c]Also 292.89 Hallucinogen Persisting Perception Disorder (Flashbacks).

Right there are four (only three are required) of the criteria for Nicotine Dependence. Because Rodney was tolerant to the effects of nicotine, his diagnosis would include the specifier With Physiological Dependence. But could he also be diagnosed with Nicotine Withdrawal? For evidence, we must look at the specific criteria for Substance Withdrawal as they relate to nicotine (Table

TABLE 14.6 *(continued)*

Sexual Dysfunction	Sleep Disorder	Disorder NOS	Dependence	Abuse	Intoxication	Withdrawal
291.8 I	291.8 I/W	291.9	303.90	305.00	303.00	291.8 PD
292.89 I	292.89 I/W	292.9	304.40	305.70	292.89 PD	292.0
	292.89 I	292.9			305.90	
		292.9	304.30	305.20	292.89 PD	
292.89 I	292.89 I/W	292.9	304.20	305.60	292.89 PD	292.0
		292.9	304.50	305.30	292.89	292.89
		292.9	304.60	305.90	292.89	
		292.9	305.10			292.0
292.89 I	292.89 I/W	292.9	304.00	305.50	292.89 PD	292.0
		292.9	304.90	305.90	292.89 PD	
292.89 I	292.89 I/W	292.9	304.10	305.40	292.89	292.0 PD

14.4). On at least two occasions he had suffered from typical withdrawal symptoms: restlessness, depression, irritability, and now slowed pulse rate. (His trouble sleeping could have been caused by his recent accident and operation.) Although these symptoms did not impair functioning when he was in the hospital, they were distressing, and they had caused a social problem with his roommate. Therefore, Nicotine Withdrawal would become an Axis I diagnosis, and it could be added to the list of symptoms supporting a diagnosis of Nicotine Dependence.

At the time of his hospitalization, then, Rodney's Axis I diagnosis would read in part:

292.0	Nicotine Withdrawal
305.10	Nicotine Dependence, with Physiological Dependence

Now we must consider the remission specifiers. For the first month after substance use stops (or decreases so that it no longer qualifies as Substance Dependence), no statement about remission is warranted. After that, two sorts of information must be considered: number of symptoms (if any) and time. A person who has completely stopped using is said to be in Full Remission; if one or two symptoms remain (remember, it takes three to qualify for active Substance Dependence), Partial Remission is diagnosed. From months 2 to 12, this person will be in Early Remission (either Full or Partial); after 1 year, Sustained Remission (of either type) can be diagnosed. Of course, upon admission Rodney was still using tobacco, so no statement at all could be made about his remission at this time.

Now let's consider Rodney's alcohol use. Rodney had never had a lot of trouble with alcohol, but he had had some. He would certainly not meet criteria for Alcohol Dependence or Withdrawal, but what about Alcohol Intoxication and Abuse? The criteria for Alcohol Intoxication are not demanding—they require only one symptom from Table 14.3. From Rodney's vignette, we can infer at least two: incoordination and loss of memory. Besides, with a blood alcohol level of 0.25, only a pedant would insist on formal criteria. As to the generic criteria for Substance Abuse (Table 14.2), he had more than once or twice failed in his obligation to attend school, so he would qualify for an additional diagnosis of Alcohol Abuse. Of course, riding a motorcycle when intoxicated was also physically dangerous, but to qualify, it would have had to occur more than once within 12 months. (Experimentation with substances is the rule in these age groups, making the conscientious use of the criteria for Substance Abuse and Dependence even more important than in adults.) No specifiers apply to the criteria for Alcohol Abuse.

Therefore, Rodney's vignette provides ample evidence to support, at the time of his hospital admission, four separate Axis I diagnoses for him. Note that the GAF score (Axis V), which for Rodney would be relatively high at admission, is not supposed to be based on any information concerning a patient's physical condition (or environmental situation).

The differential diagnosis for substance-related disorders spans the mental and physical diagnostic spectrum. Children and adolescents should also be carefully considered for those mental disorders that are often associated with the substance-related conditions, most notably the **mood** and **anxiety disorders**. **Eating disorders** have been reported with particular frequency among substance-misusing girls, and **Conduct Disorder** and **ADHD** among substance-misusing boys. Rodney's diagnosis at his admission to the hospital would read as follows:

Axis I	292.0	Nicotine Withdrawal
	305.10	Nicotine Dependence, With Physiological Dependence
	303.00	Alcohol Intoxication
	305.00	Alcohol Abuse
Axis II	V71.09	No diagnosis
Axis III	812.0	Fractured of humerus, upper end, closed
	821.11	Open fracture, shaft (middle third), right femur
Axis IV		None
Axis V	GAF = 70	(on admission)

At the time of a reevaluation 3 months later, Rodney would probably no longer be in Nicotine Withdrawal. If he had quit smoking and had no symptoms of either Dependence or Abuse, we would say that his Nicotine Dependence was in Full Remission. But because it had been only 3 months, we would also call it an Early Remission. Therefore, his diagnosis would be the following:

Axis I	305.10	Nicotine Dependence, Early Full Remission
	305.00	Alcohol Abuse
Axis II	V71.09	No diagnosis
Axis III		None
Axis IV		None
Axis V	GAF = 75	(current)

Assessing Substance-Related Disorders

General Suggestions

Especially in adolescents, obtaining information about substance use often means trying to extract private information from one who wishes to keep it private. If you interview an adolescent who is still intoxicated, you may observe classic signs, such as red eyes or slurred speech. It is far more likely, however, that you will have to depend on historical information from the patient. If this is your first contact, you may need multiple sessions to explore this area.

Some young people will be more likely than others to misuse substances: older children and adolescents; those whose parents have had substance use problems; those who have been the victims of physical or sexual abuse; and those with other mental disorders (especially mood disorders)—boys more so than girls. No young patient can be considered completely immune, of course, and the area of substance use is one of three in the mental health interview that should be considered "must cover." (The other two are sex and suicide.)

You will probably fare better if you delay asking about this and other sensitive information (misconduct, sex, history of physical or sexual abuse) until later in the interview, when you have established some rapport. Before you start, it is often wise to set some ground rules, as described in Part I of his book: "If you feel you can't talk about something, don't lie to me—just say, 'Let's talk about something else.' " You might also want to reemphasize what you have already agreed you will (or won't) tell parents. Of course, if you wait until this sensitive topic is broached, then excuse parents from the room, you may reduce the amount of relevant information you will collect. If the patient already knows that suspected substance use is the reason for the evaluation, you might acknowledge the fact: "It seems your folks are worried that [type of substance] use may be hurting you. What do you think?"

You might begin by inquiring about alcohol, tobacco, and marijuana, and by assuming that most teens have experimented with some of these socially more acceptable drugs: "What experiences have you had with alcohol [or one of the others]?" With luck, you will get a fair run of information from this open-ended question. Be alert for contradictions and ask frankly for clarification: "I'm confused. First you said . . . , but now you say. . . . Which do you mean?" Watch for body language that suggests prevarication: shifts in posture, lowered gaze, hesitation before answering.

You could also start by asking about peer involvement with drugs. The device puts some distance between the teen and the behavior, and can result in a more truthful account. Another nonthreatening introduction might be to ask about drugs that others use at the patient's school: "How hard would it be for someone to buy pot at your school?" After ascertaining some of these generalities, it is easier to inquire into the teen's own usage. Even then, you might want to start slowly with some history: "How old were you when you first had a beer?"

Of course, the patient can confound any approach at all by simply refusing to talk. Then you may have to invite a discussion of feelings: "I can see that this subject makes you [angry, sad, anxious]. I can't say I blame you . . . " Similarly acknowledge and accept profanity, which may be used as a shield against unwelcome questions. Occasionally, an adolescent may try to deflect questions about substances by offering up instances of substance use by parents or other relatives. In such a case, obtain this valuable information about family members, but then use it as a springboard back to the patient: "Now tell me about *your* experience with alcohol." If a patient minimizes (or denies) substance use in the face of evidence to the contrary, you may have to force a confrontation—after you have established a relationship solid enough to survive one. "Let's see, you say that you've never tried pot, but last week your mom found paraphernalia in your pants pocket. I don't understand that."

The information you need is extensive and varied. For each drug used, try to learn the following:

- Frequency and duration of use
- Average amount of use per episode
- The valued effect of use (e.g., to feel high, to ease social awkwardness, to promote introspection)
- The consequences of use (e.g., medical problems such as blackouts, evidence of Substance Dependence or Abuse)
- The patient's means of financing drug or alcohol use (lunch money, stealing from parents, other illegal activities)

Don't forget to ask about the abuse of prescription or over-the-counter prescriptions.

Developmental Factors

Adolescents are more likely than adults to experience severe toxicity, even in the form of coma. Intoxication in young children suggests child abuse or child neglect. Age is also associated with drug of choice: Inhalants and marijuana are more popular among young people than among adults.

CHAPTER 15 | Schizophrenia and Other Psychotic Disorders

Quick Guide to the Psychotic Disorders

As usual, the page (or table) number following each item indicates where fuller information on it may be found.

Schizophrenia

Patients with schizophrenia have been ill for at least 6 months with symptoms from at least two of these five groups: delusions, hallucinations, disorganized behavior, disorganized speech, and negative symptoms. They do not have significant manic or depressive symptoms, and both substance use and general medical conditions have been ruled out (p. 296). Five subtypes of Schizophrenia are defined:

Paranoid Type. These patients have persecutory delusions and auditory hallucinations, but no negative symptoms, disorganized speech, or catatonic behavior.

Disorganized Type. In this subtype, delusions and hallucinations are less prominent than are negative symptoms and disorganized speech and behavior.

Catatonic Type. The cardinal symptoms of this subtype are excessively retarded or excited activity and bizarre behavior.

Undifferentiated Type. Patients with this subtype will have some or all of the five basic types of psychotic symptoms. None of these symptoms dominates the clinical picture.

Residual Type. After their acute psychosis has markedly improved, these patients still seem somewhat unusual, odd, or peculiar.

Schizophrenia-Like Disorders

Schizophreniform Disorder. This category is for patients who have all the symptoms of Schizophrenia, but who have been ill for only 1 to 6 months—less than the time specified for Schizophrenia (p. 301).

Schizoaffective Disorder. For at least 1 month, these patients have had symptoms of Schizophrenia; at the same time, they have prominent symptoms of mania or depression. This condition is hard to diagnose (for one thing, the criteria keep changing), and it is rarely diagnosed in children, though it may occasionally be seen in adolescents and young adults (p. 302).

Brief Psychotic Disorder. These patients will have had at least one of the basic psychotic symptoms for less than 1 month.

Disorders with Delusions

Delusional Disorder. Although these patients have delusions that are not bizarre, they have none of the other symptoms of Schizophrenia. Such a diagnosis is unusual in children or adolescents, but it is not unheard of (p. 302).

Shared Psychotic Disorder. This condition may be diagnosed when a child or adolescent develops delusions similar to those held by a relative or other close associate (p. 302).

Other Psychotic Disorders

Catatonic Disorder Due to a General Medical Condition. A variety of medical and neurological conditions can produce catatonia and other psychotic symptoms that may not meet criteria for any of the psychotic disorders. This condition is seldom reported in children or adolescents (Table 13.1).

Psychotic Disorder Due to a General Medical Condition. A variety of medical and neurological conditions can produce psychotic symptoms that may not meet criteria for any of the conditions above (Table 13.1 and p. 303).

Substance-Induced Psychotic Disorder. Alcohol or other substances (intoxication or withdrawal) can cause psychotic symptoms that may not meet criteria for any of the conditions above (Table 14.5 and p. 303).

Psychotic Disorder Not Otherwise Specified. This category should be reserved for patients whose psychotic symptoms do not meet criteria for any of the disorders listed above (p. 304).

Disorders with Psychosis as a Symptom

Some patients have psychosis as a symptom of mental disorders that we discuss in other chapters. These disorders include mood disorders with psychosis (either severe Major Depressive Episode or Manic Episode), cognitive disorders with psychosis (dementias or deliriums), and personality disorders (patients with Borderline Personality Disorder may have transient periods of minutes or hours when they appear delusional).

Finally, some other disorders may masquerade as psychosis:

Specific Phobia. Some phobic avoidance behaviors can appear quite strange without being psychotic (p. 346).

Mental Retardation. These patients may at times speak or act bizarrely (p. 175).

Somatization Disorder. Sometimes these patients will report pseudo-hallucinations or pseudodelusions (p. 375).

Factitious Disorder. A patient (or caregiver, in the case of factitious disorder by proxy) may feign delusions or hallucinations in order to obtain hospital or other medical care (p. 382).

SCHIZOPHRENIA

The actual prevalence of psychosis in general, and Schizophrenia in particular, in children and adolescents has not been well determined. Because Schizophrenia usually begins in late adolescence or young adulthood, children and young adolescents are especially likely to exhibit only precursor symptoms. However, DSM-IV's Schizophrenia criteria are far more important for children than numbers alone would suggest: They can serve as a bulwark against an unwarranted diagnosis that, by suggesting a dismal prognosis and encouraging unwarranted therapy, can cause a lifetime of harm. The prognosis for children and adolescents validly diagnosed as having Schizophrenia appears to be even poorer than that for patients who fall ill when they are older.

In the mental health literature, Schizophrenia that begins in childhood or adolescence is termed *early-onset*; symptoms prior to age 13 are called *very-early-onset*. Note that puberty, which can occur at markedly varying ages, is no longer used as a point of reference for the beginning of a psychotic illness, though some writers still maintain that onset of DSM-IV Schizophrenia before puberty is rare. Just as in adults, the onset of Schizophrenia symptoms is most often gradual. The mean age at onset of psychotic symptoms is about 7–8 years, though the diagnosis of Schizophrenia is usually not made for another year or so (symptoms usually occur earlier in boys than in girls). In contrast to a sex ratio for adults that approaches unity, the ratio of boys to girls throughout the pediatric age range is about 2:1.

At the core of the DSM-IV Schizophrenia criteria lie two features: symptoms and time. Countless studies of adult patients have shown that chronic illness ("real Schizophrenia") is predicted by having serious symptoms and by having symptoms for a long period of time. Some writers complain that in the space of a generation, American criteria for Schizophrenia have gone from the most relaxed in the world to the most stringent. We acknowledge the truth of this assertion and applaud its intent to protect patients. However, just as some data suggest that early diagnosis and treatment are associated with a better prognosis in Autistic Disorder, early identification of Schizophrenia precursors may presage a similar improved outcome for psychotic children. Some clinicians worry that our zeal to diagnose only those children who are unquestionably ill may result in withholding treatment that could ameliorate the course in others who are in the early stages of their illness. Although this possibility exists and must be considered, we feel that the risks of casual diagnostic standards are greater by far.

The Essence of Schizophrenia: The "A" Criterion

The criteria for early-onset and very-early-onset Schizophrenia are identical to those for adults. At the core of the diagnostic criteria is the "A" criterion in DSM-IV (see the first bullet in Table 15.1, below). This criterion specifies that a spectrum (two or more) of psychotic symptoms must be present for at least 1 month for the diagnosis to be considered at all. The spectrum comprises psychotic symptoms of five types, each of which identifies a patient as being out of touch with reality.

Hallucinations

Hallucinations are false sensory perceptions; an individual perceives something when there is no actual sensory stimulus. Hallucinations are the commonest symptom in early-onset Schizophrenia. In adults, the hallucinations of Schizophrenia are usually auditory; although DSM-IV notes that visual hallucinations may occur more often in children than in adults, conclusive data have not yet been reported. It is especially important to differentiate hallucinations from *illusions*, which are misinterpretations of actual sensory stimuli. Here is an example of an illusion: Upon entering a darkened bedroom, a child misperceives a high-backed chair as a giraffe, but realizes the mistake once the light comes on. Two voices that talk with one another, or a voice that continuously comments on a patient's actions, is such a serious symptom that it alone, not two symptoms, can fulfill the "A" criterion.

Delusions

A *delusion* is a fixed, false belief not explained by a patient's education or cultural beliefs. Even when presented with evidence to the contrary, delusional patients cannot be persuaded that their beliefs are wrong. Although many types are possible, children's delusions are usually persecutory in nature—they complain of being followed, observed, or otherwise interfered with. Delusional children may also be afraid of abduction by a relative or of unusual changes occurring inside them. If a delusion can be called *bizarre* (i.e., if it is improbable, incomprehensible, and/or not based on real-world experiences), it is considered such a serious symptom that it alone can fulfill the "A" criteria.

Delusions must be distinguished from *overvalued ideas*—beliefs that, though not obviously false, cannot be proven to be correct. Usually learned from parents or peer groups, overvalued ideas include such concepts as racial superiority and gang allegiance. In young children, it is especially important not to mistake fantasies or play (such as imaginary playmates) for true delusions.

Disorganized Speech

A schizophrenic patient's thought is often marked by peculiar associations that impede communication. Such thinking, sometimes called *loose associations,* is usually reflected in a deterioration in the patient's ability to communicate (e.g., disconnected syntax, incoherence). Children with Schizophrenia are especially likely to have illogical thinking and thus disorganized speech. However, these may be hard to identify in a very young child or in any child with a communication disorder or a pervasive developmental disorder.

Disorganized Behavior

Any non-goal-directed behavior (such as making hand signals without apparent purpose) may indicate psychosis, as may some behaviors that, though goal-directed, are grossly inappropriate for the situation (taking off one's clothes in public, smearing feces). Especially in children, however, great care must be taken to evaluate competing explanations—the field of Mental Retardation provides ready examples. Again, the emphasis is on deterioration from a previous, more "normal" mode of functioning.

Negative Symptoms

All of the four foregoing symptoms are positive, in the sense that they are behaviors that can be observed as the *presence* of something. Negative symptoms are the customary aspects of interactive behavior that by their *absence* suggest something has been taken away. They include flattened or blunted affect (reduced range of emotional expression), lack of initiative (termed *avolition*), and reduced speech production, which can progress to the point of muteness.

Making the Diagnosis

The diagnosis of Schizophrenia can be made in three steps: (1) basic diagnosis, (2) subtype diagnosis, and (3) course. We consider these steps one at a time, using Tables 15.1 to 15.3.

Basic Diagnosis

A principal contribution of the DSMs has been to promote the careful distinguishing of Schizophrenia from other causes of psychosis. The basic criteria for Schizophrenia (see Table 15.1) clearly set forth several conditions that must be considered in a differential diagnosis of psychotic children and adolescents. We consider these further in the discussion that follows the single case vignette in this chapter.

Subtype Diagnosis

Once you have determined that the basic criteria for Schizophrenia have been fulfilled, examine the symptoms again to decide on subtype diagnosis. Table 15.2 presents, in a condensed format, the DSM-IV criteria for the five subtypes of Schizophrenia. A patient must meet the basic criteria plus the criteria for a particular subtype.

TABLE 15.1. Basic Criteria for Schizophrenia

- Symptoms. For much of at least 1 month (less, if effectively treated), the patient has had two or more of the following:
  ✓ Delusions (only one symptom required if delusion is bizarre, such as being abducted in a spaceship from the sun)
  ✓ Hallucinations (only one symptom required if hallucinations are of at least two voices talking to one another or of a voice that keeps up a running commentary on the patient's thoughts or actions)
  ✓ Speech that shows incoherence, derailment, or other disorganization
  ✓ Severely disorganized or catatonic behavior
  ✓ Any negative symptom, such as flat affect, reduced speech, or lack of volition
- Duration. For at least 6 continuous months, the patient has shown some evidence of the disorder. At least 1 month must include the symptoms of frank psychosis mentioned above. During the balance of this time (as either a prodrome or a residue of the illness), the patient must show either or both of these:
  ✓ Negative symptoms as mentioned above
  ✓ In attenuated form, at least two of the other symptoms mentioned above (e.g., deteriorating personal hygiene plus an increasing suspicion that people are talking behind one's back)
- Dysfunction. For much of this time, the disorder has materially impaired the patient's ability to work, study, socialize, or provide self-care. Children or adolescents may only fail to achieve the expected occupational, scholastic, or social level.
- Mood exclusions. Mood disorders and Schizoaffective Disorder have been ruled out, because the duration of any depressive or manic episodes that have occurred during the psychotic phase has been brief.
- Other exclusions. This disorder is not directly caused by a general medical condition or by the use of substances, including prescription medications and drugs of abuse.
- Pervasive developmental disorder exclusion. If the patient has a history of any pervasive developmental disorder (such as Autistic Disorder), only diagnose Schizophrenia if prominent hallucinations or delusions are also present for 1 month or more (less, if treated).

Course

Until 1 year after the onset of Schizophrenia, you cannot assign any course specifier. After that, classify its course according to Table 15.3.

PSYCHOTIC DIAGNOSES OTHER THAN SCHIZOPHRENIA

The DSM-IV criteria for Schizophrenia have intentionally been made strict to prevent misdiagnosis. A number of other diagnoses in the psychosis section of DSM-IV offer options for psychotic patients who do not fully meet the DSM-IV criteria for schizophrenia. Because several of these disorders are seen in young patients even less often than Schizophrenia itself is, we provide full criteria for Schizophreniform Disorder only. James Morrison's *DSM-IV Made Easy* (see Appendix 1 for a reference) provides criteria sets for the other disorders.

TABLE 15.2. Criteria for the Subtypes of Schizophrenia

Subtype	Patient must:	Patient must not:

295.30 Paranoid Type	• Be preoccupied with at least one delusion or with frequent auditory hallucinations	• Have *any* of the following:
		  • Disorganized speech
		  • Disorganized behavior
		  • Affect that is flat or inappropriate
		  • Catatonic behavior

295.10 Disorganized Type	• Have *all* of the following:
	  • Disorganized behavior
	  • Disorganized speech
	  • Affect that is flat or inappropriate
		• Meet criteria for Catatonic Type

295.20 Catatonic Type	• Have at least two catatonic symptoms that predominate:
	  ✓ Stupor or motor immobility (catalepsy or waxy flexibility)
	  ✓ Hyperactivity that has no apparent purpose and is not influenced by external stimuli
	  ✓ Mutism or marked negativism
	  ✓ Peculiar behaviors such as posturing, stereotypies, mannerisms, or grimacing
	  ✓ Echopraxia or echolalia	

295.90 Undifferentiated Type	• Meet basic criteria for Schizophrenia (Table 15.1)	• Meet criteria for Paranoid, Disorganized, or Catatonic Type

295.60 Residual	• Have once met criteria for Catatonic, Disorganized, Paranoid, or Undifferentiated Type
	• Still be ill, as indicated by *either* of the following:
	  ✓ Negative symptoms, such as flattened affect, reduced speech output, or lack of volition
	  ✓ An attenuated form of *at least* two characteristic symptoms of Schizophrenia, such as strange beliefs (related to delusions), distorted perceptions or illusions (hallucinations), odd speech (disorganized speech), or peculiarities of behavior (disorganized behavior)
		• Currently have any of the following:
		  ✓ Catatonic behavior
		  ✓ Delusions
		  ✓ Hallucinations
		  ✓ Disorganized speech or behavior

Disorders That Are Similar to Schizophrenia

295.40 Schizophreniform Disorder

Early clinicians observed that patients whose psychotic illnesses begin gradually often do not recover; those whose illnesses begin more abruptly are more likely to recover completely. Thus, these latter patients meet all the criteria for Schizophrenia except time—they have been ill more than 30 days and fewer than 180— and are diagnosed with Schizophreniform Disorder. This diagnosis, intended as a place holder, keeps clinicians thinking about their patients until additional time sorts out the eventual prognosis, which is usually either Schizophrenia or a mood

TABLE 15.3. Course of Schizophrenia

	Continuous	Single Episode in Partial Remission	Episodic With Interepisode Residual Symptoms	Episodic With No Interepisode Residual Symptoms	Single Episode in Full Remission	Other or Unspecified
Number of episodes	One	One	Multiple	Multiple	One	—
"A" symptoms	Continuously present	Some clinically important symptoms remain		No clinically important symptoms remain		—
If prominent negative symptoms	Add: With Prominent Negative Symptoms			Not applicable		—

disorder. This diagnosis is probably made far too seldom in children and adults alike. Table 15.4 presents the criteria for Schizophreniform Disorder.

298.8 Brief Psychotic Disorder

Patients with Brief Psychotic Disorder have had at least one "A" criterion symptom but have been ill less than 1 month. As with Schizophreniform Disorder, time is needed to see whether they recover or go on to develop schizophrenia.

295.70 Schizoaffective Disorder

As currently defined by DSM-IV, patients with Schizoaffective Disorder have had symptoms of Schizophrenia for at least 1 month; during the same time span, they have had also prominent symptoms of mania or depression. This diagnosis is rarely justified in children, but DSM-IV notes that its onset can occur in adolescence, and young adulthood is said to be the typical period of onset.

Disorders with Delusions

297.1 Delusional Disorder

As the name suggests, patients with Delusional Disorder have only one "A" list symptom: delusions. Delusional Disorder is typically diagnosed in middle to late adulthood, but an occasional case has been seen in younger patients.

297.3 Shared Psychotic Disorder

In Shared Psychotic Disorder, a relative or other close associate develops a psychotic disorder, and the symptoms are imitated by the patient. An older child

TABLE 15.4. Criteria for Schizophreniform Disorder

- Symptoms. For much of at least 1 month (less if effectively treated), the patient has had two or more of the following:
  ✓ Delusions (only one symptom required if delusion is bizarre, such as being abducted in a spaceship from the sun)
  ✓ Hallucinations (only one symptom required if hallucinations are of at least two voices talking to one another or of a voice that keeps up a running commentary on the patient's thoughts or actions)
  ✓ Speech that shows incoherence, derailment, or other disorganization
  ✓ Severely disorganized or catatonic behavior
  ✓ Any negative symptom, such as flat affect, reduced speech, or lack of volition
- Including prodromal, active, and residual phases, an episode of the illness has lasted at least 1 month but not longer than 6 months.
- Mood disorders and Schizoaffective Disorder have been ruled out, because the duration of any depressive or manic episodes that have occurred during the psychotic phase has been brief.
- Other exclusions. This disorder is not directly caused by a general medical condition or by the use of substances, including prescription medications and drugs of abuse.

A statement of prognosis should be added to the diagnosis:

With Good Prognostic Features (two or more of the following):
  ✓ Actual psychotic features begin within 4 weeks of the first noticeable change in the patient's functioning or behavior.
  ✓ The patient is confused or perplexed when most psychotic.
  ✓ Premorbid social and job (school) functioning are good.
  ✓ Affect is neither blunt nor flattened.
Without Good Prognostic Features (none or one of the foregoing)

If the diagnosis is made without waiting for recovery (which is often the case), append the term "Provisional."

---

or adolescent with a psychotic parent will occasionally develop this disorder, which is sometimes called *folie à deux*. It may also be seen in siblings, especially twins.

Other Psychotic Disorders

Psychotic Disorder Due to a General Medical Condition

Many medical and neurological illnesses can cause psychotic symptoms; see Table 13.1 in Chapter 13 for the criteria for classifying such symptoms as Psychotic Disorder Due to a General Medical Condition. (Table 13.1 also gives criteria for Catatonic Disorder Due to a General Medical Condition, which is not included in DSM-IV's section on psychotic disorders.)

Substance-Induced Psychotic Disorder

During either intoxication or withdrawal, a variety of substances can cause psychotic symptoms. In children and adolescents, it is important always to consider the possibility that psychotic symptoms have been caused by a substance of misuse, especially when the symptoms begin suddenly in an otherwise normal young person. Table 14.5 in Chapter 14 gives the criteria for Substance-Induced Psychotic Disorder, and Table 14.6 provides guidance in coding this by substance class and symptom type.

298.9 Psychotic Disorder Not Otherwise Specified

A strong minority of psychotic children and adolescents may fit none of the above DSM-IV categories. They should be provisionally diagnosed with Psychotic Disorder Not Otherwise Specified, and should be carefully observed for further developments.

DIFFERENTIAL DIAGNOSIS OF PSYCHOTIC DISORDERS IN YOUNG PATIENTS

Even the best criteria currently available can result in misdiagnosis. Longitudinal studies reveal that a large minority of children who later turn out to have Schizophrenia have been misdiagnosed as having a mood disorder; conversely, many children diagnosed as having Schizophrenia later develop mood disorders. When a child falls ill with psychosis, the clinical task is to obtain the relevant information necessary to allow a differential diagnosis. This information then provides the baseline for later follow-up and reevaluation, as in the case of Christa.

Christa

"She's always reminded me of her Aunt Pat, my other daughter." Christa's grandmother had given this history to the clinician. "Pat's still institutionalized, and Christa's mother is in jail."

Like her Aunt Pat, Christa had been a difficult child. As a baby she had been fussy and irritable, often crying with colic until late in the evening. When at the age of 18 months she still had not spoken her first word, she was taken for evaluation. A psychometrist estimated her Full Scale IQ at 95; she was diagnosed as having Pervasive Developmental Disorder Not Otherwise Specified. Her condition improved with remediation, and by her third year she was speaking sentences.

Even before she talked much, Christa appeared to socialize well; she enjoyed playing with other children and began kindergarten just after she turned 6. Because she was small for her age, she did not appear out of place, and she progressed normally through the first five grades. Her grades, though only average, did not come without effort. On her report card, her fifth-grade teacher observed: "Christa works hard and takes pride in producing the best work she can."

When Christa was 11½, her menses began; shortly after that, she complained to her grandmother of anxiety. She didn't know why she felt bad—only that her heart beat too hard and she felt "skittery." After 2 months, she started skipping classes. Several weeks of hit-or-miss attendance earned her an appointment with the guidance counselor, to whom she confided that she was frightened of a man she had seen lurking near the campus. The assistant principal investigated the story, but could not corroborate it. Despite reassurance, and despite her teacher's meeting her a block from the school grounds on several mornings, Christa would not be comforted. She complained of aches and pains; her grandmother took her to the pediatrician, who diagnosed school phobia and reassured them that she would be fine.

But Christa was not fine. Her anxiety attacks continued, and she insisted even more strongly that she was being followed. One morning, about 4 months after her first anxiety attack, she matter-of-factly told her grandmother that her face in the bathroom mirror seemed to have melted; that afternoon she was admitted to the hospital.

The admission workup revealed a thin, slightly built girl with rather scraggly hair whose physical exam, despite her sallow complexion, was completely normal. She denied feeling depressed and showed little emotion as she retold the stories of the melting reflection and the man who followed her. She felt "sure" that these events were real and not imagined. Moreover, she now admitted that for several weeks she had heard a sound just behind her ear like "crickets chirping." She thought it was trying to tell her something, but she could not make out the message.

Christa remained hospitalized for 3 months while being given trials of several neuroleptic drugs. None eliminated her symptoms, but a moderate dose of haloperidol relieved all but the faintest chirping remnants of her auditory hallucination. Although she no longer complained spontaneously of a lurking stranger, when questioned closely she would admit that he still might be there. In the hospital classroom, she sat in one corner and spent much of her time staring out the window at an empty bird feeder; her grades drifted into the C– and D range. Throughout her stay, as upon admission, she remained able to convey her thoughts in clear, goal-directed sentences.

Evaluation of Christa

The first step would be to determine whether Christa met the "A" criterion—the first bulleted item in Table 15.1. If we consider the beginning of her illness to be when she first complained of anxiety, she had been ill for about 4 months when she was hospitalized. For at least 2 months she had been delusional (a persistent idea of a man lurking about outside). For several weeks she had been having hallucinations—the chirping (auditory) and, more recently, the melting of her reflection (visual). In addition, she probably also qualified for the negative symptom of flat affect (she showed little emotion). The clinician carefully determined that Christa's beliefs were held firmly enough to qualify as delusions and hallucinations, not illusions or fantasies. She thus easily fulfilled the "A" criterion.

Christa had no prominent **mood** symptoms; if anything, as noted above, her affect was bland as she described her face melting. (However, mood symptoms are common, even usual, in children with Schizophrenia.) Her physical health was evidently good; there was no evidence of a **general medical condition** that could account for her symptoms. There is no mention of **substance use** in the vignette, though her clinician would need to press the point in additional interviews. Although she had been ill for less than the 6 months required for a diagnosis of Schizophrenia, the duration was just right for Schizophreniform Disorder.

When Schizophreniform Disorder is diagnosed, DSM-IV asks for a statement of prognosis, based on four pieces of historical and cross-sectional information (see Table 15.4). Of the Good Prognostic Features, Christa had only one: Her premorbid functioning in school had been reasonably good. However, her affect was blunted; she was never described as being confused or perplexed; and her psychotic features (delusions) apparently did not begin until she had had anxiety attacks for 2 months. Until such time as she recovered (or subsequent course necessitated a change of diagnosis), the diagnosis would have to be stated as "Provisional." Her working Axis I diagnosis at admission would therefore be Schizophreniform Disorder, Without Good Prognostic Features (Provisional).

For 3 months after her admission, Christa was treated with a variety of medications. Despite the best efforts of her treatment team, she remained psychotic even at discharge. (Had she recovered within 6 months of onset, the diagnosis would have remained as above, without the "Provisional" designation.) But as she passed the 6-month mark, time necessitated a change of diagnosis. To determine whether she would qualify for a discharge diagnosis of Schizophrenia, let us reexamine the basic criteria in Table 15.1.

- *Symptoms.* Of course, the fact that she once met the "A" criterion would not change.
- *Duration.* She had now been ill for longer than 6 months. (Christa was still psychotic at discharge, but another patient could qualify for the 6-month duration criterion by having only residual nonpsychotic symptoms of Schizophrenia, such as the negative symptom of flat affect.)
- *Dysfunction.* For children, the statement of dysfunction requires only a failure to achieve at expected scholastic levels. From the vignette, Christa's school attendance had been markedly affected; her grades actually seemed to decline during her 3 months in the hospital.
- *Mood, substance use, and general medical condition exclusions.* These have been discussed above.
- *Pervasive developmental disorder exclusion.* When small, Christa had been diagnosed as having Pervasive Developmental Disorder Not Otherwise Specified, but her current symptoms could not reasonably be ascribed to it. As required by this criterion, her psychotic symptoms had lasted longer than 1 month.

So, at her discharge from the hospital, Christa fully met the criteria for Schizophrenia. But what type? For that, we must consult the subtype diagnostic criteria given in Table 15.2. Although she was preoccupied with delusions and hallucinations, she did not qualify for the Paranoid Type because she had flat affect. She had none of the motor symptoms needed for the Catatonic Type. Despite her flattened affect and some bizarre behavior (turning away from others in the classroom), her clear and coherent speech disqualified her for the Disorganized Type. She could not have the Residual Type because her delusions and hallucinations were still prominent. The only remaining possibility would be the Undifferentiated Type—which is no more descriptive than the basic criteria.

The final diagnostic task would be to consider the course of her psychosis (Table 15.3). Even at her discharge, Christa had been ill too briefly to qualify for any statement as to the course of her psychosis. But after another 5–6 months, if we assume that her symptoms continued, she could be given a course specifier of Continuous. With improvement, this specifier could change again later. Although many psychotic patients have long-standing personality problems, none of the evidence cited suggests that this was the case with Christa, so she would not rate an Axis II diagnosis.

Her complete diagnosis at discharge would be as follows:

Axis I	295.90	Schizophrenia, Undifferentiated Type
Axis II	V71.09	No diagnosis
Axis III		None
Axis IV		None
Axis V	GAF = 35	(on admission to hospital)
	GAF = 60	(on discharge)

Assessing Psychotic Disorders

General Suggestions

Even when they cooperate, children with psychosis present a special challenge. For one thing, childhood Schizophrenia is so uncommon that clinicians are unlikely to suspect it unless the symptoms are florid. Especially when it is early in the course of illness, such a diagnosis is likely to be confounded by symptoms that may seem more typical of other conditions—mood disorders, ADHD, anxiety disorders, accidental or intentional drug ingestion, febrile illnesses, and others.

All of this underscores the importance of a twofold approach to assessing psychosis. To begin with, allow the patient plenty of time to broach and freely discuss any topics that may be causing stress, anxiety, confusion, or mere curiosity. Later in the interview, specifically request information about unusual experiences or content of thought: "Have you ever heard [seen] things other kids couldn't? What sort of things?" "Have you had thoughts that scare you or worry you?" The answers, combined with information derived from direct observation, will reveal a picture of psychosis in children that is not so very different from that in adults.

Hallucinations

Auditory hallucinations tend to be brief words or phrases. As is true with adults, they may be either friendly (e.g., the voice of God, Jesus, or the Virgin Mary) or hostile (e.g., a devil "says bad words"). The voices may give orders: A refrigerator tells the patient to "take a drink"; the voice of a dead baby sister says, "Come to Heaven"; an angel suggests that the child go play outside. When visual hallucinations are identified, they may take the form of monsters; tactile hallucinations may be reported as being "touched by the devil." Attributes of hallucinations to pursue in the interview include source, location, clarity, cause, number, identity ("Whose voices are they?"), subject ("Do they talk about you?"), and effect on the patient ("How does this make you feel?"). Similar questions will apply to hallucinations of the other senses. Remember that many young children, especially those who are socially deprived, have imaginary playmates who keep them company. Although about three-fourths of children with Schizophrenia have hallucinations, it is crucial to differentiate between a child with an active imagination (or a different mental disorder) and one who is truly psychotic.

Delusions

Though delusions are usually less well organized (systematized) in children and adolescents than in adults, they are of the same varieties: persecutory (a boy felt commanded by the devil to jump off a cliff, a girl's Wheaties were poisoned); grandiose (an eighth-grader was "the homeboy Jesus Christ"); referential (a seventh-grader felt that classmates pointed and laughed at her); and bizarre (a boy believed that he was growing hair and becoming a German shepherd). By definition, a delusion can only be diagnosed if it is firmly held and is contrary to the beliefs of a patient's culture. Assess a delusion by asking how long it has been held, what actions have been taken or are contemplated as a result, how the patient interprets its meaning, and whether it is mood-congruent (e.g., a depressed boy believes he is being punished).

Thought Disorder

Although complete incoherence is unusual, psychotic children may become distractible, dropping words from sentences or leaving sentences unfinished. Speech may appear pressured. Identifying aspects of formal thought disorder, such as reduced amount of speech, illogical speech, or neologisms, may be facilitated by getting a patient to tell a story.

Behavior

Although frank catatonia is rare, all manner of unusual and even bizarre actions may be noted—mannerisms, poor hygiene, sleeping in strange places (such as under the bed). Many authorities have noted that children who will later develop Schizophrenia have more behavioral (especially anti-social) symptoms than do other children.

Affect

Although psychotic children may react with fear to delusions or hallucinations, affect is more often blunted or flat. Expression may be blank, stare fixed; there is an absence of normal lilt (prosody) to the voice. Relatives may provide valuable historical information about these and other negative symptoms, such as loss of motivation.

Developmental Factors

Younger (school-age) children with Schizophrenia tend to develop pretty much the same symptoms as do adolescents and adults. Of course, as noted above, the content of their delusions and hallucinations will depend on their developmental stage. The prognosis for recovery tends to be worse for those patients who develop psychotic symptoms when they are very young. Because children with very-early-onset Schizophrenia grow up with their symptoms, they may regard them as ego-syntonic. If so, they may not voluntarily discuss them with parents or teachers, thus limiting collateral information available to interviewers.

| Mood Disorders

Quick Guide to the Mood Disorders

DSM-IV uses three groups of criteria sets to diagnose mental problems related to mood: (1) mood episodes, (2) mood disorders, and (3) specifiers describing most recent episode and recurrent course.

Mood Episodes

A *mood episode* refers to any period of time when a patient feels abnormally happy or sad. Mood episodes are the building blocks from which many of the codable mood disorders are constructed. By itself, no mood episode is a codable diagnosis. Most mood disorder patients will have one or more of these four types of episode:

Major Depressive Episode. For at least 2 weeks, the patient feels depressed (or cannot enjoy life) and has problems with eating and sleeping, guilt feelings, loss of energy, trouble concentrating, and thoughts about death (Table 16.1).

Manic Episode. For at least 1 week, the child feels elated (sometimes, only irritable) and may be grandiose, talkative, hyperactive, and distractible. Bad judgment leads to marked social or work impairment; patients must often be hospitalized (Table 16.1).

Mixed Episode. For as long as 1 week, the child has fulfilled the symptomatic criteria for both a Manic Episode and a Major Depressive Episode (Table 16.1).

Hypomanic Episode. This is similar to a Manic Episode, but it is briefer, milder, and does not require hospitalization (Table 16.1).

Mood Disorders

A *mood disorder* is a pattern of illness due to an abnormal mood. Nearly every child or adolescent with a mood disorder experiences depression at some time, but some also have highs of mood. Many, but not all, mood disorders are diagnosed on the basis of a mood episode.

Depressive Disorders

Major Depressive Disorder. This disorder consists of one or more Major Depressive Episodes, but no Manic or Hypomanic Episodes (Table 16.2).

Dysthymic Disorder. This form of depression is less severe but lasts much longer than Major Depressive Disorder; there are no high phases (Table 16.5).

Depressive Disorder Not Otherwise Specified. Use this category only when a patient has depressive symptoms that do not meet the criteria for the depressive diagnoses above or for any other diagnosis in which depression is a feature (p. 326).

Bipolar Disorders

Bipolar I Disorder. There must be at least one Manic Episode; most Bipolar I patients have also had a Major Depressive Episode (Table 16.2).

Bipolar II Disorder. This diagnosis requires at least one Hypomanic Episode and one Major Depressive Episode (Table 16.2).

Cyclothymic Disorder. This disorder involves repeated mood swings, but none are severe enough to be called Major Depressive Episodes or Manic Episodes (Table 16.5).

Bipolar Disorder Not Otherwise Specified. Use this category only when a patient has bipolar symptoms that do not fulfill the criteria for the bipolar diagnoses above (p. 332).

Other Mood Disorders

Mood Disorder Due to a General Medical Condition. Either highs or lows of mood can be caused by various types of physical ailments (Table 13.1 and p. 333).

Substance-Induced Mood Disorder. Alcohol or other psychoactive substances can cause highs or lows of mood that do not meet criteria for any of the above-listed episodes or disorders (Table 14.5 and p. 333).

Mood Disorder Not Otherwise Specified. Use this category only for patients whose mood symptoms do not fit neatly into *any* of the mood disorder categories listed above (p. 333).

Other Causes of Depressive and Manic Symptoms

Depressive or manic symptoms are specifically mentioned in the criteria for cognitive disorders (dementia with depressed mood), Adjustment Disorder With Depressed Mood, personality disorders, and the V-code for Bereavement. Depression can accompany many other mental disorders, including Schizophrenia, the eating disorders, Somatization Disorder, and Gender Identity Disorder. Mood symptoms are also likely in patients with an anxiety disorder (especially Panic Disorder, Obsessive–Compulsive Disorder, Social Phobia, and Posttraumatic Stress Disorder).

Specifiers

Once a mood disorder diagnosis has been made, two sets of specifiers can be added to describe (1) the most recent episode (With Atypical Features, With Catatonic Features, With Melancholic Features, With Postpartum Onset) and (2) the overall course of the mood disorder (With or Without Full Interepisode Recovery, With Rapid Cycling, With Seasonal Pattern). Their criteria are given in Table 16.3.

INTRODUCTION

Although there are many impediments to the diagnosis of mood disorders in children, we have finally overcome the biggest of them—the once-held myth that childhood, happy and inviolate, cannot sustain depression or mania. Even so, there remain other obstacles to evaluation, most notably the difficulty of evaluating the feelings of patients who communicate poorly. Infants, of course, can only be observed. Even in preschoolers, mood must largely be inferred from behavior. Very young children, for whom depression and anxiety are not well differentiated, may express depression through irritability, somatic symptoms (aches and pains), or school refusal. Manic symptoms may be mistaken for other disorders, such as ADHD. As children grow older, their mood symptoms increasingly resemble those of adult patients. While awaiting studies that will better discriminate the symptoms of mood disorders in early life, we can continue to be guided by these features:

- When you suspect either depression or mania in young patients, look for mood disorders in close relatives. (A strong family history is even more likely in depressed juveniles than in depressed adults.)
- Keep an open mind about causation. What we know now suggests that depression in early life is multifactorial, so watch out for events that could serve as environmental precipitants.
- Even more than in adults, recurrence is the rule; most children and adolescents who are so severely ill that they need inpatient care will return to the hospital within 2 years.

DSM-IV adopts a building-block approach to the diagnosis of mood disorders. With mood episodes (Major Depressive, Manic, Hypomanic, and Mixed), each of which can have a variety of modifiers based on symptoms and course of illness, dozens of mood disorders are possible. No one knows how many of these actually occur in children and adolescents, and only a handful have received much attention in the mental health literature. These include Major Depressive Disorder (Single Episode or Recurrent), Bipolar I Disorder (Single Manic Episode or Most Recent Episode Manic or Depressive), and Dysthymic Disorder. In addition, two conditions with mood symptoms that are not mood disorders per se have received some attention (Adjustment Disorder With Depressed Mood, and the V-code for Bereavement).

Clearly, the various mood episodes and mood disorders constitute a complex set of diagnostic possibilities. To provide a guide to this complexity, we begin by outlining a step-by-step approach to diagnosing and coding the mood disorders, together with a set of tables giving the criteria for the mood episodes, mood disorders, and specifiers in condensed format. We then discuss the depressive disorders, the bipolar disorders, and (briefly) the other mood disorders in turn, with case vignettes illustrating the process of differential diagnosis and coding in the first two disorder groups.

A STEP-BY-STEP APPROACH TO DIAGNOSING AND CODING MOOD DISORDERS

The following steps provide a logical approach to the diagnosis of mood disorders in children and adolescents.

1. Using the criteria in Table 16.1, identify the current and any past mood episodes: Major Depressive, Manic, Hypomanic, and Mixed. Mood epi-

TABLE 16.1. Criteria for Mood Episodes

Major Depressive	Manic	Mixed	Hypomanic
• Nearly every day in same 2 weeks, there has been a definite change from patient's usual functioning—five or more symptoms, including *depressed mood* or *decreased interest:* ✓ Most of day, depressed mood or appearance (or irritable mood for children and adolescents) ✓ Most of day, notably decreased interest or pleasure ✓ Marked weight or appetite loss or gain; children may fail to gain weight as expected ✓ Excess or insufficient sleep ✓ Speeded or slowed psychomotor activity ✓ Fatigue or energy loss ✓ Sense of being worthless, or inappropriate sense of guilt (not just about being sick) ✓ Indecision or trouble thinking or concentrating ✓ Repeated thoughts about death (not fear of dying) or suicide, or suicide attempt	• For at least 1 week (less, if hospitalized), patient's mood is abnormally and persistently high, irritable, or expansive. • During this time, persistence of three or more (four or more if mood only irritable): ✓ Grandiosity or exaggerated self-esteem ✓ Reduced need for sleep ✓ Increased talkativeness ✓ Flight of ideas or racing thoughts ✓ Easy distractibility ✓ Speeded psychomotor activity or increased goal-directed activity (social, sexual, work, or school) ✓ Poor judgment (spending sprees, sexual adventures)	• Patient has fulfilled symptom criteria for both Major Depressive and Manic Episodes nearly every day for a week or more.	• For 4+ days, patient exhibits a distinct, sustained mood that is elevated, expansive, or irritable and different from normal mood. • During this time, persistence of three or more (four or more if mood only irritable): ✓ Grandiosity or exaggerated self-esteem ✓ Reduced need for sleep ✓ Increased talkativeness ✓ Flight of ideas or racing thoughts ✓ Easy distractibility ✓ Speeded psychomotor activity or increased goal-directed activity (social, sexual, work, or school) ✓ Poor judgment (spending sprees, sexual adventures) • There is a distinct change from usual functioning. • Others notice change in mood and functioning.
• Symptoms result in clinically important distress or impair school, work, social, or other functioning. • Criteria for Mixed Episode are not fulfilled.	• Symptoms result in clinically important distress, impair school, work, or social functioning; cause psychosis; or require hospitalization	• Symptoms include psychotic features; require hospitalization; or impair school, work, or social functioning.	• Symptoms do *not* markedly impair school, work, or social functioning or cause hospitalization; no features of psychosis.

(continued)

TABLE 16.1 (*continued*)

Major Depressive	Manic	Mixed	Hypomanic
• Unless symptoms are severe, episode has not begun within 2 months of loss of a loved one.	• An episode precipitated by somatic therapy (electroconvulsive therapy, antidepressants, or bright light) cannot be used as evidence of Bipolar I or II Disorder.		

• Symptoms are not directly caused by a general medical condition or by the use of substances, including prescription medications and drug abuse.

Fifth-digit severity code applies to Major Depressive, Mixed, or Hypomanic Episode):
 .x1 Mild: Symptoms barely meet criteria.
 .x2 Moderate: Symptoms are intermediate between Mild and Severe.
 .x3 Severe Without Psychotic Features: Many symptoms or severe symptoms.
 .x4 Severe With Psychotic Features: Hallucinations or delusions.
     Mood-Congruent: Consistent with themes typical of the episode.
     Mood-Incongruent: Not consistent with themes typical of the episode.
 .x5 In Partial Remission: Symptoms formerly met full criteria, but now do not.
 .x6 In Full Remission: No symptoms for 2 months.
 .x0 Unspecified

For Major Depressive Episode: Specify chronic (if full-criteria have been met throughout past 2 years at least)

sodes are not themselves coded; they serve as building blocks for most actual mood disorder diagnoses. If your patient's symptoms do not fulfill the requirements for a mood episode, skip to step 7.

2. Use the building blocks to select the appropriate type of mood disorder. Table 16.2 gives criteria for all of the mood disorders that are based on mood episodes. If the diagnosis is Bipolar II Disorder (at least one Hypomanic Episode and no Manic Episodes), the fourth and fifth digits are already assigned, so skip to step 5.

3. If step 2 has yielded a diagnosis of Bipolar I Disorder or Major Depressive Disorder, examine the course of your patient's illness to select the appropriate fourth digit (Table 16.4). Major Depressive Disorder will be either Single Episode or Recurrent. Bipolar I Disorder will be one of these subtypes: Single Manic Episode, or Most Recent Episode Manic, Depressed, Hypomanic, Mixed, or Unspecified.

4. Choose the appropriate level of severity from Table 16.1 when the current or most recent episode is Major Depressive, Manic, or Mixed. (Because Hypomanic Episode is inherently mild, it requires no special severity criteria.) When a Major Depressive Episode has lasted continuously for 2 years or more, apply the Chronic specifier as well.

5. Although other episode specifiers are not often encountered in children, add here the wording of any that apply (see Tables 16.3 and 16.4). No special numbers apply; the verbiage is simply strung out after the main diagnosis, separated by commas.

6. Many children have a recurrence of a mood disorder within a year or two of the index episode. Therefore, again inspect Tables 16.3 and 16.4 for any course specifiers that may apply.

7. If your patient does not meet criteria for any mood episode, consider the following possible mood disorders: Dysthymic Disorder, Cyclothymic Disorder, Mood Disorder Due to a General Medical Condition, or Substance-Induced Mood Disorder. Each of them has its own set of criteria independent of any mood episode, but only Dysthymic Disorder has been often described in children. Table 16.5 gives criteria for Dysthymic and Cyclothymic Disorders; Tables 13.1 and 14.5 give criteria for Mood Disorder Due to a General Medical Condition and Substance-Induced Mood Disorder, respectively. (Note that one episode specifier, With Atypical Features, can be applied to Dysthymic Disorder; no episode or course specifiers apply to the other diagnoses.)

8. If none of the categories above seems appropriate, consider Depressive Disorder Not Otherwise Specified, Bipolar Disorder Not Otherwise Specified, or Mood Disorder Not Otherwise Specified.

DEPRESSIVE DISORDERS

Differential Diagnosis of Depressive Disorders in Young Patients

Although children, adolescents, and adults experience some depressive symptoms differently, their core depressive symptoms are so similar that, with slight modifications, the same DSM-IV criteria are used to diagnose depressive disorders at all ages. The one core symptom that may be different in children or adolescents is an important one, for it helps describe the mood abnormality itself. An adult must feel *depressed* (or express loss of pleasure), whereas a child or adolescent may express or demonstrate a mood that is either *depressed or irritable*.

For a Major Depressive Episode (Table 16.1), a patient must experience either low or irritable mood or loss of interest for most of at least 2 consecutive weeks. In addition, the patient must have four other symptoms from a list that includes appetite or weight change (for children, a failure to gain weight), problems with sleep (too little *or* too much), speeded or slowed psychomotor

TABLE 16.2. Diagnosing Mood Disorders Based on the Mood Episodes

	Major Depressive Disorder		Bipolar I and II Disorders						
	Single Episode	Recurrent	Bipolar I, Single Manic Episode	Bipolar I, Most Recent Episode Manic	Bipolar I, Most Recent Episode Depressed	Bipolar I, Most Recent Episode Mixed	Bipolar I, Most Recent Episode Hypomanic	Bipolar I, Most Recent Episode Unspecified	Bipolar II[a]
	• One Major Depressive Episode.	• Two or more Major Depressive Episodes.	• One Manic Episode, no Major Depressive Episodes.	• Most recent episode is Manic.	• Most recent episode is Major Depressive.	• Most recent episode is Mixed.	• Most recent episode is Hypomanic.	• Except for duration, patient recently met criteria for Major Depressive, Manic, Mixed, or Hypomanic Episode.	• One or more Major Depressive Episodes • One or more Hypomanic Episodes.
				• One or more previous major Depressive, Manic, or Mixed Episodes.	• One or more previous Manic or Mixed Episodes.	• One or more previous Major Depressive, Manic, or Mixed Episodes.	• One or more previous Manic or Mixed Episodes.	• One or more previous Manic or Mixed Episodes.	
	• No manic, mixed, or hypomanic episodes. If symptoms ever appear manic-, mixed-, or hypomanic-like, all are precipitated by treatment (antidepressants, electroconvulsive therapy, bright light)							• Symptoms are not caused by a general medical condition or by use of substances.	• No Manic or Mixed Episodes.

- Symptoms cause distress or impair school, work, social, or other functioning.

- Schizoaffective Disorder doesn't explain episodes better, and they aren't superimposed on Schizophrenia, Schizophreniform Disorder, Delusional Disorder, or Psychotic Disorder Not Otherwise Specified.

[a]For Bipolar II Disorder, specify whether most recent episode is Hypomanic or Depressed. See Tables 16.3 and 16.4 for other specifiers for this and other disorders.

TABLE 16.3. Criteria for Mood Specifiers

Specifiers for current or most recent episodes[a]					Specifiers for course of recurrent episodes	
With Atypical Features	With Melancholic Features	With Catatonic Features	With Postpartum Onset	With Seasonal Pattern	With Rapid Cycling	With/Without Full Interepisode Recovery
• For most recent 2 weeks of a Major Depressive Episode or predominating in most recent 2 years of Dysthymic Disorder: • Experiences mood reactivity (improved mood with something good, e.g., presence of friends). • At least two of the following: ✓ Increased appetite or weight ✓ Excess sleeping ✓ Sensation of heaviness in arms or legs ✓ Impairment of work or social relations by long-standing sensitivity to rejection—not limited to periods of depression • Patient does not meet criteria for With Melancholic Features or With Catatonic Features.	• When Major Depressive symptoms are worst, patient either or both: ✓ Loses pleasure in nearly all activities ✓ Feels no better when something good happens • Three or more of these: ✓ Perceives depressed mood as different from grief ✓ Diurnal variation of mood (mood consistently worse in a.m.) ✓ Terminal insomnia ✓ Markedly speeded or slowed psychomotor activity ✓ Appetite or weight loss ✓ Inappropriate or excessive guilt feelings	• Two or more of following: ✓ Immobility or stupor ✓ Purposeless hyperactivity ✓ Mutism or negativism ✓ Posturing, stereotypies, mannerisms, or grimacing ✓ Echolalia or echopraxia	• An episode begins within four weeks of childbirth.	• Major Depressive Episodes regularly begin at one season of the year. • Complete recovery or change of polarity occurs regularly during one season. • Seasonal changes have occurred in each of the previous 2 years, during which no nonseasonal Major Depressive Episodes have occurred. • Over patient's lifetime, seasonal Major Depressive Episodes outnumber nonseasonal episodes.	• In past year, patient has had four or more episodes that meet criteria for Major Depressive, Manic, Mixed, or Hypomanic Episode. • Boundaries of these episodes are indicated by remission or a switch between high and low.	• With: There is a full remission between the two most recent episodes. • Without: There is no full remission between the two most recent episodes.

[a]DSM-IV includes the specifiers for severity and chronicity with the episode specifiers presented here. In this book, the severity and chronicity specifiers are given in Table 16.1.

TABLE 16.4. Code Numbers and Application of Specifiers for Mood Disorder

Code number and name	Episode specifiers						Course specifiers		
	Severity	Chronicity	Atypical	Catatonic	Melancholic	Postpartum	Interepisode Recovery	Seasonal Pattern	Rapid Cycling
296.2x Major Depressive, Single Episode	×	×	×	×	×	×			
296.3x Major Depressive Recurrent	×	×	×	×	×	×	×	×	
296.0x Bipolar I, Single Manic Episode	×			×		×			
296.5x Bipolar I, Most Recent Episode Depressed	×	×	×	×	×	×	×	×	×
296.4x Bipolar I, Most Recent Episode Manic	×			×		×	×	×	×
296.6x Bipolar I, Most Recent Episode Mixed	×			×		×	×	×	×
296.40 Bipolar I, Most Recent Episode Hypomanic							×	×	×
296.7 Bipolar I, Most Recent Episode Unspecified							×	×	×
296.89 Bipolar II (Specify: Hypomanic or Depressed)	×[a]	×[a]	×[a]	×[a]	×[a]	×[a]	×	×	×
300.4 Dysthymic			×						
301.13 Cyclothymic									

Note. Adapted with permission from the *Diagnostic and Statistical Manual of Mental Disorders* (4th ed., pp. 376, 388). Copyright 1994 American Psychiatric Association.

This table can help you arrange the names, codes, and specifiers for mood disorders. Start reading from left to right in the table, putting in any specifiers that apply in the order you come to them. This applies to the two forms of Major Depressive Disorder; all forms of Bipolar I Disorder; Bipolar II Disorder; and Dysthymic Disorder. Note that no qualifier applies to Cyclothymic Disorder. Substance-Induced Mood Disorder and Mood Disorder Due to a General Medical Condition have their own lists of specifiers (see Tables 14.5 and 13.1, respectively).

[a]If depressed.

320

TABLE 16.5 Criteria for Dysthymic and Cyclothymic Disorders

Dysthymic Disorder	Cyclothymic Disorder
• Most days for 1+ years (2 for adults), the patient reports depressed mood or appears depressed to others for most of the day. (In children and adolescents, the abnormal mood may be one of irritability.)	• For at least 1 year (2 for adults), the patient has had many periods of hypomanic symptoms, as well as many periods of low mood that *don't* fulfill criteria for Major Depressive Episode.
• When depressed, the patient has two or more of these: ✓ Decreased or increased appetite ✓ Decreased or increased sleep ✓ Fatigue or low energy ✓ Poor self-image ✓ Reduced concentration or indecisiveness ✓ Hopeless feelings	
• During this period, these symptoms are never absent longer than 2 consecutive months.	• The longest the patient has been free of mood swings during this period is 2 consecutive months.
• During the *first* year (first two for adults) of this disorder, the patient has not had a Major Depressive Episode.	• During the *first* year (first 2 years for adults) of this disorder, the patient has not fulfilled criteria for a Manic, Mixed, or Major Depressive Episode.
• The patient has had no Manic, Hypomanic, or Mixed Episodes.	
• The patient has never fulfilled criteria for Cyclothymic Disorder.	
• The disorder does not exist *solely* in the context of a chronic psychosis (such as Schizophrenia or Delusional Disorder).	• Schizoaffective Disorder doesn't explain the disorder better, and it isn't superimposed on Schizophrenia, Schizophreniform Disorder, Delusional Disorder, or Psychotic Disorder Not Otherwise Specified.

• The symptoms are not directly caused by a general medical condition or by use of substances including prescription medications and drugs of abuse.

• The symptoms cause clinically important distress or impair school, work, social, or other functioning.

Specify: Early Onset (it begins by age 20)
        Late Onset (it begins at age 21 or later)

Specify if: With Atypical Features

---

activity, low energy, worthlessness or guilt, trouble thinking or concentrating, and thoughts of death or suicide. Table 16.2 gives criteria for the two types of Major Depressive Disorder that may be diagnosed (Single Episode or Recurrent), depending on whether this is the patient's first Major Depressive Episode or a subsequent one.

The symptoms required for Dysthymic Disorder (Table 16.5) are fewer and milder than those for a Major Depressive Episode. An early onset of Dysthymic

Disorder predicts a longer duration of depression and the eventual co-occurrence of Major Depressive Disorder. Although children tend to recover faster from Dysthymic Disorder than do adults, they're more likely to develop Major Depressive Disorder. Moreover, children with depression are far more likely than adults to have both Major Depressive Disorder *and* Dysthymic Disorder. Such a "double depression" diagnosis is possible if a child has qualified for a diagnosis of Dysthymic Disorder for at least 1 year (not 2, as for adults) before developing a Major Depressive Episode.

We have only begun to ascertain the incidence of depressive disorders in juveniles, and the figures given by various investigators vary widely. It should come as no surprise that these disorders are found more frequently in adolescents than in school-age children, and hardly at all in preschoolers. For what they are worth, then, our best estimate for prevalence of Dysthymic Disorder in adolescents is 3–6%. The prevalence of Major Depressive Disorder in adolescents is 3–6% (it ranges up to 28% of all adolescents, depending on the study!); for school-age children, it is 2%; for toddlers, it is essentially nil.

Merrill

"I didn't mean to hurt my little sister," was Merrill's chief complaint. Merrill was a second-grader who was being held in a children's mental health unit on the basis that he was dangerous to himself and to other people.

There had been nothing remarkable about his gestation, delivery, or developmental milestones. In fact, according to his mother he had been "a happy baby and a cheerful kid" until about halfway through kindergarten, when he was sent to live with his grandparents. Merrill's alcoholic father had deserted the family the year before, and his mother's new boyfriend earned his living selling crack cocaine. When police raided the residence, they found little in the refrigerator but drugs; Merrill's mother was jailed on a charge of child endangerment.

"So to 'protect' the kids, the judge ordered them sent to live with my mother, and my stepfather molested Merrill," Merrill's mother said with a curl of her lip. "I tried to explain going in that he had molested me, too. But who was going to pay any attention to me?"

After several months in jail, Merrill's mother was transferred to a mental facility for treatment of her Major Depressive Disorder. By the time the combined effects of legal aid and Prozac had won her release, the damage to her son had been done. Now Merrill never smiled; he always seemed either sad or angry. His sleep, appetite, and activity were about normal, but his teacher noted problems. A note sent home from first grade reported that "in class his attention wanders and on the playground he doesn't join in games—he thinks he doesn't play well."

Despite his mother's return home, Merrill did not improve. In fact, for 2 months his behavior worsened. He would scream at other children and seemed to feel that they were making fun of him. His sleep decreased to about 5 hours a night; his appetite also diminished. Two weeks before his admission to the mental health unit, he began sticking pins into the skin of his hands. The day of admission, he tried to choke his 4-year-old sister. Then, isolated in his room, he made several superficial cuts on the side of his own neck with a pocketknife.

Merrill had received all of the usual childhood vaccinations and immunizations. He had no allergies, and his only previous hospitalization was for possible asthma when he was 3. He had received treatment with prednisone at that time and had had no respiratory problems since.

Now 32, Merrill's mother had been married and divorced three times. Merrill was the second youngest of her five children, whose ages ranged from 12 to 4 years. Between pregnancies, she had earned minimum wage as a school aide. Although her depression had responded to treatment with medication, the family was currently living on Social Security disability.

Merrill was a rather thin child who was alert, made eye contact, and was reasonably cooperative. However, it took him an unusual amount of time to answer questions put to him, and he seemed less active than would be expected for an 8-year-old boy. Although his speech was slow and monotonous, his thoughts were linear and goal-directed. When asked about his mood, at first he said he felt "all right," but later admitted he had been feeling guilty because "I just keep doing bad things." He expressed remorse at having tried to harm his sister; he then admitted he wanted "to be dead," though he did not think he would try to cut himself again. "It hurt." He denied anxiety, delusions, or hallucinations; his cognitive functioning was normal for his age. On the basis that he knew that he had been admitted to the hospital because of his recent behavior, his insight seemed good. The behavior itself, however, suggested strongly that Merrill's judgment had been deficient in recent weeks.

Evaluation of Merrill

The steps mentioned in this discussion are those outlined in the section "A Step-by-Step Approach to Diagnosing and Coding Mood Disorders," on page 314.

Step 1: What symptoms would qualify Merrill for a possible mood episode? Mood change was first noted by his mother when the two were reunited after her own incarceration. He seemed sad or angry, but definitely different from his previous cheerful disposition. At first, his additional depressive symptoms seemed to include only loss of interest (wandering attention in class) and poor self-image (he didn't think he played games well), so until the few weeks prior to his admission, he could not have qualified for any mood episode diagnosis.

Recently, however, Merrill had also lost sleep and appetite and expressed death wishes and suicidal behavior; he even appeared to have psychomotor retardation. These symptoms clearly interfered with his functioning at school and at home. Before concluding that Merrill qualified for a Major Depressive Episode, his clinician would have to affirm that his symptoms had been present for most of every day, and that there was evidence of neither Bereavement nor a general health problem (in children, look especially for trauma, multiple hospitalizations, or a chronic illness such as leukemia) that could account for his depressive symptoms. Since the vignette gives no indication of bereavement or medical problems, Merrill would therefore fulfill the DSM-IV criteria for Major Depressive Episode (Table 16.1).

Step 2: Because Merrill had never had a Manic or Hypomanic Episode, a diagnosis of a bipolar disorder would not be possible (Table 16.2). His Major Depressive Episode would therefore have to be a part of Major Depressive Disorder.

Step 3: He had had only one Major Depressive Episode, so his Axis I code and diagnosis so far would be 296.2x Major Depressive Disorder, Single Episode.

Step 4: The severity code is determined from the guidelines provided for the current episode—in this case, a Major Depressive Episode (Table 16.1). Merrill's clinician regarded his depression as severe—not because he had so *many* symptoms, as the guidelines state, but because some of them (thoughts of death) were serious. (Remember, DSM-IV criteria are intended as guidelines, not shackles.) With no delusions or hallucinations, his code and diagnosis would now be 296.23 Major Depressive Disorder, Single Episode, Severe Without Psychotic Features. The chronicity specifier would not apply.

Step 5: None of the other episode specifiers (Table 16.3) would apply.

Step 6: Because this was Merrill's first episode of illness, he would have no course specifiers, either (Table 16.3). This would end the evaluation of his Major Depressive Disorder.

Step 7: However, because Merrill had had milder depressive symptoms more or less continuously for at least a year, he would also need to be evaluated for Dysthymic Disorder (Table 16.5). He had had the milder symptoms of Dysthymic Disorder more than a year before his Major Depressive Episode, so both diagnoses could be made. The Dysthymic Disorder criteria force a choice between Early and Late Onset—in Merrill's case, Early Onset. The code numbers and specifiers for the mood disorders are summarized in Table 16.4.

A number of other conditions must be included in the differential diagnosis for depressive disorders. As noted above, the Major Depressive Episode criteria require a consideration of **Bereavement**, but the vignette does not indicate that anyone close to Merrill had died within the past 2 months. Considering the trauma he had experienced, **Adjustment Disorder with Depressed Mood** seems a possibility. Adjustment Disorder is defined (p. 425) as a diagnosis of last resort, to be used only if no other Axis I disorder can explain the symptoms. (In fact, mood disorders are often misdiagnosed as Adjustment Disorder, especially in school-age children.) Patients with **Anorexia Nervosa** may look depressed and experience weight loss, but nowhere do we read that Merrill feared weight gain or had problems with his body image. Social impairment causes depression in some children who have **ADHD**; their hyperactivity may cause some to be viewed as having the mania of **Bipolar I** or **II Disorder**. Although Merrill had no phobias, compulsions, obsessions, or complaints of anxiety, in some children anxiety disorders (such as **Separation Anxiety Disorder** or **Generalized Anxiety Disorder**) may form part of the differential diagnosis. Of course, **Schizophrenia** must be considered when children or adolescents are so severely depressed or manic that they have psychotic symptoms. In those who present with somatic complaints, **Somatization Disorder** must also be considered in the differential diagnosis of Major Depressive Disorder.

Finally, let us consider disorders that may be comorbid with the mood disorders. These include **anxiety disorders** (found in about 40% of children with depression), **Conduct Disorder** (23% or more of depressed children), and **Substance Use Disorders** (especially in adolescents). Also, be alert for ADHD and eating disorders (as noted above), and for **learning disorders** such as **Reading Disorder**.

The Major Depressive Disorder prompted the current evaluation, so it would be listed first. Merrill's complete diagnosis would now be the following:

Axis I	296.23	Major Depressive Disorder, Single Episode, Severe Without Psychotic Features
	300.4	Dysthymic Disorder, Early Onset
Axis II	V71.09	No diagnosis
Axis III		None
Axis IV		Sexual abuse by grandfather
Axis V	GAF = 50	(current)

311 Depressive Disorder Not Otherwise Specified

The category of Depressive Disorder Not Otherwise Specified includes depressive disorders that are not (yet?) well enough recognized to be given code numbers of their own. They must also not fulfill the criteria for Adjustment Disorder With Depressed Mood or Adjustment Disorder With Mixed Anxiety and Depressed Mood.

Assessing Depressive Disorder

General Suggestions

Parents and teachers tend to be more accurate observers of young children's behavior, whereas the children themselves will give more accurate information about emotions. Obviously, multiple informants increase the likelihood of a complete and accurate clinical evaluation. A question about "three wishes" may yield statements as to hopelessness or, in the case of a Major Depressive Episode, even the wish for death. Throughout the interview, don't be diverted from a possible mood disorder diagnosis by the presence of somatic symptoms such as abdominal pain or headache. Although young children tend to somatize, they may acknowledge feelings of sadness, hopelessness, and wishes to die. Most children respond to simple, concrete questions from a sympathetic, patient interviewer..

Although the criteria for mood disorders are nearly identical for children and adults, we often forget that children and adolescents can have suicidal ideas and behaviors. Among young people aged 15–24, suicide is the third leading cause of death (after accidents and homicide). Even so, completed suicide is still a rare event; attempted suicide, however, is common (in one study, about 1% of school-age children reported making a recent attempt). When questioned closely, children as young as 6 who have Major

Depressive Disorder may admit to having suicidal ideas. Very young children have little comprehension that life actually terminates at death, whereas older children generally understand the consequences of suicide.

Despite admitting to feeling sad, even older children may not realize that this is a change or be able to date the change or state how long the sad feelings have been present. Because a sense of time only develops in later childhood, it is useful to relate time to important events ("Did it start before your birthday?").

Developmental Factors

Young children may appear tearful and physically slowed down, and may talk less than normally; the onset of depression may be more insidious than in older children. In school-age children and adolescents, look for somatic symptoms such as headaches and abdominal pain, as noted above. Sometimes failure to gain weight, or excessive sleepiness and inhibited overall activity level, may give the diagnosis away. Adolescents describe symptoms more precisely than younger children; they are also more likely to admit to guilt feelings and other symptoms characteristic of adult-style severe depression (psychomotor retardation, delusions, hopelessness). Of course, older children and adolescents alike may become so depressed that schoolwork and even friendships with classmates suffer. Adolescents may display their depressive illness in the form of problem behavior reminiscent of Conduct Disorder: promiscuity, petty lawbreaking, and substance use. Some young children (and even some adolescents) may not be able to specify that they feel a depressed mood; for them, irritability is an equivalent statement of mood for either Major Depressive Episode or Dysthymic Disorder. Language skills are not as well developed in very young children (perhaps to age 5), increasing the importance of such observations as slumped posture, unwillingness to play, lethargy, sad face, slow speech, and monotonous tone of voice.

BIPOLAR DISORDERS

Differential Diagnosis of Bipolar Disorders in Young Patients

If we were discussing adults, this section would consider Bipolar I, Bipolar II, and Cyclothymic Disorders more specifically. Although these disorders may occur in children and adolescents, they have been studied too little to tell us very much about *how* they occur in young patients. Here's a brief summary of what we do know.

Even Emil Kraepelin, writing a century ago, mentioned that mania can occur before puberty. In fact, late adolescence carries the greatest risk for onset of a bipolar disorder. Partly because mania is so unusual in younger patients, and partly because of symptom overlap with ADHD, clinicians do not expect it and therefore often miss it. Irritability is often the main mood change; reportedly, rapid cycling (more than four changes per year) and mixtures of mania and depression are especially common in young patients. Even before clinical symptoms appear, bipolar children and adolescents may seem different from their peers. When they are only toddlers, they may have mood or behavior problems, such as tantrums or trouble sleeping. Of course, these symptoms are also common during normal development. Early onset of mood symptoms does not in itself predict a bipolar disorder. Like adults, most children with mood disorders have only depression, but the first mood episode for many bipolar patients is depressive. Several features of depression may predict the eventual development of mania in children and adolescents:

- Rapid onset of symptoms
- Psychomotor retardation during depression
- Mood-congruent psychotic depression
- Strong family history of mood disorders
- Manic symptoms that start in response to the use of an antidepressant medication, electroconvulsive therapy, or bright light therapy

Although manic episodes occur rarely in childhood, they are more common in adolescence. Reports on bipolar disorders in these age groups remain largely anecdotal, but the underrecognition of these disorders may be considerable.

Tonya

Tonya was a 15-year-old girl whom the police brought to the hospital from her home. Her father had told them that she had threatened his life and was behaving bizarrely.

For several years she had been truant from school and had frequently run away from home. Intermittently, she had been remanded to a local alternative living center, where it was noted that her father drank heavily. A ninth-grade dropout, she had been expelled from a general equivalency diploma program several months previously for fighting.

Tonya's first real encounter with mental health professionals had occurred 6 months earlier. Then, just after breaking up with her boyfriend, she discovered that she was 2 months pregnant. She impulsively took an overdose of her father's pain pills, resulting in a rapid trip to a general hospital emergency room. She was thought not to be acutely dangerous to herself and was referred for psychotherapy. After her abortion, she seemed to have no symptoms of mood disorder.

Her father first began to notice mood swings during the past 3 months. She had told him she had lows lasting about 2 days, followed by a high of 8 or 9 hours. Because he assumed that she was "only high on crank," he did not attempt to seek help for her. Besides, he added, to prevent him from forcing her to attend school, Tonya had once threatened to accuse him of rape.

About 2 weeks before Tonya's current hospital admission, her speech became rapid and pressured; she showed increasingly labile affect, moving from tears to laughter and back within a few minutes. Her father finally called the police when she threatened him with a serrated steak knife. Although she insisted that he had raped her and three of her school friends, the police officers responding to the complaint noted her obvious mental disturbance and transported her for evaluation.

Tonya had lived with her father for nearly all of the past 9 years (except for the 6 months when he was jailed for physically abusing her 11-year-old brother). Her mother had been out of the home since Tonya was in the first grade. The mother was a known drug abuser and had been hospitalized on several occasions for psychosis.

Tonya had been a happy, easy baby who was "always talking and on the go." Her developmental milestones occurred at the normal times. She did well through eighth grade and was valedictorian of her sixth-grade graduating class. It was when she began hanging out with known drug dealers in the neighborhood that she nearly flunked the first semester of ninth grade. She also began fighting with other girls and became oppositional toward her teachers at this time, and finally dropped out of school completely.

Upon admission, she was disheveled and badly needed a shower. She seemed agitated and appeared to be in "perpetual motion." Her speech was pressured, and she admitted that her thoughts were racing. Her mood was both angry and expansive, and she told several interviewers that she thought she "had come [to the hospital] to straighten you people out." During the admission process, she had difficulty focusing her attention and frequently muttered, "What was I saying? What was I saying?" She denied having visual hallucinations, but twice claimed that she could hear "heartbeats of the love of Jesus," which meant that she was the Second Coming. She repeatedly claimed that she herself was completely well and that her father had all the problems; other than to reform the institution, she felt no need of hospitalization. She was alert and oriented, but would not cooperate further with cognitive testing. Later testing revealed a Full Scale IQ of 105 and no cognitive deficits.

Although Tonya denied having disturbed sleep or appetite, both were noted to be markedly decreased from normal during her hospitalization, which eventually stretched into 6 weeks. She remained hyperverbal and unable to focus on any task or to participate in milieu activities longer than a few seconds. When these behavioral problems were pointed out to her, she would instantly become angry and defiant.

Tonya was eventually started on lithium; within a week her activity level decreased, and she was better able to focus on the topic at hand. Her affect became much less labile as well, and her mood appeared to stabilize. At discharge she was able to state, "Now I feel pretty good inside."

Evaluation of Tonya

Hyperactivity can be encountered in several other disorders. **ADHD** typically starts at an earlier age than the usual Manic Episode, but it can be comorbid with Bipolar I or II Disorder. Tonya, however, had no history of problems with attention or hyperactivity prior to the eighth grade. The **use of drugs** such as steroids or amphetamines (either prescribed or illicit) can produce psychotic symptoms that can also be confused with mania. Tonya's symptoms persisted after she was admitted to the hospital, markedly reducing the possibility that they were drug-related. (A drug screen might have helped reassure her caregivers, however). Manic symptoms in adolescents are often accompanied by psychosis, which is too frequently misdiagnosed as **Schizophrenia**. Tonya seemed to have a few psychotic symptoms at admission, but her very considerable mood symptoms would weigh against this diagnosis. DSM-IV makes an even stronger argument in the basic criteria for Schizophrenia (see Table 15.1), which specify that the duration of any mood symptoms must be brief in relation to the duration of psychotic symptoms. Many patients in the throes of a Manic Episode may act out to such an extent that they seem to have **Conduct Disorder** or, in more extreme cases, **Antisocial Personality Disorder**. **Adjustment Disorder with Disturbance of Conduct** is also sometimes misdiagnosed, probably due to the relative infrequency with which manias are encountered in this age group. However, an Adjustment Disorder cannot be diagnosed if the symptoms fulfill criteria for another Axis I disorder.

Because Tonya's history accorded with none of the foregoing disorders, we can proceed to evaluate how well her symptoms fit the mood disorders criteria. Again, the steps mentioned here are those outlined in the Section "A Step-by-Step Approach to Diagnosing and Coding Mood Disorders" (p. 314).

Step 1: During her recent episode, which lasted far longer than the 1-week minimum for a Manic Episode, Tonya's mood seemed more angry than euphoric—not uncommon for adults, and even more likely in children or adolescents. For most of this time she talked a great deal, seemed agitated, was easily distractible, and had a decreased need for sleep and a decreased appetite. Her physical health was good. Although there was some suspicion that she might have **abused drugs** earlier, she had no opportunity to do so during her hospitalization, during which her symptoms persisted. The severity of her illness and the absence of *many* episodes precludes the diagnosis of **Cyclothymic Disorder**. She easily fulfilled the criteria (Table 16.1) for a Manic Episode.

Step 2: Coding Tonya's illness is straightforward. Because she was so ill as to require hospitalization, she had to have a form of Bipolar I (not Bipolar II) Disorder (see Table 16.2).

Step 3: Although she had had some previous depressive symptoms, she had never had a Major Depressive Episode. Moreover, the recent episode was her only Manic Episode to date.

Step 4: Tonya was at one time delusional and may have had auditory hallucinations; these psychotic symptoms were congruent with the usual manic themes of power and self-worth. Hence, the severity specifier Severe With Mood-Congruent Psychotic Features would be appropriate.

Step 5: No episode specifiers (Tables 16.3 and 16.4) would apply.

Step 6: No course specifiers (Tables 16.3 and 16.4) would apply to a single episode.

The Axis IV designation below describes a feature of Tonya's environment that might complicate her subsequent treatment. (If it were the *focus* of the current treatment, it would be coded V61.20 and placed on Axis I.) Her full diagnosis would be as follows:

Axis I	296.03	Bipolar I Disorder, Single Manic Episode, Severe With Mood-Congruent Psychotic Features
Axis II	V71.09	No diagnosis
Axis III		None
Axis IV		Parent–child relational problem
Axis V	GAF = 45	(on admission)
	GAF = 80	(at discharge)

296.80 Bipolar Disorder Not Otherwise Specified

A child or adolescent whose bipolar symptoms do not meet criteria for any better-defined bipolar disorder can be diagnosed with Bipolar Disorder Not Otherwise Specified (and should be observed closely for changes thereafter).

Assessing Bipolar Disorder

General Suggestions

Of all the patients who are brought for evaluation and who can communicate, those with mania may the most difficult to interview. They typically believe that nothing is wrong, and they *know* that they have better things to do than speaking with a clinician. When a manic patient is a child or adolescent, an added hardship may be the patient's activity level and aggressiveness, which can be physical impediments to the therapeutic alliance. Fortunately, the compulsive talking of manic patients serves as both a symptom and a vehicle for information gathering. Most manic patients will be hard-pressed to remain silent and will speak compulsively on just about any subject. Ask a question; then, by picking up on a word or phrase the patient has used, channel the subsequent barrage of speech toward the information you seek. Psychosis is a frequent accompaniment of juvenile mania—be sure to check for the presence of delusions and hallucinations. Remember that the diagnosis of a bipolar disorder is better made on the basis of longitudinal history than on an assessment of current symptoms.

Developmental Factors

Although juvenile mania strongly resembles that of adults, some differences have been noted. Children under the age of 8 may not have discrete episodes, and regular cycling is uncommon before adolescence. Young patients' illnesses often begin insidiously and sometimes appear to be chronic. Children's mood is likely to be irritable rather than euphoric, and they are more likely than adults or adolescents to have psychotic features such as hallucinations. Young children are reported to have especially troubled premorbid personalities.

When mania occurs in young children, it may resemble ADHD or Oppositional Defiant Disorder, in that the symptoms often include frequent fighting and swearing. As a check against overdiagnosis of mania in prepubertal children, you should look for a family history of bipolar disorders.

OTHER MOOD DISORDERS

293.83 Mood Disorder Due to a General Medical Condition

Many medical conditions can cause depressive symptoms; some can cause manic symptoms as well. It is always important to consider the possibility of medical problems when you are evaluating a young patient with mood symptoms. Table 13.1 in Chapter 13 lists the criteria for Mood Disorder Due to a General Medical Condition.

Substance-Induced Mood Disorder

Substance use is a common and probably underrecognized cause of mood symptoms. It is essential to consider the possibility of substance use in young patients with no history of disorder who suddenly present with mood symptoms. Table 14.5 in Chapter 14 gives the criteria for Substance-Induced Mood Disorder, and Table 14.6 provides guidance in coding this by substance class.

296.90 Mood Disorder Not Otherwise Specified

Mood Disorder Not Otherwise Specified is a category for patients whose symptoms do not clearly belong to either Depressive Disorder Not Otherwise Specified or Bipolar Disorder Not Otherwise Specified. Anyone coded here would have been evaluated too briefly or incompletely to indicate which specific mood disorder diagnosis might be more appropriate. For example, an adolescent who is currently depressed and too ill to give a complete history might not be able to state whether there has been an earlier hospitalization for mania. This code will be used infrequently; like most Not Otherwise Specified categories, it should be changed to a more specific diagnosis once you obtain the additional relevant information.

| Anxiety Disorders

Quick Guide to the Anxiety Disorders

The following conditions may be diagnosed in children and adolescents who present with prominent anxiety symptoms; comorbidity is the rule. As usual, the page (or table) number following each item tells where fuller information on it may be found.

Anxiety Building Blocks

Agoraphobia and Panic Attacks are not codable disorders in and of themselves. They are the building blocks from which several of the codable anxiety disorders are constructed.

Panic Attack. In a brief episode that begins suddenly and peaks rapidly, a child or adolescent feels intense dread, accompanied by a variety of physical and other symptoms (p. 337).

Agoraphobia. Patients fear situations or places such as entering a store, where they might have trouble obtaining help if they were to become anxious (p. 337).

Anxiety Disorders

Panic Disorder. Patients with this disorder experience repeated Panic Attacks, together with worry about having additional attacks and other mental and behavioral changes related to them. Panic Disorder With Agoraphobia is the more common form, but Panic Disorder Without Agoraphobia is sometimes diagnosed (p. 337).

Agoraphobia Without History of Panic Disorder. In this codable form of Agoraphobia related to fear of developing panic-like symptoms, the full criteria for Panic Disorder are not met (p. 337).

Specific Phobia. These patients fear specific objects or situations. Examples include animals; storms; heights; blood; airplanes; being closed in; or any circumstance that may lead to vomiting, choking, or developing an illness (p. 346).

Social Phobia. Patients imagine themselves embarrassed when they speak, write, or eat in public, or use a public urinal (p. 344).

Obsessive–Compulsive Disorder. These patients are bothered by repeated thoughts or behaviors that appear senseless, even to them (p. 352).

Posttraumatic Stress Disorder. An individual with this disorder repeatedly relives a severely traumatic event, such as a natural disaster (p. 358).

Acute Stress Disorder. This condition is much like Posttraumatic Stress Disorder, except that it begins during or immediately after a highly stressful event and lasts a month or less (p. 358).

Generalized Anxiety Disorder. Although they do not experience acute Panic Attacks, these patients feel tense or anxious much of the time (p. 348).

Anxiety Disorder Due to a General Medical Condition. Various anxiety symptoms can be caused by many medical conditions (Table 13.1 and p. 365).

Substance-Induced Anxiety Disorder. Various psychoactive substances produce anxiety symptoms that don't necessarily fulfill criteria for any of the above-mentioned disorders (Table 14.5 and p. 365).

Anxiety Disorder Not Otherwise Specified. Use this category to code disorders with prominent anxiety symptoms that do not meet criteria for any of the diagnoses above (p. 365).

Other Causes of Anxiety

Remember that Anxiety symptoms can be found in patients with almost any Axis I disorder. They are especially prevalent in patients with a Major Depressive Episode as part of a mood disorder (Table 16.1); Somatization Disorder (p. 375); or Adjustment Disorder With Anxiety (p. 425). Anxiety is response to separation from a parent or other caregiver is often found in Separation Anxiety Disorder (p. 246).

INTRODUCTION

In thinking about the anxiety disorders, keep the following points firmly in mind:

- Anxiety disorders are the most common of all mental health disorders, though their prevalence in juveniles, especially young children, is not clear. For one thing, they have only been studied for a short period of time in children and adolescents. For another, young children often lack insight that they feel anxiety, which they may express not by words but by behaviors such as clinging, crying, or freezing. Only recently have criteria insisted that symptoms produce disability or distress; older studies that omit this criterion may report a prevalence twice that of the "actual" level.

- Definitions of anxiety disorders for children and adolescents are still somewhat in flux. Overanxious Disorder of Childhood (DSM-III-R) is subsumed under Generalized Anxiety Disorder in DSM-IV, and Avoidant Disorder of Childhood (DSM-III-R) is included under Social Phobia in DSM-IV.

- The DSM-IV criteria are categorical—either you have a disorder or you haven't. (Analogy: There is no such thing as being a little bit pregnant.) However, many mental health clinicians point out the value of dimensionality in diagnosis. (Analogy: Many illnesses can be present in degrees, including diabetes, heart disease, and even cancer.)

- The typical anxious child or adolescent has at least two anxiety disorders. It is not yet clear whether this finding means multiple diagnoses (or *any* diagnosis) when this young patient grows up.

- Many anxious children and adolescents do not fully qualify for any well-defined DSM-IV anxiety disorder and must be diagnosed as having Anxiety Disorder Not Otherwise Specified.

- Although Separation Anxiety Disorder is grouped in DSM-IV with disorders usually first diagnosed in infancy, childhood, or adolescence (see Chapter 11), we believe that it really belongs with the other anxiety disorders.

- Obsessive–Compulsive Disorder is classified with anxiety disorders, but we feel that it probably belongs elsewhere, perhaps with Tourette's Disorder and the other tic disorders.

- Finally, remember that in many instances anxiety is a normal, even useful emotion that may change from one developmental stage to the next. One attraction of DSM-IV is that it takes pains to protect us from the occasional impulse to overdiagnose mental disorder.

It should be noted here that the order of our text discussion of the anxiety disorders differs somewhat from the order of their appearance in DSM-IV (which we have followed in the Quick Guide, above). First, because in our view the effects of Social Phobia are more pervasive and chronic than those of Specific Phobia, we discuss Social before Specific Phobia. Second, in DSM-IV Obsessive–Compulsive Disorder, Posttraumatic Stress Disorder, and Acute Stress Disorder precede Generalized Anxiety Disorder. In our opinion, however, the very detailed and specialized criteria for Obsessive–Compulsive Disorder and the two traumatic stress disorders set them qualitatively apart from the other anxiety disorders, and so we discuss Generalized Anxiety Disorder before going on to these three. (Acute Stress Disorder, which is new to DSM-IV and whose nature in children and adolescents is as yet unclear, is also discussed much more briefly than Posttraumatic Stress Disorder.)

PANIC ATTACKS, AGORAPHOBIA, AND DISORDERS INVOLVING THEM

As recently as a generation ago, the ability of children and adolescents to develop Panic Attacks was relatively ignored in the mental health literature. Now it is generally recognized that these symptoms can occur before puberty, even (rarely) in children as young as 5, and that the prevalences increase with age to the teen years. In one survey, 5% of high school students had had enough symptoms at some time during their lives to fulfill criteria for a Panic Attack.

In children and adults alike, Panic Attacks and Agoraphobia often develop in close association with one another. For whatever reason (both hereditary and environmental factors are implicated), a patient begins to develop panic symptoms that eventually become full-blown Panic Attacks. The fear of recurrent symptoms spawns anxiety that persists between attacks. In many cases, this anxiety ultimately generalizes to avoidance behavior that includes agoraphobia. Although the two conditions are not always linked, this sequence is thought to obtain in many instances.

Further evidence of the continuum between juvenile and adult anxiety disorders is the fact that of adults who report Panic Attacks, fully 25% first had symptoms prior to their middle teens. Although the emphasis may be different, it seems clear that the symptoms of Panic Attack and Agoraphobia are the same for children, adolescents, and adults. Their criteria are presented in Tables 17.1 and 17.2, respectively, to help clarify the picture of these common clinical conditions. But in order for a DSM-IV diagnosis to be made, they must be combined with other criteria (Table 17.3) to form one of three diagnoses: Panic Disorder With Agoraphobia, Panic Disorder Without Agoraphobia, or Agoraphobia Without History of Panic Disorder.

Hank

Hank knew exactly when his trouble began. It had been the previous year, in his seventh-grade prealgebra class. He had aced the first two questions and was just organizing his answer to a brief essay question about factoring when his test paper started swimming before his eyes.

"Like, it shimmered, you know? Like heat waves coming off a hot pavement."

"Besides the swimming, did you notice anything else?" asked the interviewer.

Hank shook his head. "No. In a few minutes it went away, and I finished the exam. But a few days later I was writing an essay during English class. My hand shook so much and my fingers felt so weak that I couldn't hold the pencil. The teacher sent me to the nurse's office. I thought I was going to faint on the way."

TABLE 17.1. Criteria for Panic Attack

- The patient suddenly develops a severe fear or discomfort that peaks within 10 minutes.
- During this discrete episode, four or more of the following symptoms occur:
  ✓ Chest pain or other chest discomfort
  ✓ Chills or hot flashes
  ✓ Choking sensation
  ✓ Derealization (feeling unreal) or depersonalization (feeling detached from self)
  ✓ Dizzy, lightheaded, faint, or unsteady feelings
  ✓ Fear of dying
  ✓ Fears of loss of control or becoming insane
  ✓ Heart pounding, racing, or skipping beats
  ✓ Nausea or other abdominal discomfort
  ✓ Numbness or tingling
  ✓ Sweating
  ✓ Shortness of breath or smothering sensation
  ✓ Trembling

TABLE 17.2. Criteria for Agoraphobia

- The patient has anxiety about being in a place or situation in which *either or both* could be true:
  ✓ Escape might be difficult or embarrassing
  ✓ If a Panic Attack occurred, help might not be available
- The patient:
  ✓ Avoids these situations or places (restricting travel), *or*
  ✓ Endures them, but with material distress (a Panic Attack might occur), *or*
  ✓ Requires a companion when in the situation
- Other mental disorders don't explain the symptoms better. These include Social Phobia (e.g., the patient avoids eating for fear of embarrassment); Specific Phobias (e.g., the patient avoids certain limited situations, such as telephone booths); Obsessive–Compulsive Disorder (e.g., the patient avoids dirt for fear of contamination); and Posttraumatic Stress Disorder (e.g., the patient avoids situations linked to a traumatic event). Children and adolescents who avoid leaving home should be evaluated for Separation Anxiety Disorder.

"Did you feel anything else during that episode?"

"I could feel my heart beating, really hard. That scared me—I guessed I was having a heart attack. The nurse said I was hypoventilating and made me breathe into a paper bag."

"Hy*per*ventilating," said the interviewer. "Did the bag breathing help?"

"Yeah, hyperventilating. It got better after a while."

Hank sat slumped a little in his chair, his forehead resting lightly on the fingers of his left hand. He had begun having attacks outside of class, too, he said. They were mostly the same—a tight chest, constricted breathing, palpitations, and the fear that he was terribly ill. Although examinations always seemed to cause an attack, more and more they would spring up any time, even when he wasn't at school. "It'll happen within seconds, right out of the blue."

From Hank's parents, the interviewer had already obtained quite a lot of information. Because he was bright and articulate, his grades hadn't suffered much at first. His parents were both professional people who hadn't delved too deeply into their son's inner feelings, or perhaps he hadn't chosen to reveal them. In any event, they hadn't noticed anything wrong until he began cutting school and "studying at home."

Hank's birth had been a full-term, normal delivery; he was the second of two planned and well-loved children. He and his sister had both done well throughout their private school education. Neither had had prior emotional difficulties, though Hank had "seemed somewhat nervous" for most of the winter and spring when he was 5. He had clung to his mother the first few days she tried to leave him at kindergarten, but was soon distracted by the playthings in

TABLE 17.3. Criteria for Anxiety Disorders That Involve Agoraphobia and/or Panic Attack

	300.22 Agoraphobia Without History of Panic Disorder	300.21 Panic Disorder With Agoraphobia	300.01 Panic Disorder Without Agoraphobia
Agoraphobia present?	• Yes, related to fear of experiencing panic-like symptoms (any Panic Attack symptom or any other that could embarrass or incapacitate patient).	• Yes.	• No.
Unexpected, recurrent Panic Attacks?	• No. Has never fulfilled criteria for Panic Disorder.	• Yes. For 1 month or more after at least one attack, one or more of these: ✓ Ongoing concern that there will be more attacks ✓ Worry as to the significance of the attack or its consequences (for health, control, sanity) ✓ Material change in behavior, such as doing something to avoid or combat the attacks	
Other	• The symptoms are not directly caused by a general medical condition or by use of substances, including medications and drugs of abuse.		
	• If there is a general medical condition, fears clearly exceed those that usually accompany it.	• The Panic Attacks are not better explained by another anxiety disorder or other mental disorder.	

the classroom. Neither of his parents had noticed any recent problems with eating or sleeping. He had had no unsavory friends, and as far as they were aware, he had never used drugs or alcohol.

Hank had been silent for some time. "So you started staying home?" the interviewer prompted.

"Yeah. I kept thinking I'd have another attack at school. Pretty soon, I couldn't stand going anywhere by myself—you know, without Mom or Dad."

Hank was pleasant to talk to, even funny as he described some of his problems. He made good eye contact with the examiner, smiled appropriately, and spoke clearly in well-constructed sentences. He had never had delusions or hallucinations, and denied ever using drugs. He readily admitted that he had a problem and said that he wished he could go back to school. "I can learn algebra at home. But heck, I'm missing sex ed."

Evaluation of Hank

The complicated DSM-IV criteria render the evaluation of any patient who has Panic Attacks a bit involved. We will take it one step at a time.

First, how did Hank's episodes of anxiety fulfill the criteria for a Panic Attack? His episodes occurred suddenly, lasted a few minutes, and then were gone (Table 17.1). They included shakiness, pounding heart, shortness of breath, chest discomfort, and feeling faint (the Panic Attack criteria require only four symptoms). But Panic Attack is not a diagnosis; for that, we must turn to the criteria for the two forms of Panic Disorder.

The criteria for both forms of Panic Disorder (Table 17.3) require recurrent attacks that are unexpected (uncued). Some of Hank's Panic Attacks were triggered (cued) by a test situation or by going to the store, but others were uncued. Hank also worried that he would have more attacks and changed his behavior to try to avoid them. The parents' report about the absence of any diagnosed general medical conditions (such as hyperthyroidism) that could cause Panic Attacks was considered accurate. Although it seemed evident that Hank did not use alcohol or drugs, the clinician wisely verified this by questioning both Hank and his parents directly.

No other anxiety or mental disorder would seem to explain Hank's symptoms better. His Panic Attacks weren't limited to social situations (such as speaking in public or asking for a date), as in **Social Phobia**, or to limited situations such as being confronted by a spider, as in **Specific Phobia**. Hank's fears also differed from those of **Separation Anxiety Disorder**, in which cued anxiety focuses on separation from parents or their surrogates. Although there were hints of separation anxiety when he was very young, it lasted only briefly. He would therefore fulfill the criteria for Panic Disorder.

Patients with Panic Attacks can have either Panic Disorder With or Panic Disorder Without Agoraphobia (Table 17.3). After he had had a number of Panic Attacks, Hank developed the fear of being away from home alone—so that was where he stayed, unless accompanied by a parent. These symptoms were no better explained by another anxiety diagnosis than were the Panic Attacks; he would fulfill the criteria for Panic Disorder With Agoraphobia. (By the way, **Agoraphobia Without History of Panic Disorder** is only rarely encountered, either in juvenile or in adult populations.)

Many patients will have more than one anxiety disorder. **Generalized Anxiety Disorder** is comorbid in many children, but Hank's worries were circumscribed rather than being about a number of different problems. In addition to one or more anxiety disorders, look carefully for evidence of mood disorder—especially **Major Depressive Disorder** or a **bipolar disorder**—in patients who develop Panic Attacks. Hank seemed to be bearing his difficulties without this sort of complication: His affect was generally good, even humorous, and there was no evidence of problems with appetite or sleep. He would need to be evaluated later for symptoms of **Avoidant Personality Disorder**, which is also sometimes comorbid in agoraphobic patients.

Hank's final diagnosis would be as follows:

Axis I	300.21	Panic Disorder With Agoraphobia
Axis II	799.9	Diagnosis deferred
Axis III		None
Axis IV		None
Axis V	GAF = 60	(current)

PHOBIC DISORDERS

A *phobia* is a fear that is triggered by something. It produces clinically important anxiety symptoms, which can be Panic Attacks (they are cued) or more general symptoms of anxiety. Now let us consider the two main types of phobias, Specific and Social. Specific Phobia is a fear of situations (e.g., acrophobia—fear of heights) or objects (e.g., spiders or thunderstorms). Social Phobia is a fear of some kinds of social or performance situations (such as speaking in public). The symptoms of Specific and Social Phobias are nearly identical and can be quickly summarized:

- A defined condition triggers fear.
- The patient almost always feels anxiety when exposed to the trigger.
- Although adults usually have insight that their anxiety is excessive, children (and some adolescents) may not.
- A patient avoids the feared condition, or endures it with severe distress. (Children and adolescents are often less able than adults to avoid the stimulus.)
- The phobia seriously affects the patient's life or causes marked distress.
- Anyone under 18 must have had the symptoms for at least 6 months. This requirement helps to compensate for the fact that some fears, such as fear of strangers or the dark, can be developmentally normal (they may even have survival value).
- The symptoms aren't better explained by another anxiety disorder diagnosis. However, phobic children and adolescents usually have other Axis I disorders, especially anxiety disorders.
- A final point applies only to Social Phobia: Patients with medical or mental conditions that are disfiguring or cause unusual behavior may fear

the scrutiny of other people. This criterion prevents us from diagnosing, for example, Social Phobia in a child or adolescent with Trichotillomania if the only concern is that people notice the hair pulling.

Although the symptoms of phobias may be somewhat different in juveniles (especially young children) than in adults, the criteria are fundamentally the same (see Table 17.4). Many phobic adults first develop their symptoms during childhood or adolescence. Of all the anxiety disorders, phobias are the most common, affecting about 10% of general child and adult populations.

TABLE 17.4. Criteria for Social and Specific Phobias

Social Phobia	Specific Phobia
• The patient strongly, repeatedly fears at least one social or performance situation that involves facing strangers or being watched by others. The patient specifically fears showing anxiety symptoms or behaving in some other way that will be embarrassing or humiliating.	• The patient experiences a strong, persistent fear that is unreasonable or excessive. It is set off (cued) by a specific object or situation that is either present or anticipated.
• Children cannot receive this diagnosis unless they have demonstrated the capacity for social relationships. The anxiety must occur not just with adults, but with peers.	

- The phobic stimulus almost always brings on an anxiety response, which may or may not be a situation-linked Panic Attack. Children may express the anxiety response by clinging, crying, freezing, withdrawing, or having tantrums.
- The patient realizes that this fear is unreasonable or out of proportion. A child may not realize this.
- The patient either avoids the phobic stimulus or endures it with severe anxiety or distress.
- Either there is marked distress about having the phobia, or it markedly interferes with the patient's usual routines or social, school, job, or other functioning.
- Patients under the age of 18 must have the symptoms for 6 months or longer.

• The symptoms are not directly caused by a general medical condition or by use of substances, including medications and drugs of abuse. If the patient has another mental disorder or a general medical condition, the phobia is not related to it.	• The symptoms are not better explained by another mental disorder.

Specify whether: Generalized. The patient fears most social situations.	Specify type (include all that apply):
	  Situational Type (e.g., airplane travel, being closed in)
	  Natural Environment Type (e.g., thunderstorms, heights)
	  Blood–Injection–Injury Type
	  Animal Type (e.g., spiders, snakes)
	  Other Type (situations that might lead to illness, choking, vomiting; in children, this can include avoiding loud noises or people in costumes)

300.23 Social Phobia

Youngsters with Social Phobia so fear the scrutiny of others that they may have difficulty reciting in class, asking for a date, going to a party, or even using a public restroom. The disorder typically begins in the early teenage years and tends to become chronic. These children often grow up without friends and tend to develop depressive and substance use disorders; as adults, they may not marry. Note that this diagnosis cannot be given unless a child has developed sufficiently to have social relationships, and that the symptoms in children must occur with *peers*, not just with adults. Children with Social Phobia lack self-confidence and are excessively and age-inappropriately timid, perhaps to the point that they perform poorly in school or avoid playing with other children. One way DSM-IV tries to sort out clinically important distress from developmental phases is to require a duration of at least 6 months in patients under the age of 18 years. As many as 1% (some clinicians say more) of children and adolescents may have Social Phobia.

It is important to note the difference between Social Phobia and Agoraphobia. In either condition patients may avoid social situations, but in Social Phobia the object is to avoid embarrassing encounters, whereas in Agoraphobia it is to avoid the symptoms of anxiety themselves.

Rita

When she was 12, Rita was referred for evaluation by her Sunday school teacher, whose report read in part: "Rita is a lovely little girl who seems to have a problem. She was to play a Wise Man in the Christmas pageant, but froze up completely when it came time to say her line." Although the Virgin Mary stage-whispered the line several times, Rita never could say it. The pageant finally went on without her verbal participation; afterward, she cried.

According to her mother, Rita had been a normal, happy infant and toddler. Although she made "about average" grades in school, she had never enjoyed school. When the other children went out to play at recess, she would stay in her seat, drawing or reading a storybook. In fourth grade, she complained that she hated to write on the chalkboard when the class did math. At first her teacher made her go up to the board anyway; eventually she was allowed to do most of her work at her seat.

The previous summer, Rita had attended camp for 2 weeks. She made nine whistle cords in the crafts tent, but no new friends. For 5 days after she returned, her lonely letters home continued to arrive.

At home, Rita played normally with her sister, who was almost 2 years younger than she. When her mother tried to start her in Brownies, she spent nearly all of the meetings she attended standing off to one side "looking completely miserable," though the Brownie leader repeatedly tried to engage her in singing and planning a field trip. Eventually her mother gave up the struggle, and she stopped attending.

Within a few sessions, Rita formed a close, warm relationship with her clinician, to whom she confided a wish to be more like the other kids. But her self-consciousness continued to get in her way. "I can't stand to have everyone looking at me," she told the clinician. "It makes me feel like I'm burning up."

Evaluation of Rita

With nine main criteria, Social Phobia is one of the more complicated diagnoses in DSM-IV (see Table 17.4). Rita feared not just social situations (appearing in a play, playing with others at camp or Brownies) but the embarrassment that they entailed. The criteria state that the feared situation must almost always cause anxiety, which in Rita's case seems likely from the history (though it was not yet proven). She responded principally by withdrawing, and avoided these situations whenever possible. Her distress and impaired social functioning were palpable.

Note that Rita fulfilled several criteria that differentiate children from adults: The manner of response may be different in a child (clinging, crying, freezing, withdrawing, or having tantrums); the child must have advanced far enough developmentally to be able to form social relationships (Rita interacted normally with her younger sister); the anxiety must occur not solely with adults, but with peers (Rita avoided camp activities and playground games); children must have symptoms for at least 6 months; and insight is not strictly required for children (but at age 12, would Rita still qualify as a child?). Although the vignette is a little unclear, Rita probably recognized that her fears were unreasonable.

Before making a definitive diagnosis, her clinician would have to ascertain that Rita's symptoms cannot be explained better by a **general medical condition** or by a **different mental disorder**. Because her symptoms persisted despite long acquaintance (e.g., the classroom situation), Rita's problem could not be explained as a **temperamental variant**—a case of a timid child who warmed up slowly. The differential diagnosis also often includes **Generalized Anxiety Disorder**, which frequently accompanies Social Phobia, and **Separation Anxiety Disorder**. Rita felt anxiety, but her distress was never expressed as actual Panic Attacks, ruling out a diagnosis of **Panic Disorder**.

Rita's complete diagnosis would be as given below. Whereas we would make no personality disorder diagnosis at this time, her Axis II code would remind the clinician to reevaluate Rita when she was older. **Avoidant Personality Disorder** has been associated with Social Phobia, and the two conditions show some overlap.

Axis I	300.23	Social Phobia
Axis II	799.99	Diagnosis Deferred on Axis II
Axis III		None
Axis IV		None
Axis V	GAF = 55	(current)

300.29 Specific Phobia

Fears are nearly ubiquitous in children, but in only a few children and adolescents (perhaps 2–3%) do they cause a clinical level of distress. Still, with many lasting fears having their onset in early childhood, Specific Phobia is among the most commonplace of the childhood anxiety disorders. For instance, animal phobia typically begins at about the age of 7, fear of blood at 9, and dental phobia at 12. Specific environmental phobias, such as claustrophobia, typically begin much later—perhaps at about age 20. Fears of animals or environmental phenomena such as thunderstorms usually occur in females. DSM-IV notes that some children especially fear loud noises or costumed characters (e.g., Goofy and Ronald McDonald).

The vignette that follows describes one of Sigmund Freud's best-known patients. Our source is "Analysis of a Phobia in a Five-Year-Old Boy," in the *Standard Edition* of Freud's works (Vol. 10, pp. 5–149).

Little Hans

When Hans was not quite 5 years old, he developed a fear that "a horse would bite him in the street." That Sigmund Freud associated this terror with Hans's fear of big penises and a desire to possess his mother sexually need not concern us here. In brief, here is the story.

Beginning in early January of 1908, Hans would cry whenever he saw a horse. When taken to the park, he would grow "visibly frightened"; even when accompanied, he was reluctant to go out of doors. He "always ran back into the house with every sign of fright if horses came along." This fear appeared to apply to any horse, whether it was being ridden or pulling a carriage or cart. When traffic was light and no horses were visible, however, Hans did not appear to be frightened. "How sensible!" he said. "God's done away with horses now." Other than when he was confronting a horse, he appeared to be a cheerful, healthy boy.

By May of that year, Hans's anxiety symptoms when he encountered a horse had largely disappeared. At follow-up 14 years later he remained asymptomatic, even through the divorce and remarriage of his parents.

Evaluation of Little Hans

How does this classic Specific Phobia stack up against DSM-IV criteria? The presence of horses (specific object) nearly always triggered (cued) fearful crying and "every sign of fright" (unreasonable anxiety response). Hans avoided proximity to horses whenever possible. There is no clear evidence that Hans ever realized his fears were disproportionate, but the presence of insight is not necessary for a diagnosis of childhood phobia.

So far, so good—several of the bulleted criteria for Specific Phobia in Table 17.4 were met. But did his distress reach the level of clinical significance? To be sure, Hans cried when taken to the park, but that hardly constituted a clinically important event. He didn't attend school, and we read nothing of his interactions with friends. He didn't appear to be at odds with his family (with the possible exception of his father, whom he allegedly wanted to replace in his mother's affections). Fear of horses disrupted his activities only to the extent that he didn't go to the park much. Although he felt distress, DSM-IV specifies that the distress should be about having the phobia—not about the mere prospect of encountering, for example, horses.

Finally, the evidence suggests that Hans's fear of horses had dissipated in less than the minimum 6 months' duration DSM-IV requires for this diagnosis in children or adolescents. Some might suggest that Freud's consultation had in some way shortened the duration of illness. It is as plausible, and perhaps more likely, that Hans never suffered from a "disorder" at all, but rather a simple childhood fear that vanished with further development. This conclusion is somewhat strengthened by Freud's observations that Hans apparently had none of the conditions so often comorbid with phobic disorders.

Could Freud have mistaken Hans's condition for some other mental disorder? His fear was not of being away from home in general, as would be expected from **Agoraphobia**; nor were his spells of anxiety (we are not sure whether he ever had true Panic Attacks) uncued, as would be the case for **Panic Disorder**. We don't learn of other fears (robbers, kidnappers, train accidents) that could harm the family, as might be true in **Separation Anxiety Disorder**.

With the benefit of DSM-IV criteria, at the time of first evaluation Freud might have felt he needed more data or time before a definitive diagnosis could be made. In the interim, he might have diagnosed something on the order of the following:

Axis I	300.9	Unspecified Mental Disorder (nonpsychotic)
Axis II	V71.09	No diagnosis
Axis III		None
Axis IV		None
Axis V	GAF = 60	(upon first evaluation)

But Freud could not have diagnosed Specific Phobia in Little Hans.

300.02 GENERALIZED ANXIETY DISORDER

Children with Generalized Anxiety Disorder (abbreviated GAD in this section only) worry about a variety of situations or events. They have worry they cannot control—worry that is out of all proportion to the objective seriousness of the situation. They may feel anxiety when anticipating situations in which their behavior or performance will be assessed by others.

As applied to children and adolescents, DSM-III-R called this behavior Overanxious Disorder of Childhood (abbreviated OAD here) and included it in the chapter on disorders usually first diagnosed in infancy, childhood, or adolescence. However, researchers came to realize that OAD is similar to, and probably on a continuum with, adult GAD; therefore, the two diagnoses were combined. As of this writing, most of our information on childhood GAD comes from studies of OAD.

A large minority of children will at one time or another have enough symptoms to meet the old DSM-III-R criteria for GAD (or OAD). But with the DSM-IV criterion (see Table 17.5) requiring that symptoms be important enough clinically to cause distress or impair functioning, the prevalence of GAD in general child populations falls to about 3% (6% for adolescents). These figures are still substantial, and GAD probably accounts for about half of childhood anxiety dis-

TABLE 17.5. Criteria for Generalized Anxiety Disorder

- For more than half the days in at least 6 months, the patient experiences excessive anxiety and worry about several events or activities.
- The patient has trouble controlling these feelings.
- Associated with this anxiety and worry, the patient has three or more (only one is required for children) of the following symptoms, some of which are present for over half the days in the past 6 months:
  - ✓ Feelings of being restless, edgy, keyed up
  - ✓ Tiring easily
  - ✓ Trouble concentrating
  - ✓ Irritability
  - ✓ Increased muscle tension
  - ✓ Trouble sleeping (initial insomnia or restless, unrefreshing sleep)
- Aspects of another Axis I disorder do not provide the focus of the anxiety and worry (see Coding Note, below).
- The symptoms cause clinically important distress or impair school, work, social, or other personal functioning.
- The disorder is not directly caused by a general medical condition or by use of substances, including medications and drugs of abuse.
- It does not occur only during a mood disorder, a psychotic disorder, Posttraumatic Stress Disorder, or a pervasive developmental disorder.

Coding Note: Aspects of another Axis I disorder include worries about the following: weight gain (Anorexia Nervosa); contamination (Obsessive–Compulsive Disorder); having a Panic Attack (Panic Disorder); separation from home or relatives (Separation Anxiety Disorder); public embarrassment (Social Phobia); or having physical symptoms (somatoform disorders).

order diagnoses. GAD begins at an average age of about 9 years, with boys and girls fairly equally affected. The prognosis is unclear.

Gerald

Gerald's parents said that he'd always been a "worrywart," and everything about Gerald seemed to confirm their opinion. Last year, he told the interviewer, he had worried that he was too short to play basketball; he had grown quite a bit in the fifth grade, but he still couldn't shoot very well. He was also afraid that he wasn't very popular: He'd been elected class vice-president, but not president. His dad had told him that vice-president was a responsible position, but Gerald wasn't having any of that. "He's always trying to reassure me," said Gerald. "Besides, I think he and Mom are getting a divorce. They fight an awful lot." Recently, he had decided not to join the Boy Scouts—he knew he could never learn to tie knots.

Gerald was the second of three brothers. The other two had always seemed pretty normal, rough-and-tumble kids, according to their parents, both of whom worked as clerks at a Veterans Affairs medical center. Gerald was just as healthy as they, but he was "the most cautious kid in six counties." When all three boys got skateboards for Christmas one year, Gerald was the one who put his in the closet after a couple of trial rides. He never touched it again.

Although Gerald had always been a good student, his fifth-grade teacher had lately remarked that his mind seemed elsewhere. "Something seems to be troubling him," she had said that fall at a parent–teacher conference. "Some days he's just cranky with everyone; other days he gets up and wanders around the room. He wasn't like that last year at all."

Gerald denied that he was depressed or on drugs. "But," he said, "I know I worry too much—everyone says so. I can't help it. I've tried closing the door in my mind on these problems, but it keeps popping open again." Although he denied having somatic symptoms typical of a Panic Attack, he did admit to feeling "wired" when he thought about his problems. Then moving around would sometimes help him feel better.

Evaluation of Gerald

Gerald's worries were numerous. They included his physical abilities, his schoolwork, his popularity, and even the integrity of his own family. That's the point of GAD: A patient finds plenty to worry about. Even though Gerald struggled for control, it cost him considerable distress. The vignette implies that his schoolwork was about to suffer, too. Gerald's anxiety symptoms included inattention, restlessness, and irritability. DSM-IV criteria require only one of these symptoms for children and adolescents, but three or more for adults. Neither drug use nor medical illness could account for Gerald's symptoms.

The criteria for GAD include the usual long list of anxiety disorders that must be ruled out as a focus of anxiety: **Panic Disorder** (Gerald had no Panic Attacks), **Social Phobia** (his fears were multiple and varied), **Obsessive–Compulsive Disorder** (his worries only concerned everyday problems), **Separation Anxiety Disorder** (his anxiety was not limited to concerns about separation from parents), and **Posttraumatic Stress Disorder** (there had been no traumatic event). Other disorders that must be ruled out include **Anorexia Nervosa** (anxiety about being fat) and **Somatization Disorder** (anxiety about physical complaints). Of course, some of these same disorders may be comorbid with GAD. The vignette provides no evidence that another diagnosis might explain Gerald's symptoms better than GAD. His five-axis diagnosis would thus be as follows:

Axis I	300.02	Generalized Anxiety Disorder
Axis II	V71.09	No diagnosis
Axis III		None
Axis IV		None
Axis V	GAF = 70	(current)

Assessing Disorders Involving Panic, Agoraphobia, Other Phobias, and Generalized Anxiety

General Suggestions

Young children will not understand the term *anxiety*, so you will need to ask, "Are there things that frighten you?" The responses will be quite varied, ranging from the dark to germs to snakes or strangers or visits to the dentist. Depending on the history given by parents, it may be necessary to run through a list of other possibilities: animals, bee stings, being lost or teased, burglars, death, inability to breathe, making errors, or poor grades. Not all of these will constitute phobias—some young patients will worry about competence in school or sports, the future, and various physical complaints, whether real or imagined. What do the patients fear as dire outcomes for themselves, for family members, for close friends, or for pets? Be sure to ask whether a child is afraid of water (water phobia was reported in 98% of phobic children in one study).

Behavioral traits that suggest an anxiety disorder include avoidance, clinging, crying, and school refusal. Some children may become restless or have difficulty concentrating. Even a long latency before speaking can suggest an extremely cautious child who may ultimately develop an anxiety disorder. Children tend to express anxiety by physical symptoms. Stomachaches (also called recurrent abdominal pains), headaches, and diffuse limb/muscle aches ("growing pains") are the most common.

Children and adolescents with Panic Disorder probably won't spontaneously mention their panic symptoms; you will have to ask. They are most likely to report tremors, palpitations, dizziness or faintness, trouble breathing, sweating, and fear of losing control or dying. An 8-year-old child should be able to answer questions about anxiety symptoms. Older children and adolescents can keep diaries to record the nature, timing, precipitation, and duration of their anxieties. They can also usually express the imagined consequences if exposed to the object of fear. For example, ask,

"What do you think will happen if a dog runs into the room?" Those who become phobic in adolescence may experience a decline in functioning, just as adults do. However, you may have to compare a young child's actual school progress with expected progress, based on testing or estimation of teachers.

Developmental Factors

Young children often respond timidly to new situations. Indeed, caution is normal in children of any age and may have self-protective value. Phobic youngsters will show even more reluctance than usual to interact in new situations, perhaps hugging the wall at a birthday party or demanding that a parent remain for the entire time.

A patient's age will to some extent determine the content of a phobia: Younger children will be afraid of the dark or animals, whereas older children or adolescents may fear nuclear disaster or other social calamities. Panic Attacks are unusual before puberty, but are increasingly encountered after adolescence. Adolescents will typically report Agoraphobia or fears relating to sex or failure.

Although insight into the irrationality of the fear is a hallmark in adults, young children often don't recognize that their fears are unreasonable. For that reason, the criterion is specifically not required for children by DSM-IV, though the manual does not specify age limits.

300.3 OBSESSIVE–COMPULSIVE DISORDER

For generations, mental health clinicians have known of Obsessive–Compulsive Disorder (abbreviated OCD in this section). What we have not recognized is that, far from being rare in juveniles (as it was once thought to be), OCD is actually relatively common, occurring in perhaps 1–2% of all teenagers. We have also failed to appreciate until recently just how often this debilitating condition begins in early childhood. Part of the explanation is that children may keep their obsessive thinking and compulsive behavior secret. They may control repetitive rituals relatively well when in public (such as at school), only letting down their guard at home. Even parents are sometimes surprised to learn the extent of a child's disability. With parents' ignorance and children's reluctance to ask for help, many youngsters with OCD remain undiagnosed and untreated for months or years.

Like adults, children and adolescents exhibit compulsions more frequently than obsessions. Though the sexes are about equally likely to develop OCD, boys' symptoms begin earlier than girls' (ages 9 and 11, respectively). OCD is sometimes episodic, but it more commonly runs a chronic course: At several years' follow-up, most patients still have symptoms.

Young children often don't have obsessional thinking that accompanies their compulsions—just "an urge to do it." This would technically seem to fly in the face of the criterion for compulsions (see Table 17.6) that specifies: "The aim of these behaviors is to reduce or eliminate distress or to prevent something that is dreaded." Even some adults don't meet this criterion, which may be eliminated or substantially revised in the future.

Corey

When he was 15, Corey tried to buy a gun. He was tall and had been shaving for a couple of years, and he might have succeeded if he hadn't written his actual telephone number on the form for the 5-day waiting period. The clerk thought he looked depressed, and called Corey's mother after he left the shop.

"That's how I ended up here instead of the morgue," Corey told his clinician the day after he was admitted to a locked mental health unit. "Anything seemed better than feeling rotten all the time."

Information from a number of sources supported a diagnosis of a mood disorder. Several teachers had noticed that Corey's concentration had been impaired for a month or more; his grades had plummeted. His mother had worried that he wasn't eating; his father observed that he had seemed to lose interest in the basement color photo-processing lab they had worked on all winter. Corey himself complained of several weeks' sleeplessness and chronic fatigue; he said he felt guilty that he had let his father down about the lab, which he "knew he enjoyed." His family doctor had said he was physically healthy.

After a diagnosis of Major Depressive Disorder and 10 days' treatment with imipramine, Corey improved enough that his name came up in a discharge-planning conference. "What about the compulsions?" asked the evening nurse, who had doubled back that morning to fill in.

"What compulsions?" everyone else wanted to know.

The nurse hadn't known about them either, until Corey's roommate had finally spilled the beans during group therapy. It took Corey 3 hours to get ready for bed. Everything had to be done in a certain order—teeth first, 10 strokes per tooth from top to bottom, beginning with the left upper molars. If

TABLE 17.6. Criteria for Obsessive–Compulsive Disorder

- The patient has obsessions or compulsions, or both.
  - ✓ **Obsessions.** *All* of the following must be present:
    - Recurring, persisting thoughts, impulses, or images inappropriately intrude into awareness and cause marked distress or anxiety.
    - These ideas are not just excessive worries about ordinary problems.
    - The patient tries to ignore or suppress these ideas or to neutralize them by thoughts or behaviors.
    - There is insight that these ideas are products of the patient's own mind.
  - ✓ **Compulsions.** *All* of the following must be present:
    - The patient feels the need to repeat physical behaviors (checking the stove to be sure it is off, washing hands) or mental behaviors (counting things, silently repeating words).
    - These behaviors occur as a response to an obsession or in accordance with strictly applied rules.
    - The aim of these behaviors is to reduce or eliminate distress or to prevent something that is dreaded.
    - Either these behaviors are not realistically related to the events they are supposed to counteract, or they are clearly excessive for that purpose.
- During some part of the illness, the patient recognizes that the obsessions or compulsions are unreasonable or excessive. (This is not applicable to young children.)
- The obsessions and/or compulsions do at least one of these:
  - ✓ Cause severe distress
  - ✓ Take up time (more than an hour per day)
  - ✓ Interfere with the patient's usual routine or social, school, work, or other functioning
- If the patient has another Axis I disorder, the content of obsessions or compulsions is not restricted to it.
- The symptoms are not directly caused by a general medical condition or by use of substances, including medications and drugs of abuse.

Specify if: With Poor Insight. During most of this episode, the patient does not realize that these thoughts and behaviors are unreasonable or excessive. (This specifier does not apply to young children.)

Coding Note: DSM-IV specifies preoccupations typical of other Axis I disorders that must be ruled out: appearance (Body Dysmorphic Disorder); food (eating disorders); being seriously ill (Hypochondriasis); guilt (mood disorders); sexual fantasies or urges (paraphilias); drugs (substance use disorders); and hair pulling (Trichotillomania).

he lost count, or if he thought he did, he started over. Toothbrushing alone sometimes occupied 45 minutes.

"If I don't get it right, I feel awful. I squirm." Corey admitted that he didn't know what would happen if he didn't get it right, but he thought it would be pretty terrible. "It even sounds dumb to me. Like, rationally, what could possibly happen? But being rational doesn't seem to have much to do with it."

After Corey finally finished brushing his teeth, he would shower—scrubbing away with his washcloth for 100 strokes per body part at a time, until the hot water ran out. He mentally divided his towel into four segments: the first for his face and neck, the second for his arms and legs, the third for his upper body, and the fourth for "everything that's left over." There had been a few times 6 or 8 months ago, not long after his rituals began to get out of hand, when he became confused about which part of the towel he had used and commenced the whole showering process again. But cold showers and soggy towelings had taught him to pay close attention to the details of his drying process. Other rituals would follow—how many steps to take, which objects to touch (or untouch if he got it wrong), how to arrange his slippers, how to take off his bathrobe—as he physically got, or tried to get, into bed.

Although Corey's bedtime rituals had begun only about a year ago, even as a small child he had had a variety of fears and obsessional thoughts. "Mainly, I'd count things. You know—how many steps it took to get from one block to the next; how many breaths; how many ceiling tiles, or holes in ceiling tiles, in the classroom. There's nearly 10,000 in my room here."

From the time Corey was 5, his mother noted, he had been afraid of nuclear attack. When he would open his eyes in the morning, it would sometimes seem so bright outdoors that he would start counting seconds as he waited for the blast that seemed sure to come. She added that the family history was negative for mental disorders—except for her husband's brother, who had developed a facial tic when he was a teenager. It had lasted until he committed suicide when he was 31.

Evaluation of Corey

Corey's current OCD symptoms were largely limited to compulsions; obsessions by themselves would also qualify him for this diagnosis. All of the required components were present. He felt that he had to repeat behaviors (primarily his bedtime rituals, although his earlier behavior of counting was also still present). He carried out these behaviors according to strict rules (number of strokes, arranging his slippers, touching), and he felt that if he didn't follow the rules, something awful would happen. It didn't matter that he couldn't define the consequence; this simply underscored the fact that there could be no realistic relationship between the behaviors and the consequences they were intended to avert. The symptoms were important, in that they both caused him distress and wasted a lot of time. The family doctor found no evidence of a **medical condition**; this would be important to rule out, since obsessive–compulsive behavior has been reported in Lyme disease and streptococcal infections. Although as a younger child he might not have had insight into the excessive or unreasonable nature of his symptoms, he did now. (If he did not

The condition known as PANDAS has only been described in the past few years. The acronym stands for "pediatric autoimmune neuropsychiatric disorders associated with streptococcal infection." Following a streptococcal infection such as a sore throat, these child (or, occasionally, adolescent) patients abruptly develop obsessions and/or compulsions that may be accompanied by tics. The symptoms wax and wane, often recurring with repeat infections. Many patients also exhibit labile emotions, fears or rituals at bedtime, anxiety at separation from parents, and distractibility. PANDAS children typically fall ill at age 6–7, at least 3 years younger than the average age at onset for childhood OCD. Many of them also meet criteria for ADHD. Although the exact cause is not known, one postulated mechanism of action is that in genetically susceptible individuals, infection-induced antibodies cross-react with areas of the brain (such as the basal ganglia) that have been implicated in the development of OCD.

have insight currently, but had had it at one time, the specifier With Poor Insight would apply.)

Depressions like Corey's are frequently encountered in OCD and are often the reason why patients come for evaluation. Corey had more than enough symptoms for a Major Depressive Episode (see Table 16.1 in Chapter 16): depressed mood, poor concentration, decreased appetite, loss of interest, insomnia, fatigue, and a suicide plan. They caused him much distress and interfered with school; because he was not psychotic and had no history of prior mood disorder, he would be diagnosed as having Major Depressive Disorder, Single Episode, Severe Without Psychotic Features (Table 16.2). Because his guilt feelings were consistent with the general themes of depression and he did not try to suppress them, they would not be considered obsessional.

Corey had not reported **Panic Attacks**, and his fears were of some vague retribution that could occur, not of those typical of the more **Specific Phobia** or **Social Phobia**. Patients with **Generalized Anxiety Disorder** also worry a lot, but about a variety of situations that seem realistic (see, e.g., the history of Gerald given earlier). Obsessive–compulsive symptoms are often encountered in patients with **Tourette's Disorder**, which should have been considered (and quickly rejected) in Corey's case.

Because it more urgently required attention, Corey's Major Depressive Disorder would be listed first in his five-axis diagnosis:

Axis I	296.23	Major Depressive Disorder, Single Episode, Severe Without Psychotic Features
	300.3	Obsessive–Compulsive Disorder
Axis II	V71.09	No diagnosis
Axis III		None
Axis IV		None

Axis V   GAF = 45   (on admission)
            GAF = 70   (on discharge)

Assessing Obsessive–Compulsive Disorder

General Suggestions

Due to shame or embarrassment, neither children nor adults are likely to mention obsessions and compulsions spontaneously. You will probably have to ask young patients a question like this: "Have you ever felt you had to do something, or had certain habits, that might seem senseless to you but that you just *had* to keep on doing?" Be prepared to give some examples, as of dressing or bathing routines that must be done a certain number of times, or rituals that involve repeatedly checking the stove or oven to be sure it is off. Be sure to query family members to learn whether they are involved in carrying out rituals; because these demands are insatiable, siblings and parents sometimes become enmeshed in trying to help an affected child or adolescent cope.

Obsessions tend to concern contamination (germs, dirt), danger (self or others), the drive for symmetry, and morality (scrupulosity). Compulsions include washing for cleanliness, carefully drawing numbers or letters until they are perfect, and ordering things into appropriate groupings. Rituals, often quite elaborate, are much more likely to be reported by parents than to be observed in the clinician's office. Symptoms tend to change over time, so that in the course of a year or two a young patient may have washing, checking, and ordering rituals.

Developmental Factors

OCD symptoms also tend to change with increasing age. Preoccupation with counting and symmetry is especially prevalent in grade school children; concerns about cleanliness become more prominent during adolescence. It is important not to diagnose OCD in children who are merely experiencing normal developmental rituals of childhood, such as games with stringent rules ("Step on a crack and break your mother's back") and hobbies that require careful attention to detail (collecting stamps, match covers, and the like).

309.81 POSTTRAUMATIC STRESS DISORDER
(AND 308.3 ACUTE STRESS DISORDER)

Most DSM-IV diagnoses do not postulate a particular etiology. When the cause of mental symptoms is known, it is usually something physical like cocaine use or a brain tumor. In the case of Posttraumatic Stress Disorder (abbreviated PTSD here), however, the cause is an emotion—fear, helplessness, or horror—evoked by an overwhelming event. For children and adolescents, those events are pretty much the same as for adults: physical or sexual abuse, violence (especially prevalent wherever drugs are readily available), and the disruption caused by war or by environmental catastrophes (fires, earthquakes, or tornadoes). Even events that are only "near-misses," such as leaving the shelter of a tree moments before it was struck by lightning, can qualify as the precipitant.

Of course, it takes more than a traumatic event to create PTSD. Otherwise, how can we explain the fact that the same stressor may produce symptoms in one individual but not in another? Several factors may be involved:

- Duration and severity of the stress and the duration of the evoked terror
- The emotional stability of the child or adolescent
- Reactions shown by parents and extended family members
- The community's social network
- Cultural and political factors (e.g., national struggles)

The frequency of PTSD may be increasing in children and adolescents, especially those who live in the inner city, where stressors are abundant. One study found that 40% of inner-city teenagers had experienced at least one such event by the age of 18. In another study, nearly half of children involved in traffic accidents developed PTSD. Although juvenile PTSD may be among the most underrecognized of mental health disorders, there is also some evidence that young patients can recover quickly: Perhaps two-thirds recover within the first 18 months of developing symptoms. However, some remain symptomatic well into adulthood.

DSM-IV has introduced criteria for a new disorder, Acute Stress Disorder (abbreviated ASD in this discussion) to cover instances where symptoms like those of PTSD develop rapidly and persist for a month or less. Any patient whose symptoms last longer than 1 month will have to be rediagnosed as having PTSD. The criteria for both disorders are given in Table 17.7. However, very little is known as yet about ASD, especially in young patients.

Monica

When Monica was 5, she nearly died in an earthquake. With her best friend, Erin, she had been riding in a car driven by Erin's mother. Coming home from an after-school party for a classmate's birthday, they were just ready to leave the expressway when the car began to pitch from side to side. Monica, buckled into the right side of the rear seat, glanced at her friend just as a piece of the overpass fell onto the left half of the car. That was the last she ever saw of either Erin or her mother.

It was nearly 2 days before rescuers could get to the car. They found Monica physically unhurt, though hungry and cold. When a metalworker finally cut through the side of the car with an acetylene torch and brought her out, the television reporters took to calling her the "miracle girl."

After a physical checkup at the hospital, Monica went home with her father. Of course, she had been reunited with both her parents, but her mother was too distraught to care for her; besides, it was her father's week to have her. Since the parents' trial separation began, Monica and her sister, Caroline, had spent that summer and fall shuttling between their parents. Although her mother was still heavily sedated, she agreed that Monica should return to after-noon kindergarten as soon as possible. "We both thought she should get back on the horse," as her father put it.

The following Monday she was back in class, but right away her teacher noticed that something was wrong. Monica had always loved the rhythm band, but now she would leave the circle and roam aimlessly. She couldn't even be enticed by her favorite instrument, the triangle. At times she would put her forearm across her eyes. "It looked just like she was trying to shut out the light," her teacher told the clinician. "I tried to talk to her about it, but she'd wander off. It seemed as if we just didn't have her with us any more."

Her father had noticed the change, but he kept thinking, "She'll come out of it." Besides, he said, he only saw her for a week at a time, and he and his wife didn't talk much about anything, even the children. He knew that Monica had begun wetting the bed once again, after nearly 2 years of being dry at night, and now she nearly always cried whenever she had to go anywhere in the car. But it was 9-year-old Caroline who finally tipped him off to the extent of Monica's dete-rioration. Monica had trouble falling asleep, and nearly every night she awakened screaming about some dream she'd had—"monsters, or something," Caroline explained. Several times she had been observed playing "earthquake" with a set of blocks, which she repeatedly tumbled onto her dolls.

TABLE 17.7. Criteria for Posttraumatic Stress Disorder and Acute Stress Disorder

Posttraumatic Stress Disorder	Acute Stress Disorder
• The patient has experienced or witnessed, or was confronted with, an unusually traumatic event that has *both* of these elements: • The event involved actual or threatened death or serious physical injury to the patient or to others. • The patient responded with intense fear, horror, or helplessness. (Children may respond with agitated or disorganized behavior.)*	
• The patient repeatedly relives the event in at least one of these ways: ✓ Intrusive, distressing recollections (thoughts, images); in children, repetitive play centered around trauma-related themes may occur* ✓ Repeated, distressing dreams; children's dreams may be frightening, but without recognizable content* ✓ Through flashbacks, hallucinations, or illusions, acting or feeling as if the event were recurring (includes experiences that occur when intoxicated or awakening); young children may reenact the trauma* ✓ Marked mental distress in reaction to internal or external cues that symbolize or resemble the event ✓ Physiological reactivity (such as rapid heartbeat, elevated blood pressure) in response to these cues	• The patient repeatedly relives the event in at least one of these ways: ✓ Recollections (dreams, flashbacks, illusions, images, thoughts) ✓ The sense of reliving the event ✓ Mental distress as a reaction to reminders of the event
• The patient avoids trauma-related stimuli and has numbing of general responsiveness (absent before the traumatic event), as shown by three or more of these: ✓ Tries to avoid thoughts, feelings, or conversations concerned with the event ✓ Tries to avoid activities, people, or places that recall the event ✓ Cannot remember an important feature of the event ✓ Shows a marked loss of interest or participation in important activities ✓ Feels detached or isolated ✓ Has a restricted affective range or ability to feel strong emotions ✓ Views future life as brief or unfulfilled	• The patient strongly avoids activities, conversations, feelings, people, places, or thoughts reminiscent of the trauma. • During the event or just after, the patient exhibits three or more symptoms of dissociation: ✓ Numbed or detached feelings, or lack of emotional responses ✓ Diminished awareness of surroundings, as in a daze ✓ Derealization ✓ Depersonalization ✓ Amnesia for important aspects of the event
• The patient has at least two of the following persistent symptoms of hyperarousal that were not present before the traumatic event: ✓ Insomnia (initial or interval) ✓ Angry outbursts or irritability ✓ Poor concentration ✓ Excessive vigilance ✓ Increased startle response	• There are marked symptoms of anxiety or hyperarousal, such as excessive vigilance, insomnia, irritability, poor concentration, restlessness, or increased startle response.

(continued)

TABLE 17.7 (continued)

Posttraumatic Stress Disorder	Acute Stress Disorder
• These symptoms cause clinically important distress or impair school, work, social, or other functioning.	• The symptoms cause clinically important distress; impair school, work, social, or other functioning; or block the patient from doing something important, such as getting help or relating the experience.
• Symptoms have lasted longer than 1 month.	• Symptoms begin within 4 weeks of the trauma and last from 2 days to 4 weeks. • The symptoms are not directly caused by a general medical condition or by use of substances, including medications and drugs of abuse. • They are not better explained by another Axis I or Axis II disorder, including Brief Psychotic Disorder.

Specify whether:
    Acute: Symptoms have lasted less than 3 months.
    Chronic: Symptoms have lasted 3 months
        or longer.
 	
Specify if:
    With Delayed Onset: The symptoms did not appear
        until at least 6 months after the event.	

Coding Note: The PTSD criteria marked with an asterisk (*) may be experienced differently by children than by adults. It is not clear whether they should apply to ASD as well.

Caroline had tried to talk to their mother, who was still somewhat in shock herself. "She just shakes her head when I try to tell her about Monica," Caroline said. "She cries a lot."

During his third week with the children after the earthquake, their father took Monica for an evaluation. He reported that she had been born after a full-term, normal pregnancy, and that as far as he could remember, her developmental milestones had been normal. "No use asking their mother. She insists that both girls are perfect, have never been sick a day in their lives. Not even a cold." But he was pretty sure that Monica had had no previous health problems or allergies. The only family history of mental disorder he knew of was in some of his wife's relatives—her father had been a serious alcoholic, and her older brother had shot and killed himself for unknown reasons when he was quite young.

Monica would only enter the playroom accompanied by her father. She was an almost-pretty, dark-haired child who, with his urging, spent several minutes surveying the contents of the room before carefully seating herself on the edge of a wooden chair and adjusting her dress so it fell well below her knees. Throughout the interview, she never made a single spontaneous comment, though she would respond to questions from the interviewer. On two occasions, she said that she "didn't know" or "didn't remember" about what happened in the car the day of the earthquake. Toward the end of the session, the interviewer placed the doll house squarely in front of Monica and began to play with it. Monica showed her first spark of enthusiasm when she took the little girl doll and stuffed it into the pink plastic toilet. "We don't need her any more," she explained. "She died."

Evaluation of Monica

Monica's event was traumatic by anyone's standards. Not only did it threaten her own life, but in her presence it took the lives of Erin and her mother. We could surmise Monica's emotional reaction, but she also showed disorganized behavior in response, thus fulfilling the second DSM-IV requirement about the event itself.

She relived the event in three ways: through distressing dreams (some children may sleepwalk), the content of which was unclear (as is typical); by playing "earthquake" (traumatic play) with her dolls; and by crying whenever she had to take a car ride, which seemed to symbolize the event to her. She showed avoidance and numbing through refusal to talk, aversion to car rides, and reduced interest in her schoolwork. (Could the patently obvious play with the "dead" doll also be a child's version of fear of a brief life?) Her insomnia and poor concentration suggested hyperarousal. Her symptoms caused serious distress and impaired school functioning.

At the time of her interview, Monica had been symptomatic for just over 5 weeks, so her diagnosis would be PTSD. If she had been evaluated several weeks earlier, might she have been diagnosed as having ASD? The stressors required for ASD are the same as for PTSD, but the time frame is compressed to 30 days or less. And, though their number can be fewer, the same symptom elements must be present: reexperiencing the event, avoiding reminders of it, and experiencing anxiety or hyperarousal. So far, Monica would seem to have filled the bill. But did she show at least three symptoms of dissociation (required for ASD, not for PTSD)? The vignette suggests only that she was detached, but ASD is such a new diagnosis in DSM-IV that we don't know yet how children experience the dissociative symptoms usually found in adults.

Prominent among the symptoms found associated with PTSD are those of depression and anxiety; these are the categories of diagnoses that usually form the backbone of the differential diagnosis. Monica had too few depressive symptoms to warrant an independent diagnosis of **Major Depressive Disorder** (though future clinicians would need to watch for suicide attempts), and no symptoms of any other **anxiety disorder** (especially **phobias**). An **Adjustment Disorder** would be diagnosed only if the stressor were milder (not life-threatening) and if the specific PTSD symptoms were not present—and if no specific Axis I diagnoses were appropriate.

Because comorbidity is the rule with juvenile PTSD, clinicians must also ask about symptoms related to the **misuse of substances,** as well as the additional symptoms that might allow an additional diagnosis of **Reactive Attachment Disorder of Infancy or Early Childhood** and **Separation Anxiety Disorder.** Preexisting **learning disorders** may be exacerbated. Other possible comorbid disorders include **Panic Disorder**, **Generalized Anxiety Disorder**, **Sleep Terror Disorder**, and **Sleepwalking**. None of these was evident in Monica's case.

Note that the criteria for PTSD allow the stressor to be one that has been vicariously experienced. Could Monica's mother, whose inability to provide emotional support may have contributed to Monica's symptoms, have been suffering from a degree of PTSD herself?

A variety of environmental factors that could complicate treatment would be listed on Axis IV of Monica's full diagnosis:

Axis I	309.81	Posttraumatic Stress Disorder, Acute
Axis II	V71.09	No diagnosis
Axis III		None
Axis IV		Earthquake survivor; death of friend; parents separated
Axis V	GAF = 50	(current)

Assessing Posttraumatic Stress Disorder (and Acute Stress Disorder)

General Suggestions

Of all the DSM-IV diagnoses, PTSD (as well as ASD) presents some of the greatest challenges to interviewers. One impediment consists in the diagnostic criteria, which are more numerous and more complicated than for most other commonly diagnosed mental disorders. Even when children or adults do remember what happened to them, they often try to forget either the actual incidents or their feelings at the time.

Permit a cooperative child or adolescent to report the entire event spontaneously. To facilitate recall, you may have to mention a number of possible stressors, such as natural disasters or physical or sexual trauma. Drawing or dramatizing trauma can facilitate communication and data gathering in a younger child. Of course, history obtained from parents or other informants will guide your emphasis. Some clinicians ask a child or adolescent to imagine once again actually being in the traumatic situation. This tactic requires extensive preparation for anxiety or other emotional reactions on the patient's part. Also, beware of inducing false memories in suggestible individuals; some authorities recommend audiotaping or even videotaping interview sessions, to preserve the exact feeling-tone of questions and answers for later possible legal challenges. We emphasize that some of these data-gathering methods are extremely controversial and will be rejected by many child mental health professionals.

The abuse of trust that accompanies sexual or physical abuse may cause some children or adolescents to have difficulty expressing their feelings, even to the most sympathetic of interviewers. Accurate information may be especially difficult to obtain in cases of suspected parental abuse. Whenever possible in such a case, interview each informant separately and alone.

The length of time since the trauma occurred may affect the symptom picture you observe. Immediately after the incident, there may be acute anguish and the appearance of shock—the patient moves slowly, as if dazed. Later, there may be gradual withdrawal that, accompanied by other symptoms, can be mistaken for depression. It is easy to diagnose a mood disorder and ignore the PTSD.

Developmental Factors

Young children are especially likely to develop PTSD symptoms. Young children may talk less than before, complain of physical symptoms (headache or abdominal pains), or repetitively act out their anxieties. Such play may specifically reenact the causative trauma: For example, a 6-year-old who had fallen out of a boat repeatedly "drowned" a GI Joe doll in the bathtub as he worked through his anxiety. Others may regress to muteness, bedwetting, thumb sucking, or immature speech. Older children develop anxiety or depressive symptoms; they, too, may regress to an earlier developmental stage (crying when frustrated, "forgetting" what they have already learned well, doing chores to the standards of a younger child). Adolescents may engage in dangerous counterphobic play that may come to light only as historical material. Whereas adults may relive the traumatic incident in flashbacks or dreams, most children have only the latter, which may take the form of monsters or other frightening images.

OTHER ANXIETY DISORDERS

293.89 Anxiety Disorder Due to a General Medical Condition

Many medical conditions can cause symptoms of anxiety. Usually these will be similar to the symptoms of Panic Disorder or Generalized Anxiety Disorder, but occasionally they take the form of obsessions or compulsions. In general, anxiety symptoms in a young patient will not be caused by a medical disorder, but it is most important to identify those that are. Table 13.1 in Chapter 13 lists the criteria for Anxiety Disorder Due to a General Medical Condition.

Substance-Induced Anxiety Disorder

Many substances can produce anxiety symptoms. These may occur during either intoxication (or heavy use, in the case of caffeine) or withdrawal, and they may take the form of panic, generalized anxiety, obsessions or compulsions, or phobias. As always in young patients, it is important to consider the possibility of substance use when symptoms develop suddenly and when no history of such symptoms exists. Table 14.5 in Chapter 14 gives the criteria for Substance-Induced Anxiety Disorder, and Table 14.6 provides guidance in coding this by substance class.

300.00 Anxiety Disorder Not Otherwise Specified

In many adult patients, anxiety symptoms are the predominant features of distress, but they do not qualify for any specific DSM-IV diagnosis. Although the data are still lacking, we have no reason to believe that this finding will be different for children and adolescents. This category can be used for those whose symptoms are too few, too many (such as a mixture of anxiety and depressive symptoms), too confusing, or too poorly delineated to permit a more exact diagnosis. Before assigning a child or adolescent to this category, be sure to consider Adjustment Disorder With Anxiety or With Mixed Anxiety and Depressed Mood.

CHAPTER 18 | Somatoform Disorders

Quick Guide to Somatic Symptoms

As usual, the page (or table) number following each item indicates where a more detailed description of it can be found.

Somatoform Disorders

Somatization Disorder. The young patient (usually an adolescent) has multiple, unexplained symptoms (including pain and three other groups of symptoms) that affect multiple areas of the body. It is found almost exclusively in females (p. 375).

Conversion Disorder. These patients complain of isolated symptoms that resemble neurological or other medical conditions (*not* pain, although they may experience pain as well), but the symptoms have no identifiable physiological or anatomical cause. DSM-IV requires the clinician to presume a psychological cause (p. 368).

Pain Disorder. Either the pain in question has no apparent physical or physiological basis, or it far exceeds expectations suggested by a patient's objective physical condition (p. 372).

Hypochondriasis. An otherwise healthy patient who has the unfounded fear of a serious, often life-threatening illness such as cancer or heart disease may warrant this diagnosis. It has not been studied in children.

Body Dysmorphic Disorder. In this rare disorder, physically normal patients believe that parts of their bodies are misshapen or ugly. Body

Dysmorphic Disorder typically begins in adolescence, but it is uncommon to the point of rarity.

Somatoform Disorder Not Otherwise Specified. This is a catch-all category of unexplained somatic symptoms that fail to meet criteria for *any* of the DSM-IV somatoform disorders (p. 379).

Other Causes of Somatic Complaints

Before any somatoform disorder can be diagnosed in a young patient, medical illness must be carefully excluded. An adolescent who complains of abdominal pain may be evaluated for appendicitis and ulcerative colitis; if no physical cause for the pain is found, Somatization Disorder or Pain Disorder may be diagnosed.

Pain with no apparent physical cause is characteristic of some patients with a major Depressive Episode (Table 16.1). Patients who use substances may complain of pain or other physical symptoms that result from the effects of Substance Intoxication or Withdrawal (Tables 14.3 and 14.4), or they may represent efforts to obtain the substance of choice. Complaints of pain or other somatic symptoms also characterize the Malingering (p. 443) and behavior of parents who want to occupy the sick role in factitious disorder by proxy (p. 382).

INTRODUCTION

DSM-IV describes six somatoform disorders—Somatization Disorder, Undifferentiated Somatoform Disorder, Conversion Disorder, Pain Disorder, Hypochondriasis, and Body Dysmorphic Disorder—as well as the ubiquitous Not Otherwise Specified diagnosis. Although these disorders often have their roots in childhood and adolescence, they have been little studied in juveniles, especially young children. Indeed, most DSM-IV somatoform disorders apply poorly to children, partly because the criteria were not written with them in mind. For example, although Somatization Disorder is frequently encountered in adult mental health populations, its very low frequency in children may be due to criteria that emphasize behaviors that can only be expected after puberty. With a single possible exception (Body Dysmorphic Disorder), the somatoform disorders are typically chronic illnesses, beginning so early and enduring so long that some regard them as closely related to the personality disorders.

As in some other chapters of this book, we have been selective in our choice of disorders discussed in this chapter. We have omitted Undifferentiated Somatoform Disorder because it is a residual category badly crippled by its overly broad definition (it requires only one physical complaint) and because there is no evidence for its applicability to child populations. Hypochondriasis has also not been studied in young patients. Although Body Dysmorphic Disorder typically begins in adolescence, we omit it, too, because it is so rare. In addition, we have departed from DSM-IV's order of presentation for the remaining somatoform disorders. DSM-IV describes Somatization Disorder before Conversion and Pain Disorders, but we have moved the latter two disorders up to precede Somatization Disorder. We do so to describe the bases for these two disorders (conversion or pseudoneurological symptoms and pain symptoms, respectively) in some detail before introducing Somatization Disorder, which includes symptoms from these two groups as criteria.

300.11 CONVERSION DISORDER

A *conversion symptom* occurs when there is (1) a change in how the body functions (2) in the absence of apparent physical or physiological malfunction and (3) under the influence of an emotional conflict. Conversion symptoms (named because they supposedly convert anxiety into physical manifestations) suggest the presence of neurological deficits when none exist. They are sometimes called *pseudoneurological symptoms.* Examples include patients who complain of total deafness but jump when a paper bag is burst behind them, or who indicate inability to speak but are still able to whisper. The criteria for Conversion Disorder (see Table 18.1) require the clinician to postulate that psychological factors are related to the development of at least one pseudoneurological symptom in a patient who is not malingering.

Both motor and sensory deficits can be experienced as conversion symptoms. Although the list of possible symptoms is long, only a few have been much reported in young children. They include fatigue, muscle stiffness and pains, upset stomach, and pseudoseizures. (Patients may also complain of headache, abdominal pain, and other bodily pains. When *only* pain symptoms occur, however, in DSM-IV these are given a diagnosis of Pain Disorder.) Older children and adolescents may report classical pseudoneurological symptoms, such as numbness or tingling of extremities (paresthesias), partial paralysis, and trouble walking. Other conversion symptoms can include blindness, dou-

TABLE 18.1. Criteria for Conversion Disorder

- At least one symptom or deficit of sensory or voluntary motor function indicates a neurological or other general medical condition.
- The deficit or symptom is not limited to pain or sexual dysfunction.
- It is serious enough to produce at least one of these:
  ✓ It warrants medical evaluation
  ✓ It causes distress that is clinically important
  ✓ It impairs social, school, work, or other functioning
- Appropriate investigation cannot identify a neurological or other general medical condition, or the direct effects of substance use, as a full explanation for the deficit or symptom.
- Conflicts or other stressors that precede the onset or worsening of this symptom suggest that psychological factors are related to it.
- The patient doesn't consciously feign the symptom for material gain (as in Malingering) or in order to occupy the sick role (as in Factitious Disorder).
- The symptom is not a culturally sanctioned behavior or experience.
- It does not occur solely during Somatization Disorder, and no other mental disorder better explains it.

Specify type of symptom or deficit:
  With Motor Symptom or Deficit
  With Seizures or Convulsions
  With Sensory Symptom or Deficit
  With Mixed Presentation

---

ble vision, deafness, inability to speak (aphonia), difficulty urinating, difficulty swallowing (possibly due to the sensation of a lump in the throat), loss of consciousness, amnesia, and hallucinations—in fact, any of the symptoms specifically listed in the pseudoneurological symptom group for Somatization Disorder (see Table 18.3, below).

The diagnosis of Conversion Disorder is rarely made in young children. Paradoxically, this may result from the seeming ubiquity of conversion symptoms in children. For example, think of the child who complains of feeling nauseated prior to a dreaded arithmetic test. Such a child is *not* malingering and truly feels ill. Most often, because the stress underlying such a complaint is patently obvious, the child is sent to school anyway. Only in extraordinary circumstances do such complaints cause enough distress to require clinical attention or interfere with functioning; hence the rarity of this diagnosis in children.

Under what circumstances is Conversion Disorder likely to occur? In adults, it is more often found among those who are economically deprived, poorly educated, and medically unsophisticated. Similar factors might well be expected in children and adolescents. It may also be facilitated in families where illness is used as a form of communication or as metaphor. In a large minority of cases, conversion symptoms develop in those who earlier have experienced genuine somatic disease. Although no accurate prevalence data exist for children or adolescents (or adults for that matter), Conversion Disorder is one of the few DSM-IV diagnoses that may actually be declining in frequency in the Western Hemisphere.

Diane

When Diane was only 4, she was started on valproic acid for petit mal epilepsy, which had been diagnosed by EEG. A therapeutic dose was achieved within a few weeks, and her staring spells abruptly stopped. For the next 10 years, Diane took her medicine religiously twice a day; only once or twice, as she neared adolescence, did she ever look at the videos her parents had made of her during one of her spells.

Diane's sister, Deirdre, was 3 years older. Deirdre was a honey blonde, senior class president, and chairperson of the school science fair. Diane had stringy, carrot-red hair and little scholastic aptitude. Her freshman year was the first time the two sisters had ever attended the same school together. On the evening of the homecoming dance, to which Deirdre had been invited by several boys and Diane by none, Diane had the first in a series of staring episodes that continued throughout that year.

Her valproic acid level was reassessed and found to be within clinical limits; nonetheless, the dose was gradually raised almost to the point of toxicity, without effect. Next she was tried on a series of other anticonvulsants, then on combinations of these medications. Several times she improved temporarily, only to relapse into staring episodes (which now occurred as often as four or five times a day). To her distress, she was almost completely unable to participate in extracurricular activities.

Near the end of her freshman year, Diane was admitted to a neurology unit for inpatient observation with continuously monitored EEG. On none of the seven episodes of staring did her EEG show the 3-cycles-per-second, spike-and-wave pattern of discharges that had been present during her episodes years earlier. During each episode she was unresponsive when nursing staff or family members spoke to her, but twice the neurology resident aborted the episode by tickling the bottom of her foot. Subsequently, when a therapist observed that her pseudoseizures probably served to remove her from competition with her older sister, Diane remarked, "Deirdre's beautiful and smart, and I'm nothing!"

Evaluation of Diane

Ruling out **general medical** or **neurological disease** is a cardinal task for any clinician evaluating a patient suspected of Conversion Disorder. Diane's case was confounded by the fact that she had both pseudoseizures and genuine epileptic seizures, as is true of about 70% of patients with pseudoseizures and 20% of those with epileptic seizures. However, even had no physical cause been found, this would not have been sufficient for a diagnosis of Conversion Disorder: Many apparent conversion symptoms later turn out to be caused by physical disease or a different Axis I disorder.

The fact that Diane's seizures could be aborted by a noxious stimulus (tickling) suggested that they were conversion symptoms. Some writers recommend the further test of bringing on an episode through suggestion, but we worry about this procedure's implications for trust and therapy. Of course, a *sine qua non* of the diagnosis is the identification of a probable psychological stressor, because by definition Conversion Disorder occurs when the patient is under stress. No evidence was given to suggest that Diane was consciously feigning her seizures (she seemed upset when she couldn't engage in after-school activities), as would be the case in **Malingering**.

Pain symptoms can occur in the context of Conversion Disorder, but not if they are the *only* symptoms, when a diagnosis of **Pain Disorder** is more appropriate. Diane would also need to be carefully investigated for other somatic symptoms to rule out **Somatization Disorder**, which is by far the better-defined common diagnosis. Somatic symptoms can also occur in patients who have **Major Depressive Disorder** or **Posttraumatic Stress Disorder**. The case vignette provides no evidence concerning any abnormal character traits, but Diane would need to be watched carefully for the development of a **personality disorder**; hence the cautious Axis II designation. Her full diagnosis would be as follows:

Axis I	300.11	Conversion Disorder With Seizures
Axis II	799.9	Diagnosis deferred
Axis III	345.00	Petit mal epilepsy, well controlled
Axis IV		Envious of sibling
Axis V	GAF = 70	(on admission)

307.8X PAIN DISORDER

We think of pain as having a clear-cut cause. Most of the time, for most humans, the etiology is something that can be seen, felt, or deduced from medical tests—an infected thumb, a sore throat, a twisted loop of bowel. Such pain is not a mental disorder; DSM-IV calls it Pain Disorder Associated with a General Medical Disorder, and lists it only to help in the differential diagnosis. But a substantial number of individuals experience pain that has either no identifiable physical cause at all, or no physical cause that is adequate to explain the degree of pain. When either of these is the case, and when *psychological* factors can be identified that help to explain the pain, the diagnosis is Pain Disorder. There are two subtypes of Pain Disorder, coded according to whether or not a general medical condition is also involved (see Table 18.2).

Both Pain Disorder and Conversion Disorder present clinicians with a puzzle: Just how clearly must the putative psychological factor have created, worsened, or maintained the physical symptoms in question? And what constitutes evidence of psychological causation? Although none of the following factors can be considered definitive, they can suggest psychological causation:

- Pain begins after psychological trauma.
- Stressful events increase the pain.
- Disability is worse than seems reasonable for the cause.
- There is evidence of secondary gain (such as avoiding school or punishment).

Some children have episodes of pain for which inadequate medical cause can be found. In one survey, about one-fourth of second-graders were reported to have recurrent abdominal pain. Of course, the number of children for whom this finding was clinically important may have been much lower, but the results suggest the frequency of the complaint. In another study, in only about 10% of children with recurrent abdominal pain could a biological cause be identified.

The experience of pain is subjective, so its measurement relies on the judgment of the sufferer. This is a difficult enough task for an adult; it approaches the Herculean for a young child, who has fewer experiences that can serve as reference points of severity. Response to a placebo is often positive, regardless of whether a patient suffers from organic pain or Pain Disorder.

The origins of Pain Disorder are still not known. Both children and

TABLE 18.2. Criteria for Pain Disorder

• The patient's presenting problem is clinically important pain in one or more body areas.

• The pain causes distress that is clinically important or impairs school, work, social, or other functioning.

• Psychological factors seem important in the onset, maintenance, severity, or worsening of the pain.

• Other disorders (mood, anxiety, psychotic) do not explain the symptoms better, and the patient does not meet criteria for Dyspareunia.

• The patient doesn't consciously feign the symptoms for material gain (as in Malingering) or in order to occupy the sick role (as in Factitious Disorder).

Code according to the predominant cause of pain:
307.80 Pain Disorder Associated With Psychological Factors. If a general medical condition is present, it does not play the major role in the cause, maintenance, severity, or worsening of the pain. Do not use this code if the patient also meets criteria for Somatization Disorder.
307.89 Pain Disorder Associated With Both Psychological Factors and a General Medical Condition. Both of these types of factors seem important in the onset, maintenance, severity, or worsening of the pain.

For either of these, specify whether:
Acute: Has lasted less than 6 months.
Chronic: Has lasted 6 months or longer.

Coding Notes: Also code the general medical condition or site of the pain on Axis III, if the diagnosis is Pain Disorder Associated With Both Psychological Factors and a General Medical Condition. The site is coded only if the exact general medical condition is not yet known. The following Axis III code numbers for sites of pain are included for your convenience:

Site	Code	Site	Code
Abdominal	789.0	Joint	719.4
Back	724.5	Limb	729.5
Back, low	724.2	Pelvic	625.9
Bone	733.90	Renal	788.0
Breast	611.71	Sciatic	724.3
Chest	786.50	Shoulder	719.41
Ear	388.70	Throat	784.1
Eye	379.91	Tongue	529.6
Facial	784.0	Tooth	525.9
Headache	784.0	Urinary	788.0

Pain Disorder Associated With a General Medical Condition is the term used for any patient who has pain that is mainly caused, worsened, or maintained by a general medical condition, so long as any psychological factors play at most a minor role. This is not considered to be a mental disorder and is coded only on Axis III. The Axis III code numbers for sites are as given above.

adults may use pain and other physical symptoms to communicate emotional distress or a need for comfort; certainly the family pattern of illness behavior can influence a child's or adolescent's response to pain. The roots of Pain Disorder may ultimately be found in a young patient's genetic predisposition, but factors specific to the patient's own social circumstances—school problems or lack of social support from the parents, for example—may also play a role.

Jordan

On a Saturday afternoon in October, during the second period of his team's soccer match against a rival third-grade class, Jordan gradually became aware that his stomach was hurting him. At the time he was tending goal—his favorite position—and he didn't tell anyone until after the match, but that evening his parents took him to the urgent care department at their HMO. After X-rays and lab tests proved entirely normal, he was sent home. He soon recovered, but intermittently during the following weeks, he experienced abdominal pain. Now it was nearly Christmas, and Jordan had spent nearly 10 days (off and on) at home, complaining of cramping pain. Several more visits to the doctor and a variety of increasingly complicated laboratory and radiological tests revealed no pathology. In desperation, the pediatrician referred them to the HMO's mental health department.

On the surface, Jordan's was a "Dick and Jane" sort of family, according to the social worker who interviewed them. They lived in a quiet suburb, owned a dog and a cat, and (as could best be determined) had no serious social or financial problems. His dad's job entailed reasonable hours, good pay, and no travel out of town. Jordan's mother hadn't taught school since just before Jordan and his twin sister, Sarah, were born. Now she stayed home to care for them and their 3-year-old sister. A dour woman who looked older than her 38 years, during the interview she complained of her own ill health. Over the years she had evidently consulted a variety of physicians and other clinicians, but the social worker knew of no definitive diagnosis that had ever been made.

Jordan was a good student who liked school, and his grades had not yet suffered. He had cried when told that he couldn't finish the soccer season with his team, but his mood had otherwise remained good throughout the fall. He always fussed when his pain kept him home from school, and he carefully followed the regimen his doctor advised.

Evaluation of Jordan

In most respects, Jordan's history would seem to qualify him for a diagnosis of Pain Disorder. It had resulted in numerous episodes of treatment (clinical importance) and had caused him to miss a number of days of school (impaired functioning). No **general medical disorder**—such as abdominal migraine or ulcerative colitis, both of which can cause recurrent abdominal pain—had been identified. Always described as cheerful, Jordan did not appear to have another Axis I condition, such as **Major Depressive Disorder**. There was no evidence of a desire to be sick or intent to deceive, which would suggest **Factitious Disorder** or **Malingering**, respectively; indeed, he enjoyed school and objected to remaining at home when stricken. There was no evidence that even suggested a **personality disorder.** Had a diagnosis of Pain Disorder been warranted, the relatively brief duration (less than 6 months) and lack of a defined general medical condition would force its classification as Pain Disorder Associated with Psychological Factors, Acute.

For Jordan, however, there was as yet no clear evidence that psychological factors had caused, worsened, or maintained his pain. Therefore, no Pain Disorder Diagnosis was warranted at this time. DSM-IV does not define the degree of relationship a presumed psychological factor must bear to the pain, so one could argue that Jordan's mother's somatizing behavior served as a model. But his clinician regarded that relationship as too tenuous and instead used the Somatoform Disorder Not Otherwise Specified diagnosis, which would help all future clinicians maintain an open mind about the etiology of Jordan's pain.

Axis I	300.81	Somatoform Disorder Not Otherwise Specified
Axis II	V71.09	No diagnosis
Axis III	789.0	Abdominal pain, unknown etiology
Axis IV		None
Axis V	GAF = 70	

300.81 SOMATIZATION DISORDER

Somatization Disorder is the latest iteration of *hysteria*, a mental diagnosis that dates to the time of the ancient Egyptians and Greeks. It has more recently been called *Briquet's syndrome*, for the 19th-century French physician who first described the typical presentation of multiple physical and mental symptoms.

These symptoms often last for many years, perhaps a lifetime, and have a variety of undesirable sequelae: unnecessary surgical procedures, loss of time from work or school, prescription of harmful medications. At its worst, the disorder can result in alienation of patients from their families; suicides have been reported.

According to the criteria (see Table 18.3), Somatization Disorder must begin by the age of 30, but in nearly every case the onset is far earlier—sometimes as young as 4 or 5. Although this condition is rare in men, it affects about 1% of women in the general population. Somatization Disorder tends to run in families; it is probably transmitted through both genes and the environment.

Despite the fact that Somatization Disorder may account for as many as 8% of mental health clinic visits by women, clinicians often overlook it. Perhaps this is because comorbid Axis I disorders are more obvious, or perhaps it is the complicated nature of the criteria: For each of a list of symptoms, either tests show that it cannot be fully explained by organic illness or substance use, or if there *is* an organic condition, the symptom exceeds what would normally be expected. Determining all this requires more time than some clinicians can devote to such meticulous history taking.

Wilma

Although Wilma was only 17 when she was hospitalized for suicidal ideas, she and her mother agreed that she had been sickly and hypochondriacal most of her life. By the time she was 16, she had had two laparotomies for abdominal pain, retention of urine that required catheterization, headaches for which she had consulted a neurologist, and menstrual periods so heavy and painful that she had to stay out of school 3 days a month. The only positive finding had been a cervical polyp, which her gynecologist said could not have caused her trouble. Her attacks of anxiety produced wheezing and chest pain, which her family physician had pronounced "no big deal." When she was only 14 she had had an episode of visual blurring, but the ophthalmologist could find no medical cause for it. Recently she had also been evaluated for vomiting spells, which

The major precursor to the DSMs, the Washington University Criteria for Mental Disorders (popularly called the Feighner criteria), included mood symptoms in the criteria for Somatization Disorder. They were dropped in DSM-III, allowing clinicians to make multiple Axis I diagnoses (e.g., Somatization Disorder plus Major Depressive Disorder). An unintended consequence is that the change allows clinicians to forget that mood and anxiety symptoms are often integral parts of Somatization Disorder.

TABLE 18.3. Criteria for Somatization Disorder

- Starting before age 30, the patient has had many physical complaints occurring over several years.

- The patient has sought treatment for these symptoms, or they have materially impaired social, school, work, or other functioning.

- The patient has at some time experienced a total of at least eight symptoms from the following lists, distributed as noted. These symptoms need not be concurrent.
  - Pain symptoms (four or more) related to different sites, such as head, abdomen, back, joints, extremities, chest, or rectum; or related to body functions, such as menstruation, sexual intercourse, or urination.
  - Gastrointestinal symptoms (two or more, excluding pain), such as nausea, bloating, vomiting (not during pregnancy), diarrhea, or intolerance of several foods.
  - Sexual symptoms (at least one, excluding pain), including indifference to sex, difficulties with erection or ejaculation, irregular menses, excessive menstrual bleeding, or vomiting throughout all 9 months of pregnancy.
  - Pseudoneurological symptoms (at least one), including impaired balance or coordination, weak or paralyzed muscles, lump in throat or trouble swallowing, loss of voice, retention of urine, hallucinations, numbness (to touch or pain), double vision, blindness, deafness, seizures, amnesia or other dissociative symptoms, or loss of consciousness (other than with fainting). None of these is limited to pain.

- For each of the symptoms above, one of these conditions must be met:
  ✓ Physical or laboratory investigation determines that the symptom cannot be fully explained by a general medical condition or by use of substances, including medications and drugs of abuse.
  ✓ If the patient does have a general medical condition, the impairment or complaints exceed what you would expect, based on history, laboratory findings, or physical examination.

- The patient doesn't consciously feign the symptoms for material gain (as in Malingering) or in order to occupy the sick role (as in Factitious Disorder).

Coding Note: In each of the four symptom categories above, the specific symptoms are listed in approximate descending order of frequency.

---

she thought might be related to severe food intolerance (for several years she had been nauseated by the very thought of coconut, celery, and peanut butter); again, however, no pathology had been found. Frequent, dramatic mood swings and numerous claimed suicide attempts had led to a diagnosis of Bipolar I Disorder. For several months she had taken lithium until she became "allergic" to it.

The second of four siblings, Wilma described her family life as "a disaster." Her mother had a long-standing drinking problem; her father gambled; a cousin had accidentally died from an overdose of heroin.

In the hospital, Wilma was at first tearful and distraught. Within a few hours, however, she became interested in a college freshman who had been admitted to deal with his cocaine addiction. In the evening they were seen giggling together in a corner of the dayroom; later that night they eloped from the hospital.

Evaluation of Wilma

As for nearly every other mental disorder, a first order of business is to rule out possible physical causes for the symptoms. That requirement has been embodied in the next-to-last bulleted criterion in Table 18.3. With the minor exception of an isolated cervical polyp, medical investigation had found no causes for Wilma's many complaints.

The DSM-IV version of Somatization Disorder is far simpler than the original Briquet's syndrome criteria (which required some 25 symptoms in nine categories; partly due to its complexity, the diagnosis was infrequently made). Wilma easily fulfilled the following criteria for Somatization Disorder (note that the symptoms do not have to be concurrent): *pain*, in head and abdomen and with menstruation and urination; *gastrointestinal*, food intolerance and vomiting spells; *sexual*, excessively heavy menses; and *pseudoneurological*, urinary retention. There is no evidence that over the years she had intentionally faked her symptoms, which might warrant a diagnosis of **Malingering**, or that she was consciously trying to occupy the sick role, as in **Factitious Disorder**.

In addition, like so many other patients with Somatization Disorder, Wilma had been treated for severe **mood disorder**. Should she also receive a mood disorder diagnosis? To some degree, this would be a matter of judgment. Although she might at one time have met strict criteria for a Major Depressive Episode, the added diagnosis of a mood disorder could encourage a subsequent clinician to use inappropriate somatic treatment when behavioral management might be more appropriate. In any Somatization Disorder patient, it is vital to ask about other disorders and behaviors that often co-occur: **substance-related disorders** and **personality disorders** (especially **Histrionic Personality Disorder**, though **Borderline** and **Antisocial Personality Disorders** are also sometimes diagnosed). For now, diagnosis would be deferred on Axis II. Wilma's full diagnosis would thus be the following:

Axis I	300.81	Somatization Disorder
Axis II	799.9	Diagnosis deferred
Axis III		None
Axis IV		Inconsistent parenting
Axis V	GAF = 65	(on admission)

300.81 SOMATIZATION DISORDER NOT OTHERWISE SPECIFIED

The Somatoform Disorder Not Otherwise Specified category should be reserved for patients who do not meet criteria for *any* of the somatoform disorders described in DSM-IV (including Undifferentiated Somatoform Disorder, Hypochondriasis, and Body Dysmorphic Disorder, as well as those discussed above). Examples of conditions that might be assigned this diagnosis include pseudocyesis (false pregnancy), transient hypochondriacal states, chronic fatigue syndrome, total environmental allergy syndrome, and unexplained physical symptoms lasting less than 6 months; however, it is doubtful whether the first three of these would ever apply to young patients. The case of Jordan (described above in regard to Pain Disorder) illustrates the application of the Not Otherwise Specified diagnosis to a child.

Assessing Somatoform Disorders

General Suggestions

A clinical interview is not usually the appropriate venue for validating physical complaints. Volumes could be (and indeed have been) written describing tests for discriminating conversion symptoms from physically or neurologically based pathology. (For example, genuinely blind patients comply when asked to sign their names; pseudoblind patients may just scribble; any conversion symptom may decrease when a patient is being distracted.) Although many mental health practitioners don't routinely perform such tests, they can look for a complicated medical history (multiple hospitalizations and many trials of medication) and for patterns of behavior and personality characteristics that distinguish patients with a tendency to somatize.

The affective tone used to describe the physical complaints can provide useful information in a teenager who giggles or otherwise appears unconcerned when describing serious symptoms. This characteristic is called *la belle indifférence,* which means "lofty indifference." (Rather than responding with indifference, most young patients with mental or physical illness are frightened by their symptoms.)

The following features include some of the characteristics typical of Histrionic Personality Disorder, which often accompanies Somatization Disorder:

- A presentation that may be either overly dramatic or, paradoxically, blasé
- A seductive manner toward the examiner
- Constant attention seeking
- Excessive emphasis on the patient's own physical attractiveness
- Vagueness when recounting historical data
- An apparent need for frequent praise or reinforcement

On the other hand, remember that, although the following factors can *suggest* a somatoform disorder, they are *not* diagnostic:

- A given patient's anxiety or somatic symptom is increased by stress (stress or conflict can worsen physical symptoms, too).
- The symptoms seem too intense for real illness (individuals vary tremendously in their reactions to pain or dysfunction).
- The patient seems sensitive or dramatic (many histrionic people—and others with Axis II disorders—are physically healthy).
- The presenting symptom seems bizarre (physical illness and other Axis I disorders can begin with highly unusual symptoms).

Because somatoform disorders and childhood abuse are strongly correlated, it is especially important to consider the possibility of sexual or physical abuse in young patients with these disorders. Above all, when assessing any of the somatoform disorders, always be alert for the possibility of organically caused disease.

Developmental Factors

It is developmentally normal for a young child temporarily to react to a minor injury by limping or complaining of pain. In the normal course of events, a few hours or days of diminishing parental attention to the injury will be repaid when the child, too, shifts attention elsewhere. When children do develop conversion symptoms, they tend to have numbness or tingling of extremities (paresthesias), paralyses, pseudoseizures, and trouble walking. Among young children, boys and girls are about equally likely to develop conversion symptoms; after puberty, they occur several times more often in girls. Other studies find that fatigue, back pain, and blurred vision can be experienced by children of any age. Adolescent concern with normal body parts and functioning is developmentally appropriate, and should be considered pathological only when it endures and causes clinically important distress or impairs functioning.

The way children react to pain changes as they mature. Very young children may request hugging or other maneuvers as a distraction from severe, recurrent pain. Older children are often better able to understand and rationalize the need for painful procedures. Tolerance to pain also increases as a child grows; an 8-year-old can shrug off an injury that would make a toddler howl. The physical complaints most frequently reported by prepubertal children are headache and recurrent abdominal pain. Older children and adolescents will complain of extremity pain, muscle aches, and neurological symptoms.

| Factitious Disorder and
Factitious Disorder by Proxy

Quick Guide to Factitious Symptoms

As always, the page number following each item indicates where further information can be found.

Conditions Involving Manufactured Symptoms

Factitious Disorder. In DSM-IV language, these patients make up symptoms for the purpose of assuming the "sick role." They do *not* appear to have material gain in mind (p. 383).

Factitious Disorder by Proxy (Factitious Disorder Not Otherwise Specified). In the proposed DSM-IV diagnosis of factitious disorder by proxy, it is a caregiver who complains of factitious symptoms in a patient. In such a case, the actual DSM-IV diagnosis given must be Factitious Disorder Not Otherwise Specified (p. 383).

Malingering. These people devise symptoms for material gain—obtaining money or drugs, avoiding work or punishment. Malingering is only infrequently diagnosed in adolescents and *never* in young children (p. 443).

Conditions Involving Symptoms That May Look Manufactured

Conversion Disorder. These patients complain of isolated symptoms that seem to have no physical cause (p. 368).

Somatization Disorder. Multiple, unexplained symptoms (including pain and three other groups of symptoms) characterize this chronic disorder, found almost exclusively in women (p. 375).

300.1X FACTITIOUS DISORDER

Patients with Factitious Disorder feign symptoms not for financial or other gain, as is the case with malingerers, but to obtain sympathy or attention for themselves. DSM-IV calls this occupying the "sick role." This condition has borne a variety of other names—most prominently *Münchausen's syndrome*, after the storied 18th-century Baron von Münchausen, who wandered Europe concocting tall tales about his adventures.

Because Factitious Disorder is thought to begin early in life, and because it is occasionally (though not often) diagnosed in older children and adolescents, criteria for it are provided in Table 19.1. However, we do not discuss it further or provide a case vignette for it here, because our emphasis in this chapter is on a particularly troubling condition involving factitious symptoms in young patients—in this instance, symptoms manufactured by their caregivers.

TABLE 19.1. Criteria for Factitious Disorder

- The patient intentionally feigns or produces physical or mental symptoms or signs.
- The patient's apparent motive for this behavior is to occupy the sick role.
- There are no other motives, such as those found in Malingering (financial gain, revenge, or evading legal responsibility).

Code based on predominant symptoms:
  300.16 With Predominantly Psychological Signs and Symptoms
  300.19 With Predominantly Physical Signs and Symptoms
  300.19 With Combined Psychological and Physical Signs and Symptoms (if both are present but neither predominates)

FACTITIOUS DISORDER BY PROXY (300.19 FACTITIOUS DISORDER NOT OTHERWISE SPECIFIED)

Some people attempt to occupy the sick role not by affecting illness in themselves, but by inducing its appearance in others. DSM-IV calls this *factitious disorder by proxy* and includes it in Appendix B as a criteria set proposed for further study (see Table 19.2 for the proposed criteria). (Because it is not yet a formal diagnosis, the DSM-IV code assigned in such a case must be that for Factitious Disorder Not Otherwise Specified.) Usually the mother of a child is responsible for the behavior, but occasionally it will be a father, grandparent, babysitter, or other caregiver who has primary responsibility for the child. Only rarely is the perpetrator of factitious disorder by proxy psychotic; usually there is a personality disorder, substance use disorder, or other Axis I pathology (such as an eating disorder). Many perpetrators have a background in health care, and some have had a personal history of Factitious Disorder.

A caregiver may feign or produce symptoms in a child by various means:

- Parental description only (especially seizures or apnea by smothering)
- Parental description plus false specimens or falsified charts
- Poisoning, smothering, or withholding of food or medicine
- Fabrication of psychiatric disorder
- Factitious signs of pregnancy (in adolescents)
- Embellishment of a genuine physical illness

Suspicion may be raised when a parent seems unconcerned about a seriously ill child, when the child's physician cannot make sense of the symptoms, or when the child remains ill despite apparently adequate treatment. The medical and emotional havoc such a family wreaks may come to light only at the end of a long and frustrating clinical course. The injurious behaviors usually continue until one of three outcomes occurs: The perpetrator is apprehended; increasing age of the child causes the perpetrator to move on to a younger child; or the child dies. In one survey, over 70% of 117 patients sustained permanent disability or disfigurement.

A notorious example of suspected factitious disorder by proxy involves some victims of sudden infant death syndrome (SIDS), in which apparently healthy infants are found dead in their cribs. Some writers hypothesize that up to 10% of SIDS babies are actually murdered. In 1995, one mother was finally convicted in the deaths of five of her own children in the late 1960s. As a result of his experience with this family, the treating pediatrician had speculated in a 1972 journal article about a genetic predisposition to sleep apnea. Although clearly duped, this physician may have influenced a generation of doctors to overlook the suspicious deaths of many children.

Melissa

It all started when she was 8, with an ankle twisted during soccer practice. Melissa fell while driving toward the net and had to sit out the rest of the practice session. Her family doctor diagnosed a mild

TABLE 19.2. Criteria for Factitious Disorder by Proxy

- A person intentionally feigns or produces mental or physical signs or symptoms in someone else who is under the first person's care.
- The person's apparent motive is by proxy to occupy the sick role.
- There are no other motives, such as those found in Malingering (financial gain, revenge, or evading legal responsibility).
- No other mental disorder better explains the behavior.

sprain, and recommended ice and a few days of "taking it easy." Though this prescription seemed to help at first, the pain limited her mobility to the point where she eventually had to stay in bed and receive home tutoring. But it wasn't until her toes turned blue and she complained of prickly numbness in her left leg that Melissa was admitted to the hospital. There she was seen by a sports medicine orthopedist and a neurologist.

Despite the devoted attendance of her mother and increasingly heroic therapeutic efforts, the pain became so severe that Melissa couldn't move her foot and wouldn't let anyone touch it but her mother. MRI, EMG, and sophisticated studies of body chemistry all were normal. The change in the leg's color and temperature alarmed her physicians enough that they transferred her to the intensive care unit. There, separated from her mother, Melissa began to improve almost miraculously. After a week, she had recovered enough that she was returned to the pediatric floor. The day before her scheduled discharge, however, the pain and discoloration returned.

More consultants were called in, but after 2 weeks Melissa's condition again deteriorated. She developed myoclonic jerks of her left leg and spasms of her foot, causing her to kick uncontrollably. Her mother, distraught, begged for more consultants. Increased use of pain medication dulled Melissa's senses so that she slept most of the time; when awake, she was often disoriented and spoke with a thick tongue. The diagnoses ranged from degenerative spinal cord disease to psychogenic myoclonus.

Finally, a neurologist suggested surreptitious video monitoring of Melissa's bed. The following day, the treatment team watched the video replay in horrified fascination as Melissa's mother soothed her daughter and stroked her hair as she gently tightened a tourniquet around the damaged leg. Before the authorities could be notified and protective measures established, Melissa and her mother left the hospital and disappeared.

Evaluation of Melissa

At the top of the list of differential diagnoses belongs every possible **general medical condition** that could cause the symptoms. It was only after the members of Melissa's treatment team had seemingly considered them all that they suspected foul play. For adults with Factitious Disorder (*not* factitious disorder by proxy), **Malingering** should be considered in the differential diagnosis. However, we know of no instances of young children who have inflicted pain or trauma upon themselves, or even, for that matter, falsified other signs or symptoms of physical or mental disease. We will never know exactly why Melissa herself did not disclose the reason for her descent into the medical vortex. Her silence undoubtedly hinges on the strength of the family bond and the reluctance of children, even when they suffer the most grievous forms of abuse, to reveal secrets about parents and others who love and harm them.

Note that in a case of factitious disorder by proxy, it is the perpetrator who receives the diagnosis of Factitious Disorder Not Otherwise Specified. In the case of Melissa's mother, as in most where the patient is merely the vehicle for the perpetrator's behavior, an Axis I V-code for Physical Abuse of Child (V61.21) would also be given. (If a victim is the subject of clinical attention, note that the code number will be different: 995.5.)

Unfortunately (as so often happens), Melissa's mother bolted before her motives could be determined and before her daughter's well-being could be safeguarded. Of course, due to the lack of information, a **personality disorder** could only be suspected, as indicated below on Axis II. Similarly, other Axis I diagnoses, though possibly warranted, could not be made. Not even a GAF score could be assigned. The five-axis diagnosis for Melissa's mother would therefore have to be the following:

Axis I	300.19	Factitious Disorder Not Otherwise Specified
	V61.21	Physical Abuse of Child
Axis II	799.9	Diagnosis deferred
Axis III		None
Axis IV		None
Axis V	GAF = 0	Inadequate information

Had Melissa helped her mother produce false signs or symptoms of a physical disease, she herself could have been diagnosed as having Factitious Disorder With Predominantly Physical Signs and Symptoms (see Table 19.1). Such is sometimes the case for older children, adolescents, and adults who are the victims, but it would rarely be warranted in a child as young as Melissa. If an actual diagnosis of Physical Abuse of Child had not been warranted on Axis I, the fact of abuse could be mentioned on Axis IV. Melissa's GAF score would be high (remember that this score is determined only by mental state, not impairment due to physical or environmental limitations). Melissa's complete diagnosis would be as follows:

Axis I	995.5	Physical Abuse of Child
Axis II	V71.09	No diagnosis on Axis II
Axis III	333.2	Myoclonus
Axis IV		
Axis V	GAF = 85	

Assessing Factitious Disorder by Proxy

General Suggestions

Factitious disorder by proxy is a situation that defies the skills of the most experienced interviewer, for the perpetrators themselves are highly experienced at concealment, and their victims—whether out of fear, love, or simple failure to perceive anything amiss—may remain silent about maltreatment. When faced with possible factitious disorder by proxy, focus on behaviors and personality characteristics of the principal caregiver, who will almost invariably be the perpetrator. These adults are rarely psychotic but may have a history of Somatization Disorder. They will almost certainly have an Axis II disorder, with a personality style that may be bizarre, boisterous, demanding, histrionic, or vague. Some of their characteristics include the following:

- Effusive praise of the providers they are attempting to deceive
- In a caricature of good parenting, excessive attentiveness to a sick child, refusing even to leave the bedside for days at a time
- Lack of appropriate concern for a child who does not respond to treatment and may be desperately ill
- A sometimes remarkable fund of knowledge about a child's medical condition
- Often, a close association with one of the health care professions

Developmental Factors

These children present with all sorts of factitious symptoms, but age helps determine a few basic patterns. Infants and toddlers may present with apnea, cyanosis (blue skin), and seizures, whereas older children are likely to have gastrointestinal symptoms such as diarrhea and vomiting. Other symptoms can include ataxia, headache, paralysis, or weakness.

Young children will be able to provide little information about their own health status. Most adolescents and older children will have the knowledge (and perhaps even the judgment) that something is amiss, but will they divulge information that is critical of a parent or other caretaker? For some, an approach that emphasizes trust and truth between patient and clinician may help. You might say, for example, "It is terribly important that we figure out what's happening here. I'm going to ask you some questions about your problem. If you feel you can't answer truthfully, don't lie—that will confuse us. Just say, 'I'd rather not talk about that right now.' OK?" For others, you will have to rely on covert observation and medical detection.

CHAPTER 20 | Dissociative Disorders

Quick Guide to Dissociation

As in other Quick Guides, the page (or table) number following each item tells where fuller information on it can be found.

Dissociative Disorders

DSM-IV describes four dissociative disorders (Dissociative Amnesia, Dissociative Fugue, Dissociative Identity Disorder, and Depersonalization Disorder) plus the usual Not Otherwise Specified diagnosis. However, for various reasons that are discussed in the chapter introduction, we have chosen to describe only one of these in this chapter.

Dissociative Amnesia. The patient cannot remember important information that is usually of a personal nature and related to stress (p. 391).

Dissociative Fugue. The patient suddenly travels away from home and cannot remember important details about the past.

Dissociative Identity Disorder. One or more additional identities intermittently seize control of the patient's behavior.

Depersonalization Disorder. The patient has episodes of detachment without memory loss, as if observing the patient's own behavior from outside.

Other Disorders Involving Dissociation

Memory loss and other dissociative symptoms can also occur in Posttraumatic Stress Disorder and Acute Stress Disorder (p. 358), substance-induced disorders (Tables 14.3 and 14.4), Conversion Disorder (p. 368), Somatization Disorder (p. 375), and Sleepwalking Disorder (p. 414).

INTRODUCTION

Dissociation a term that originated 400 years ago, but only during the 20th century has it been applied to thought. It occurs when a group of normal mental processes is cut off from the rest; we will define it as a loss of the normal relationships between the different groups of mental processes, so that one or more of consciousness, identity, memory, or perception appear to function independently. The phenomenon of dissociation is found in a variety of mental illnesses, including the somatoform disorders and Posttraumatic and Acute Stress Disorders. When dissociative symptoms are encountered in the course of other mental diagnoses, a separate diagnosis of a dissociative disorder is not ordinarily given.

In fact, authorities still vigorously argue about the DSM dissociative disorders: Do they deserve their own category, or should they be combined with Somatization Disorder and even Histrionic Personality Disorder? Dissociative Identity Disorder, famous in its DSM-III-R incarnation as Multiple Personality Disorder, is especially controversial: Many clinicians feel that the disorder is sometimes induced in susceptible patients by (largely North American) therapists who are particularly interested in this strange condition.

In all dissociative disorders but one, patients experience memory loss that is not caused by physiological or structural disorders of the brain. The fourth, Depersonalization Disorder, constitutes episodes of detachment in which individuals feel as if they are third persons observing their own behavior. Theoretically, a child or adolescent can have any of these disorders, but none has been extensively reported in young patients. Dissociative Identity Disorder and Depersonalization Disorder may begin in childhood but are usually not diagnosed until adulthood, and very few instances of Dissociative Fugue have been reported in juveniles. For this reason, and because of the controversy surrounding the status of the dissociative disorders in general and Dissociative Identity Disorder in particular, we have chosen not to discuss these disorders extensively. We focus here on Dissociative Amnesia, the one dissociative disorder that DSM-IV notes can be presented by any age group from young children upward (although it is still not common in youngsters).

300.12 DISSOCIATIVE AMNESIA

The most frequent cause of amnesia is a medical condition, such as the use of substances, a blow to the head, or the effects of a brain operation. However, in patients with Dissociative Amnesia, no such medical condition can account for the inability to remember certain important events that have occurred in either one or multiple episodes over a period of time. This loss of memory is sufficiently serious to cause distress or to interfere with functioning in some important way. Table 20.1 gives the criteria for this disorder.

Dissociative Amnesia usually begins suddenly, and the time "lost" to the amnesia can be brief or extended—a matter of hours or days to several months. The cause most frequently given is emotional stress or trauma, such as the sense of betrayal a child might feel at being forced into a sexual relationship with a trusted parent. Some of these incidents have come spectacularly to light when an adult, an adolescent, or an older child finally recalls the event and accuses a parent or other adult. In many of these cases, the accused adult has successfully challenged the allegation as factitiously induced by an overzealous therapist. Organizations are now devoted to supporting victims of this so-called *false-memory syndrome,* though sorting out victims from perpetrators has sometimes occupied courtrooms for months.

Rosalind

In her junior year of high school, at age 17, Rosalind tipped the scales at nearly 300 pounds. Despite 3 years of faithfully attending Weight Watchers, she had recently gained another 35 pounds. That had prompted the referral for psychotherapy.

TABLE 20.1. Criteria for Dissociative Amnesia

- The patient's main problem is at least one episode of inability to recall important personal information. This information usually concerns trauma or stress, and it is more extensive than can be explained by common forgetfulness.
- These symptoms cause clinically important distress or impair school, work, social, or other functioning.
- It does not occur solely during Dissociative Identity Disorder, Dissociative Fugue, Posttraumatic Stress Disorder, Acute Stress Disorder, or Somatization Disorder.
- The symptoms are not directly caused by a general medical condition or by the use of substances, including medications and drugs of abuse.

Rosalind proved an excellent candidate for therapy: she was intelligent, clear in her thinking, and unafraid to disagree with an authority figure. Although she didn't lose an ounce, within a couple of months she made real progress in understanding her problems. "It really spooked me," she said during one session. "I had just been watching TV when an image occurred to me and I shut off the sound with the remote. I could see myself in bed with my father, back when I was about 6. He was lying on top of me, with his pants down, and I had a lot of pain between my legs."

Over the next few weeks, Rosalind reported more such memories. She was now sure that her father had repeatedly had intercourse with her over a 3-year period. At this point, her therapist got her permission to interview others in her family. The additional information was shocking, even to a clinician who had spent decades working with mental patients. Her brother Bert (older by 7 years) confirmed not only that he had had suspicions about Rosalind's relationship with her father, but that in fact he had been involved at the same time in an incestuous affair with their mother. Both relationships had lasted until their father was jailed on unrelated charges; he later died in a knife fight in the prison yard. Before long, their mother found a boyfriend and lost interest in Bert.

At no time since the age of 10 had Rosalind experienced any sense of lapses in time; nor had she ever "awakened" to find that she had wandered from home. Other than a lifetime of obesity, her history was unremarkable. Her overall physical and mental health were both good, and she denied any use of drugs or alcohol. A physical exam revealed no neurological cause for concern.

Evaluation of Rosalind

Rosalind's lack of memory for a prolonged period of incest would easily qualify for a diagnosis of Dissociative Amnesia. The absence of alternative personalities or travel from home during any of these periods would rule out **Dissociative Identity Disorder** and **Dissociative Fugue**. Of course, the repeated sexual attacks by her father would qualify as severely traumatic incidents; nevertheless, **Posttraumatic Stress Disorder** and **Acute Stress Disorder** would be eliminated from consideration, in part because she did not reexperience the incidents in flashbacks or dreams.

Rosalind's age and intact cognitive abilities would rule out **dementia** as a possible cause of memory loss. She denied **substance use** and **general medical problems** such as head trauma, and she did not complain of multiple physical problems, as would be the case in **Somatization Disorder**. There was no evidence at all to suggest a **Factitious Disorder**. The fact that her brother corroborated the memories she developed while in therapy militated strongly against her story's being an example of false-memory syndrome. Her diagnosis would thus be as follows:

Axis I	300.12	Dissociative Amnesia
Axis II	799.9	Diagnosis Deferred on Axis II
Axis III	278.01	Morbid obesity
Axis IV		None
Axis V	GAF = 80	(current)

Assessing Dissociative Disorders

General Suggestions

Assessing memory and other dissociation-related mental functions in anyone can be a challenge, but doing so in a child can be especially difficult. As DSM-IV points out, young children normally have memory gaps, due to either inattention or brain immaturity. Because children are acutely aware of the desires of adults, it is all too easy for an interested, sympathetic clinician inadvertently to influence the direction of a child's narrative. Whenever you are attempting to assess apparent amnesia or other dissociative symptoms in a child or teenager, you need to be doubly careful to enter into the project with no agenda or expectation beyond learning the truth.

Besides maintaining an open mind, you should adopt a casual approach, ask open-ended questions, and try to minimize the opportunity for distortion. Avoid penetrating glances and repeated questions about sensitive areas. Material that seems significant and needs exploration in depth may be more safely assessed in multiple interviews. When the possibility of sexual or physical abuse exists, consider obtaining permission to audiotape or videotape interviews, as documentation that you have not led or otherwise unduly influenced answers. Finally, watch for behaviors that may be associated with dissociative disorders in children or adolescents. These include excessive daydreaming, forgetting names of familiar people, losing track of time, having vivid imaginary playmates, and talking to oneself frequently.

Developmental Factors

Younger children typically go spontaneously into trances, during which they may be oblivious and unresponsive to their surroundings. Even at the age of 7 or 8, a child playing with dolls or toys may imbue them with personalities and other qualities that help them form a reciprocal relationship. Of course, this statement holds for any diagnosis and is the basis for using play materials and fantasy in evaluations with a young child. The symptoms of dissociating adolescents closely resemble those of adults.

CHAPTER 21 | Gender Identity Disorder

Depending on the principal type of pathology, DSM-IV divides the sexual and gender identity disorders into three groups: (1) sexual dysfunctions; (2) paraphilias; and (3) Gender Identity Disorder (abbreviated GID in this brief chapter) and GID Not Otherwise Specified. (Because GID Not Otherwise Specified is applied even more rarely than other Not Otherwise Specified diagnoses—it is used primarily for patients with certain congenital endocrine conditions, which DSM-IV refers to as *intersex conditions*—it is not discussed here.) For obvious reasons, the first two groups are not relevant to most juveniles. GID occurs when the assigned genetic sex, as determined by the appearance of the external genitalia, does not accord with the patient's own self-perception as to masculinity or femininity. This results in two features common to all those with GID: identification with the opposite sex, and profound discomfort with one's own sex. The variable manifestations of these two fundamental features differ for children and adults and are listed in the diagnostic criteria for GID (see Table 21.1). The symptoms of an adolescent who presents with the disorder may tilt toward either child or adult manifestations, depending on the patient's maturity.

GID begins surprisingly early—often by the age of 2 and usually by the age of 4. The symptoms are well detailed in the criteria. Note that for children, fulfillment of strong identification with the opposite gender (the first bulleted item in Table 21.1) requires 80% of the check-marked criteria; this is the strictest requirement of any criteria set in DSM-IV. This underscores the importance of ascertaining a child's strong desire to be of the opposite gender.

As is true for so many other disorders, no one knows the cause of GID. And as is true for nearly every disorder where this is the case, each possible

TABLE 21.1. Criteria for Gender Identity Disorder

- The patient strongly and persistently identifies with the other sex. This is not simply a desire for a perceived cultural advantage of being a member of the other sex.

  Children who are younger than adolescent age must have four or more of the following signs of identity with the other sex:
  - ✓ The child reiterates a desire to be, or insistence that the child is, the other sex.
  - ✓ A boy prefers cross-dressing or simulating female garb; a girl insists on wearing only male clothing.
  - ✓ The child persistently and strongly prefers cross-sex roles in fantasy play or repeatedly fantasizes about being the other sex.
  - ✓ The child badly wants to participate in games and pastimes of the other sex.
  - ✓ The child strongly prefers to play with children of the other sex.

  In **adolescents and adults**, this desire may be manifested by any of the following:
  - ✓ Stated wish to be the other sex
  - ✓ Often passing as the other sex
  - ✓ Wish to live or be treated as the other sex
  - ✓ Belief that the patient's feelings and reactions are typical of the other sex

- There is strong discomfort with the patient's own sex or a feeling that the gender role of that sex is inappropriate for the patient.

  A **boy's** discomfort with his assigned sex may be shown by any of these:
  - ✓ Disgust with his genitals
  - ✓ Assertion that his genitals will disappear or that it would be preferable not to have a penis
  - ✓ Rejection of rough-and-tumble play and male activities, games, and toys

  A **girl's** discomfort with her assigned sex may be shown by any of these:
  - ✓ Rejection of urinating in a seated position
  - ✓ Desire not to develop breasts or menstruate
  - ✓ Claims that she will have a penis
  - ✓ Pronounced dislike for usual female clothing

  In adolescents and adults, this is shown by any symptoms such as these:
  - ✓ Preoccupation with hormones, surgery, or other physical means to change one's sex characteristics
  - ✓ Patient's belief in having been born the wrong sex

- The patient does not have a physical intersex condition.

- These symptoms cause clinically important distress or impair school, work, social, or personal functioning.

Assign code number according to current age:
    302.6   Gender Identity Disorder in Children
    302.85   Gender Identity Disorder in Adolescents or Adults

For patients who are sexually mature, specify whether:
    Sexually Attracted to Males
    Sexually Attracted to Females
    Sexually Attracted to Both Males and Females
    Sexually Attracted to Neither Males nor Females

cause has its adherents. The effects of heredity are surmised from studies that find an excess of brothers in families of GID boys. A social etiology is suggested by studies that find GID girls less attractive and GID boys more attractive than their respective nonaffected peers. Findings of depression or Borderline Personality Disorder in over half the mothers of GID children can be used to support either a biological or a psychological etiology. Clinical populations are heavily weighted toward boys (ratios range from 4:1 to 6:1), but this finding

GID occupies an unusual—perhaps unique—niche in DSM-IV: At least as applied to children, it is a diagnosis with a virtually guaranteed lack of stability. In fact, not only do nearly all patients given a childhood diagnosis of GID not receive the diagnosis on follow-up, but most are found to have a lifestyle (homosexuality) rather than a disorder. The problems of construct validity were less apparent in DSM-III-R, which considered Gender Identity Disorder of Childhood a separate diagnosis. Furthermore, a diagnosis called Transsexualism (involving the desire to rid oneself of secondary sex characteristics) was discussed at some length in DSM-III-R but is not even mentioned in DSM-IV. Now, to eliminate the need for developmental cutoffs that may seem arbitrary, all three DSM-III-R diagnoses are combined in DSM-IV: Transsexualism, Gender Identity Disorder of Childhood, and Gender Identity Disorder of Adolescence and Adulthood.

may be skewed by the fact that North American society tolerates effeminate males less well than it does masculine females.

Although there are no solid population-based figures, estimates put the prevalence of GID at about 1 in 1,000 children. The ultimate fate of GID children is known with somewhat greater certainty, for only a tiny minority retain their opposite-sex identification much past puberty. (DSM-IV estimates the rate of GID in the adult population, based on European data for adults seeking sex change surgery, at about 1 in 30,000 for men and 1 in 100,000 women.)

Stanley

"I wasn't very comfortable with myself when I was a child, that's for sure," Stanley admitted to the interviewer. "Fact is, I must have been a pretty strange little kid."

At age 19, Stanley was being interviewed for a follow-up research project. He had been evaluated 12 years earlier at a community child guidance center. That information, recorded in neatly checked boxes and tight paragraphs, revealed the following:

Back then, his mother had reported that he had frequently played dress-up, donning her clothing or that of his older sister. She had noticed that he refused to wrestle or engage in other typical "boy" activities; he usually preferred to play with girls. On one occasion, she heard him and a neighbor girl arguing over which of them would get to be the mother when playing house; she had thought it was cute. The year before, he had asked for a doll for his birthday. His father, who worked two jobs and couldn't be present for any of the diagnostic or subsequent therapy sessions, reportedly worried about his son's cross-dressing but had taken no action because his wife assured him that "it would be all right." Stanley had hated team sports and had preferred jacks to baseball. For this and his other mannerisms, he took an unmerciful ribbing almost from the time he first entered school. During her third interview, his mother admitted that she had been disappointed when Stanley, her fourth and final child, had turned out to be yet another boy.

A physical exam and laboratory tests had been normal, and Stanley had been given a DSM-III diagnosis of Gender Identity Disorder of Childhood. But at follow-up, the young adult Stanley rejected the notion that he was anything but male. "I outgrew it, that wanting to be a girl, years ago," he told the interviewer. "Maybe it was the therapy, but for quite a while now I've been happy being a guy. I'm a *gay* guy you understand, but I am a guy."

Evaluation of Stanley

As a young child, Stanley seemed uncomfortable with being a boy—he hated team sports and other activities typical for boys. He also clearly, strongly, and persistently identified with girls, as shown by cross-dressing, wanting to play the mother's role in a game, playing with dolls and jacks, and preferring girls as playmates. The social ostracism and absence of physical or laboratory indications of an intersex condition would complete the requirements for the diagnosis by DSM-IV criteria; we have already seen that Stanley met the less stringent DSM-III criteria. Of course, at the age of 7, no specifier for sexual attraction would apply. Among sexually mature individuals, nearly all females will be sexually attracted to females. However, only about 75% of males will have a homosexual orientation; the rest will be heterosexual or bisexual.

DSM-IV carefully notes that the diagnosis of GID indicates serious pathology and should be carefully discriminated from mere **lack of conformity with typical sex role behavior**. Thus "tomboy" behavior in a girl or effeminate behavior in a boy, absent the inclusion criteria of the first two bulleted items in Table 21.1 and the clinical significance as required by the fourth, would not qualify. If gender identity problems are found in association with adrenal hyperplasia (as they are in 1 of 5,000 male births), androgen insensitivity, or other intersex conditions, the appropriate diagnosis would be **GID Not Otherwise Specified**. Some adolescents who cross-dress to achieve sexual arousal may be showing early symptoms of **Transvestic Fetishism**, not GID.

Social isolation is a complication that especially affects boys who maintain effeminate speech or physical mannerisms. Other mental conditions that can especially affect GID children include **Generalized Anxiety Disorder, depressive disorders,** and **Separation Anxiety Disorder**. Stanley's childhood diagnosis (according to DSM-IV criteria) would be as follows:

Axis I	302.6	Gender Identity Disorder in Children
Axis II	V71.09	No diagnosis
Axis III		None
Axis IV		Discord with classmates
Axis V	GAF = 71	(age 7)

Stanley's diagnosis at age 19 would be the following:

Axis I	V71.09	No diagnosis or Condition
Axis II	V71.09	No diagnosis
Axis III		None
Axis IV		None
Axis V	GAF = 85	(current)

Assessing Gender Identity Disorder

General Suggestions

Whether treated or not, the vast majority of children with GID will not retain this diagnosis as adults, so their evaluation challenges clinicians to find reasons to reject the diagnosis. As of this writing, no constellation of symptoms (certainly not cross-dressing or effeminate behavior alone) reliably predicts which children will retain the GID diagnosis through adolescence and into adulthood. Of course, the possibility of an intersex condition must be evaluated by physical exam and endocrinological tests. DSM-IV notes that prolonged evaluation may be necessary, especially of adolescent patients, who may be ambivalent or guarded in their presentation.

Although there isn't much objective evidence about its value, some clinicians look to doll play with family figures as a clue to abnormal gender identification in younger children. If, for example, a girl elects neither parent doll when asked which one she would prefer to be, a suspicion of gender identity confusion may be entertained. A child who chooses the opposite-sex doll should be asked to explain the reason for the choice. An answer couched in terms of a perceived social advantage of that sex (e.g., "Only men can be President") doesn't qualify as GID. Children can also be asked to draw the parent they would like to be. Or you can ask, "What do you like about being a [boy or girl]? What don't you like about it?" An older child can understand and respond to the question "Do you ever feel more like [the opposite sex] than like [the child's actual gender]?"

Developmental Factors

Children aged 5 or under may state that they will grow up to be persons of the opposite sex. Older children may display this sort of wish fulfillment in the form of fantasies or play.

Quick Guide to the Eating Disorders

This page (or other) number following each item indicates where a fuller discussion can be found.

Primary Eating Disorders

Each of the primary eating disorders is defined by abnormal eating behaviors, and they have a number of other features in common. Both patients with Anorexia Nervosa and those with Bulimia Nervosa may binge-eat, purge with laxatives, and exercise excessively. Both conditions are encountered mainly in girls and young women; onset is usually during the teenage years.

Anorexia Nervosa. Despite the fact that they are severely underweight, these patients see themselves as fat (p. 402).

Bulimia Nervosa. These patients eat in binges, then prevent weight gain by self-induced vomiting, purging, and exercise. Although appearance is important to their self-evaluations, these patients do not have body image distortion (p. 402).

Eating Disorder Not Otherwise Specified. This category is used for disorders of eating that do not meet the full criteria for either Anorexia Nervosa or Bulimia Nervosa, as well as for binge-eating disorder, a condition proposed for further study that is included in Appendix B of DSM-IV (p. 406).

Other Causes of Abnormal Eating

Changes in weight and appetite are characteristic of Manic and Major Depressive Episodes (Table 16.1) and of Somatization Disorder (p. 375). Patients with Schizophrenia and other psychoses may develop bizarre eating habits (see Chapter 15).

307.1 ANOREXIA NERVOSA

307.51 BULIMIA NERVOSA

As recently as DSM-III-R, Anorexia Nervosa and Bulimia Nervosa were included in the section on disorders usually first diagnosed in infancy, childhood, or adolescence. Despite the fact that these two disorders do usually begin in the teen years, they bear no kinship to the other feeding/eating disturbances included in that section, so DSM-IV gives them their own section.

Anorexia Nervosa and Bulimia Nervosa typically arise in early to middle adolescence and are especially prevalent in young women. Males constitute 10% or fewer of patients with either condition. Although case reports of Anorexia Nervosa have appeared in the literature for at least 200 years, Bulimia

TABLE 22.1. Criteria for Anorexia Nervosa

- The patient will not maintain a minimum body weight—for example, 85% of expected weight for height and age. A child who is still growing may fail to *attain* 85% of weight normal for height and age.
- Despite being underweight, the patient intensely fears becoming fat.
- Self-perception of the body is abnormal, shown by at least one of these:
  ✓ Unduly emphasizes weight or shape in self-evaluation
  ✓ Denies seriousness of low weight
  ✓ Has a distorted perception of own body shape or weight
- Due to weight loss, a female patient who has previously begun menstruating has missed at least three consecutive periods (or periods occur only when she is given hormones).

Specify whether:
    Binge-Eating/Purging Type. During an anorectic episode, the patient often purges (vomits, uses laxatives, or uses diuretics) or eats in binges.
    Restricting Type. No bingeing and purging occur during an anorectic episode. This is the more usual type.

Coding Note: Don't adhere too strictly to the 85% figure in the first bulleted item; it is only a rough guide.

Nervosa has been described only recently; however, the latter is now the more common of the two, affecting perhaps 1–2% of adult women. Perhaps 4% of adolescent girls have bulimic symptoms at one time or another. The reason for the recent upsurge in prevalence is unclear.

These two disorders (see Tables 22.1 and 22.2 for their full criteria) have a number of features in common. The patients have unusual eating habits and place strong emphasis on body weight and shape. They control weight by inappropriate means (purging, fasting, or inappropriate exercising). Either disorder can entail serious consequences for health. Although most Anorexia Nervosa patients remit spontaneously or with treatment, about 5% of them will eventually succumb to complications of their disease. The prognosis for life is better for patients with Bulimia Nervosa, who may nonetheless suffer from malnutrition or electrolyte imbalances due to loss of body fluids. The two disorders often occur at different times in the same individual, as illustrated in the vignette of Camilla.

Camilla

"This thing has gotten beyond me. Even when my weight is normal, I'm still all lumpy."

For the past 4 years, Camilla had had problems with eating. They began

TABLE 22.2. Criteria for Bulimia Nervosa

- The patient repeatedly eats in binges. In a binge episode, the patient does *both* of these:
  - Consumes much more food than most people would in similar circumstances and in a similar period of time
  - Feels that the eating is out of control
- The patient repeatedly controls weight gain by inappropriate means, such as fasting, self-induced vomiting, excessive exercise, or abuse of laxatives, diuretics, or other drugs.
- On average, both of the behaviors above (binge eating and inappropriate control) have occurred at least twice a week for at least 3 consecutive months.
- Weight and body shape unduly affect the patient's self-evaluation.
- These symptoms do not occur solely during episodes of Anorexia Nervosa.

Specify whether:
   Purging Type: The patient often induces vomiting or misuses diuretics or laxatives. This is the more common type.
   Nonpurging Type: The patient fasts or exercises excessively, but does not often induce vomiting or misuse diuretics or laxatives.

when she was a high school sophomore, and to one degree or another, they still persisted.

In gym class, she'd noticed that she seemed fatter than most of the other girls. Even when she was older, she believed that there had been some truth to this—she could remember being teased about "love handles." Whatever the truth of the situation, when she was 15 she resolved never again to risk being called fat. She joined the Health Club, an organization of girls at her school who exchanged diet tips and supported one another for weight loss. Several years earlier, the club had been driven underground after several members were found passing around diet pills. Once the club was banned, parents and teachers had no control at all over the use of medications and other aids to weight loss some girls used.

Camilla had been an extraordinarily successful dieter. From her highest-ever weight of 135 pounds (she stood only 5 feet, 3 inches tall), through strict dieting and vigorous exercise she had lost nearly 40 pounds. Even then, she thought the "love handles" still showed, so she began using laxatives and diuretics supplied by one of her classmates. Although she managed to lose another 10 pounds, her mirror confirmed her worst fears: She still looked fat. By this time she was eating only about 400 calories a day, and even some of that she would throw up—she had learned the trick of vomiting at will.

As Camilla's weight dipped to 85 pounds, her parents finally became sufficiently alarmed to admit her to a hospital. Six months of treatment, education, and fear (while she was there, another anorectic patient about her age died of malnutrition) had their effect. She was discharged weighing a healthy 117 pounds, and her periods, absent for nearly a year, had started again. To protect her from the adverse consequences of further association with other girls in the Health Club, Camilla's parents moved to the opposite end of the county. Camilla eventually graduated from the high school there, but she never lost the feeling that something was terribly wrong with the shape of her body.

After high school, Camilla took a business course and went to work in the secretarial pool of an insurance company. As soon as she could afford it, she moved into a tiny studio apartment. Now that she was free from the watchful eyes of her parents, her eating habits quickly deteriorated.

About 1 year prior to her present evaluation, she began consuming large quantities of food within a remarkably short period of time. At the movies, she might eat a "family-size" tub of popcorn and a giant cola drink; at home, she would consume a quart of frozen yogurt during a single 1-hour episode of *Law and Order*. Because she was still morbidly fearful of becoming overweight, she usually regurgitated most of what she had eaten. In recent weeks, these binge episodes were occurring as often as two or three times a week and were extending beyond snack time into her regular meals. She told the interviewer, "When I eat alone, I've put away as much as a 1-pound package of spaghetti and two cans of sauce. I don't binge every day, but once I start, I can't seem to stop."

Evaluation of Camilla

When Camilla was 15, she developed the unreasonable and intense fear of being overweight, despite the fact that she was losing so much weight that others worried about her health. At 135 pounds she had probably been a little overweight for her height, but a drop of 50 pounds—over one-third her previous weight—clearly far exceeded what was safe. At that point, when she refused to regain weight, she had to be hospitalized. Despite her pronounced emaciation, her self-perception continued to be distorted, and her menses ceased for nearly a year. She thereby fulfilled the criteria for Anorexia Nervosa.

During the later phase of her illness, Camilla became bulimic. No one can doubt that she consumed far more food than normal for a given time period; she admitted feeling that she had lost control of her eating habits. Occurring several times a week, these episodes had persisted throughout the previous year. She controlled her weight by vomiting; others might exercise excessively or abuse laxatives or other drugs. Although Camilla's perception of her own body shape was still unrealistic and dominated her self-perception, it no longer had the near-delusional quality that had characterized her anorectic phase. Therefore, at age 19 she no longer qualified for a diagnosis of Anorexia Nervosa, thus fulfilling the final criterion for Bulimia Nervosa.

Disordered appetite occurs in a number of other physical and mental disorders. Some rare **organic disorders** (e.g., pituitary tumors) are associated with voracious appetite and other abnormalities of eating. Patients with **mood disorders** may eat either too much or too little, but they don't usually have the abnormal self-perception typical of the primary eating disorders. Patients with **Schizophrenia** or **other psychoses** can have peculiar eating habits, but usually without fearing weight gain, and patients with eating disorders don't have hallucinations or delusions. Camilla's clinician would need to ask further about **anxiety** and **depressive disorders**, as well as about a **personality disorder**—comorbidity is the rule. **Abuse of stimulant medications** should also be suspected in patients who control their weight through misuse of those drugs.

In the coding of both Camilla's Anorexia Nervosa and her Bulimia Nervosa, the subtype would be determined by the fact that she controlled her weight by purging (specifically, forced vomiting). Because her clinician thought that Camilla's Anorexia Nervosa had been especially serious, a generic severity specifier would be used there. Camilla's full diagnosis at age 15 would be:

Axis I	307.1	Anorexia Nervosa, Binge-Eating/Purging Type, Severe
Axis II	V71.09	No diagnosis
Axis III	783.2	Abnormal loss of weight
Axis IV		None
Axis V	GAF = 41	(age 15)

And, at age 19, it would be as follows:

Axis I	307.51	Bulimia Nervosa, Purging Type
	307.1	Anorexia Nervosa, Prior History
Axis II	V71.09	No diagnosis
Axis III		None
Axis IV		None
Axis V	GAF = 60	(current)

307.50 EATING DISORDER NOT OTHERWISE SPECIFIED

The Eating Disorder Not Otherwise Specified diagnosis should be reserved for patients who have problems related to appetite, eating, and weight, but who do not meet the criteria for either Anorexia Nervosa or Bulimia Nervosa. Many such problems (e.g., anorexia with normal menses, anorexia in which weight is low but remains within the normal range, bulimia with infrequent binges, bulimia without swallowing food) will meet many of the criteria for one or the other of these two diagnoses. Eating Dis-

Several DSM-IV diagnoses have different criteria for females than for males. Nearly all of these are in the section on sexual and gender identity disorders, and have little relevance for young children. The physiological requirement that female Anorexia Nervosa patients have no menstrual periods has no counterpart for males with this disorder, making Anorexia Nervosa the only mental disorder whose criteria show a gender bias in their rigor.

order Not Otherwise Specified is also used when patients meet the criteria for a newly proposed diagnosis, binge-eating disorder, in which binges occur but the patients do not try to compensate for them by purging, exercising, or using medications. Proposed criteria for this condition are given in Appendix B of DSM-IV.

Assessing Eating Disorders

General Suggestions

The patient with Anorexia Nervosa, whether adult or adolescent, is in denial and may refuse to discuss eating behaviors frankly. You may have better success with questions about mood (which is likely to be depressed), though these patients are often vague about their own feelings. They probably won't perceive themselves as thin—a judgment you should avoid contradicting. They may express disgust at their own physical appearance or reluctance to eat. You can screen for Anorexia Nervosa by asking, "Have you ever lost so much weight that people said you were too thin?" For Bulimia Nervosa, ask, "Have you ever eaten so much at one time that it made you sick?"

If possible, observe for suspicious behavior at mealtime: pushing food around on the plate, taking excessively small portions, and/or using the bathroom immediately after meals. In addition, be alert for vigorous activity in the face of marked weakness and wasting. You will probably encounter denial of behaviors a patient knows are frowned upon, such as self-induced vomiting and purging. Also ask about frequent weighing, about making and following rules about when and where to eat, and about maintaining lists of forbidden foods. Bulimic patients may express a feeling of tension release after vomiting or purging; such patients should also be asked about feelings of loss of control (similar to those experienced in other addictions) over their eating binges.

Developmental Factors

In anorectic patients under the age of 14, severe weight loss can halt puberty. Indeed, failure to grow to full height may also result.

Quick Guide to the Sleep Disorders

Both in this Quick Guide and in the chapter text, the approach taken to the sleep disorders differs considerably from that in DSM-IV. The majority of the sleep disorders in DSM-IV are grouped into two categories, the dyssomnias and the parasomnias; two further groupings—sleep disorders related to another mental disorder, and other sleep disorders—are also presented. However, because most of the dyssomnias and both of the sleep disorders related to another mental disorder are much rarer in children and adolescents than in adults, they are not discussed here. This chapter describes three parasomnias, one dyssomnia, and (briefly) two other sleep disorders, in that order. As usual, the page (or table) number following each item tells where further information on it can be found.

Parasomnias

In a *parasomnia*, the timing, duration, and quality of sleep are essentially normal, but unusual behaviors occur during sleep or when the person is falling asleep or waking up. Three of the four parasomnias included in DSM-IV are described in this chapter (Parasomnia Not Otherwise Specified is omitted).

   Nightmare Disorder. Bad dreams trouble some youngsters much more than others (p. 410).

   Sleep Terror Disorder. These young patients cry out in apparent fear during the first part of the night. Often they don't really wake up at all (p. 410).

Sleepwalking Disorder. Persistent sleepwalking usually occurs early in the night (p. 414).

Dyssomnias

Someone with a *dyssomnia* sleeps too little, too much, or at the wrong time of day, though the sleep itself is pretty normal. DSM-IV describes several dyssomnias, including Primary Insomnia and Primary Hypersomnia (the word *primary* in this context means that no cause can be found). Narcolepsy (in which brief but refreshing sleep intrudes into wakefulness, causing patients to fall asleep abruptly), Circadian Rhythm Sleep Disorder (in which there is a mismatch between a patient's sleep–wake pattern and environmental demands), and Dyssomnia Not Otherwise Specified. However, only one dyssomnia is found with any frequency in children and adolescents:

Breathing-Related Sleep Disorder. Although most patients with breathing problems such as sleep apnea complain of hypersomnia, some instead have insomnia (p. 415).

Other Sleep Disorders

Sleep Disorder Due to a General Medical Condition. Some medical problems can result in sleep disturbances (Table 13.1 and p. 418).

Substance-Induced Sleep Disorder. Most psychoactive substances commonly misused, as well as various prescription medications, can interfere with sleep (Table 14.5 and p. 418).

DISTINGUISHING AMONG PARASOMNIAS

Two sleep disorders commonly found in juveniles (especially young children) are Sleep Terror Disorder and Sleepwalking Disorder, both of which DSM-IV classifies as arousal parasomnias. They are manifestations of central nervous system arousal that usually occur in the first 1–3 hours after sleep onset. Arousal episodes have many features in common: automatic behavior; relative nonreactivity to external stimuli; absent or fragmentary dream recall; mental confusion and disorientation when awakened; and amnesia for the episode the next morning. Arousal parasomnias tend to run in families and are more common in males than in females; children with one type of arousal parasomnia are likely also to have symptoms of another.

Arousal parasomnias, which occur during non-REM sleep, must be distinguished from the much more common REM parasomnia, or nightmare. (REM, or rapid-eye-movement sleep, occurs especially during the last part of the night, when most of the dreams we remember occur.) Nightmares are anxiety-laden dreams that cause awakening with detailed recall. Various stressors, especially traumatic experiences, increase the frequency and severity of nightmares. They usually start between the ages of 3 and 6, and they affect a strong minority of children severely enough to disturb their parents. Table 23.1 presents a "nutshell" comparison of Sleep Terror Disorder and Nightmare Disorder, to clarify the differences between the two.

TABLE 23.1. Comparison of Sleep Terror and Nightmare Disorders

	Sleep Terror Disorder	Nightmare Disorder
Occurrence in sleep period	First few hours (non-REM sleep)	Last third (REM sleep)
Arousability	Difficult	Easy
Dream imagery	No	Yes
Episode recalled in morning	No	Yes

307.47 NIGHTMARE DISORDER

As an aid in making the distinction between full-fledged, codable Nightmare Disorder and the occasional occurrence of nightmares in children and adolescents, we present the criteria for Nightmare Disorder in Table 23.2. However, because nightmares in and of themselves are well-known phenomena to clinicians (and most parents, for that matter), we do not discuss this disorder further here or present a vignette for it.

307.46 SLEEP TERROR DISORDER

Approximately 60–90 minutes after falling asleep, a young patient with Sleep Terror Disorder suddenly sits up, screams, and stares with glassy, unseeing eyes. Manifestations of autonomic discharge—palpitations, sweating, and irregular respiration—are obvious. The patient is inconsolable and difficult to

TABLE 23.2. Criteria for Nightmare Disorder

- The patient repeatedly awakens with detailed recall of long, frightening dreams. These usually occur in the second half of the sleep or nap period and concern threats to security, self-esteem, or survival.
- The patient quickly becomes alert and oriented upon awakening.
- These experiences (or the resulting sleep disturbance) cause clinically important distress or impair school, work, social, or other functioning.
- They don't occur solely during another mental disorder (such as Posttraumatic Stress Disorder or a delirium).
- The symptoms are not directly caused by a general medical condition or by the use of substances, including medications and drugs of abuse.

awaken, and if awakened, is disoriented and confused. If there is no awakening, after 30 seconds to 5 minutes the patient calms down and drifts back into normal sleep. In the morning, the patient has no recollection of the event. Table 23.3 gives the full criteria for Sleep Terror Disorder.

Paul

Paul was a 3-year-old only child brought for evaluation by his parents, who were distraught by attacks of screaming and agitation that for the past 6 months had interrupted his sleep two to three times a week. Most days Paul's babysitter cared for him in his own home, but 2 days a week he attended a well-staffed preschool with 30 other toddlers.

His mother described their bedtime routine as follows. After getting ready for bed, she would read him stories for 5–10 minutes. Then Paul would kiss

TABLE 23.3. Criteria for Sleep Terror Disorder

- On numerous occasions the patient awakens abruptly, usually during the first third of sleep and usually with a scream of panic.
- During each episode the patient shows evidence of marked fear and autonomic arousal, such as rapid breathing, rapid heartbeat, and sweating.
- The patient responds poorly during the episode to others' efforts to provide comfort.
- The patient cannot recall any dream in detail at the time and cannot recall the episode later.
- These symptoms cause clinically important distress or impair school, work, social, or other functioning.
- These symptoms are not directly caused by a general medical condition or by the use of substances, including medications and drugs of abuse.

her goodnight, clutch his teddy bear, and fall asleep easily at about 9:00 P.M. Between 11:30 P.M. and midnight, Paul would sit bolt upright in bed and begin screaming. His eyes would be open, but he would not seem to see anything. He would perspire, breathe rapidly with pounding heart, and seem to be in great distress. His parents would try unsuccessfully to awaken and console him, but Paul would not speak coherently or respond to questions. After 3–5 minutes, the attack would end spontaneously, and he would quickly return to normal sleep. Some nights a second attack would occur 60–90 minutes later. In the morning, Paul would awaken refreshed, with no recollection of the previous night's event.

Paul was a planned baby whose intrauterine and postnatal development were normal. He had reached all of his motor, sensory, and social milestones to date on time. During the day he was a curious, energetic, bright, happy 3-year-old who brought his parents much pleasure. However, his parents had noted that his attacks seemed more likely to occur after a day in the child care center, and they feared that he was being overwhelmed by his day care experience. The center's staff assured them that Paul was flourishing there, though during his days there he usually missed his nap. Those were often the nights when he had attacks. Paul's mother also worried that her working away from the home during the day might be responsible. Paul's paternal uncle was an occasional sleepwalker as a child.

While his mother related the history, Paul curiously explored the available toys in the examination room. His attention seemed focused, and he checked in with his mother whenever he moved to a new activity. He formed an appropriate relationship with the examiner, and soon they were comfortably playing together while the examiner continued to question the mother. After requesting Paul's permission, the examiner asked the mother to step out of the room for a few minutes. Paul tolerated the separation without distress; upon her return, he greeted her warmly.

Evaluation of Paul

Paul's arousal 2–3 hours after sleep onset, his agitation, his autonomic arousal (pounding heart and sweating), and his unresponsiveness to his parents' attempts to awaken and console him were all reactions typical of Sleep Terror Disorder. Paul played hard at his day care center, and without his usual nap, it was likely that he was more exhausted on those nights (arousal parasomnias are more likely to occur after periods of excessive fatigue). Nightmares are associated with stressful daytime experiences, but episodes of **Nightmare Disorder** generally occur later, after 4–5 hours of sleep, when REM sleep predominates. Then the patient is wide awake, well oriented, and usually able to relate a vivid and coherent narrative. Paul showed no evidence suggesting either **Panic Disorder** or **psychomotor epilepsy**, either of which can produce fear, even in the middle of the night. Paul's five-axis diagnosis would be as follows:

Axis I	307.46	Sleep Terror Disorder
Axis II	V71.09	No diagnosis
Axis III		None
Axis IV		None
Axis V	GAF = 85	(current)

307.46 SLEEPWALKING DISORDER

Sleepwalking usually occurs during the first third of the night, perhaps following excessive fatigue or unusual stresses during the day before. The individual first sits up and makes some sort of random movement (such as picking at the bedclothes). Apparently purposeful behavior such as dressing or using the toilet may follow, but these behaviors are usually poorly coordinated and incomplete. Facial expression is usually blank; speech, if it occurs at all, is typically garbled. An episode can last from a few seconds to 30 minutes, and will usually be followed with amnesia for the episode. If the sleepwalker awakens at all, it is usually to a brief period of disorientation. The condition affects 1–5% of all children, who usually outgrow it by age 15. It is not usually considered pathological in children, though it can be in adults. Table 23.4 provides the full criteria for Sleepwalking Disorder.

Contrary to the myth that sleepwalkers never harm themselves, Sleepwalking Disorder is dangerous. Body movements are clumsy and purposeless. The sleepwalker may be injured by falls or by bumping into objects, so it is important to make the environment as safe as possible. Sealed windows, locked doors, and alarms that are triggered when the sleepwalker rises from bed may also help prevent injury.

George

The examination of 16-year-old George was prompted by his father's concern that George might have Sleepwalking Disorder. At 2 A.M. earlier that month,

TABLE 23.4. Criteria for Sleepwalking Disorder

- On numerous occasions, the patient arises and walks about, usually during the first third of sleep.
- During sleepwalking, the patient stares blankly, can be awakened only with difficulty, and responds poorly to others' attempts at communication.
- Although there may be a brief period of confusion upon first awakening from the episode, within a few minutes the patient's behavior and mental activity are unimpaired.
- After the episode or the next morning, the patient has no memory of the episode.
- These symptoms cause clinically important distress or impair school, work, social, or other functioning.
- The symptoms are not directly caused by a general medical condition or by the use of substances, including medications and drugs of abuse.

George had been discovered sound asleep in his girlfriend's bedroom. Though he must have walked a mile or more through suburban streets, and must have used a ladder taken from her garage to climb through the bedroom window, he claimed not to know how he had gotten there. It was unclear whether such episodes had occurred previously. George had not had a history of sleep terror attacks at a younger age, nor was the family history positive for arousal parasomnias.

George had had occasional struggles with his parents, who didn't like some of his recent friends. Until the past year or two he had been a good student, but lately he had put little effort into his studies and had had a number of unexplained absences from school. He admitted to the use of marijuana, which he claimed helped him with his "insight." During the interview, he seemed neither depressed nor anxious.

Evaluation of George

Because sleepwalkers are poorly coordinated and disoriented during their episodes, it is highly unlikely that Sleepwalking Disorder could explain George's well-organized, goal-directed behavior. Sleepwalking must also occur on many occasions, not just one.

Sometimes sleepwalking attacks resemble sleep **seizures,** and an EEG is required to differentiate the two. **Dissociative disorders** may also resemble sleepwalking attacks, but they usually last longer, and the episodes carry on into the waking state. George's age of onset was wrong for **Sleep Terror Disorder,** with which sleepwalking can be associated; the vignette also specifically mentions that he had no previous history of sleep terrors. Although marijuana does not typically cause sleepwalking, further evaluation would be needed to rule out **Substance-Induced Sleep Disorder, Parasomnia Type**, which might be caused by drugs such as psychotropic medications.

The vignette does not permit a definitive DSM-IV diagnosis. Because several possibilities remained to be explored, his Axis I diagnosis would have to be deferred. The changes in George's behavior over the past couple of years did suggest that there might be a personality disorder; hence the similarly cautious statement on Axis II.

Axis I	799.9	Diagnosis deferred
Axis II	799.9	Diagnosis deferred
Axis III		None
Axis IV		None
Axis V	GAF = 65	(current)

780.59 BREATHING-RELATED SLEEP DISORDER

Table 23.5 gives criteria for the one dyssomnia discussed this chapter, Breathing-Related Sleep Disorder. The principal type of Breathing-Related Sleep Disorder that afflicts children and adolescents is *sleep apnea,* a condition in which breathing is noisy or discontinuous for periods throughout the night. The cause is usually obstruction of the airway due to mechanical features of the mouth, nose, or throat; hence the complete formal name, *obstructive sleep apnea syndrome* (OSAS). The mildest, most obvious symptom of this disorder is snoring, which by itself is a common enough occurrence in childhood and

---

TABLE 23.5. Criteria for Breathing-Related Sleep Disorder

- The patient experiences disruption of sleep that causes excessive insomnia or sleepiness.
- The clinician judges this disruption to be caused by a breathing problem related to sleep such as central or obstructive sleep apnea or central alveolar hypoventilation syndrome.
- Another mental disorder does not better explain this behavior.
- The symptoms are not directly caused by a general medical condition or use of substances, including medications and drugs of abuse.

Coding Note: On Axis III, also code a sleep-related breathing disorder.

adolescence (10–12% of school-age children snore). But 1–3% of young children actually stop breathing for brief periods, resulting in physical, behavioral, and even cognitive symptoms of varying severity.

Complete cessation of breathing for 10 seconds or longer results in a struggle to breathe that is obvious to an observer. The child becomes restless, may sweat, and awakens frequently during the night. Although most children do not suffer from daytime symptoms (which are common in adults with OSAS), some children may complain of morning headache and excessive sleepiness. Some become hyperactive and oppositional; more severely ill children may experience learning difficulties. At worst, physical consequences can include pulmonary hypertension, developmental delay, short stature, and even death.

OSAS may be especially common in children who have allergies or multiple ear or throat infections. Other risk factors include obesity, abnormalities of the face or cranium, and oral pathology such as large tonsils or tongue. Clinical history and physical exam alone may not discriminate OSAS from simple snoring. A definitive diagnosis requires an overnight stay in a sleep lab for polysomnography.

OSAS is relatively common even in young children, but its incidence actually increases in adults. Sex incidence is about equally distributed between boys and girls, and between men and women after the age of menopause; in younger adults, males are more often affected.

Johann

When Johann was 28 months old, his mother requested an evaluation because he was so small. Although both his height and weight were below the 3rd percentile for his age, a comprehensive endocrine, neurological, metabolic, and gastrointestinal workup had revealed no physical cause for his size. Despite a history of repeated ear infections and upper respiratory illnesses, hearing tests and a chest X-ray were normal. Suspecting stress-related, nonorganic failure to thrive, the pediatrician referred Johann and his mother to the mental health clinic. There, the clinician learned the following:

Before antibiotics, fear of chronic infection routinely prompted removal of tonsils and adenoids. Now only about one-fourth as commonplace as it once was, tonsillectomy is performed most often for problems with breathing. Then sleeping improves in up to 75% of children. Although only a few controlled outcome studies have been performed to date, these children may experience significant reductions in aggression, hyperactivity, and inattention. The procedure can be helpful in children with underlying conditions as diverse as Down's syndrome, asthma, cerebral palsy, and severe obesity.

Although she had been single with few social supports and only 22 years old, Johann's mother had taken good care of herself throughout her uneventful pregnancy. Johann had weighed 7 pounds, 6 ounces at birth, with Apgar scores of 8 and 10. He and his mother had left the hospital on the second day following his birth, and at 1 month and 1 year of age, his development seemed on track. At 1 year of age, his weight was 19½ lbs. Then, because his mother had begun began working in a distant city and they'd moved away, the clinic had lost track of him until the present.

Johann's mother seemed to be a reliable reporter. Parent–child relations seemed warm and appropriately sensitive. Aside from his small stature, Johann seemed normal; his mental status examination and play interactions with the evaluator were unremarkable. When a history of snoring was elicited, a more detailed sleep–wake history was obtained. It revealed that he went to bed easily at 8:00 P.M. and slept until awakened at 6:30 A.M. Excessive daytime somnolence was not present, though his mother reported that Johann sometimes lacked energy by the end of the day. At the day care center, he did not nap.

Johann slept in the same room as his mother, who reported that mouth breathing and expiratory snoring had been present over the past year. She made an audiotape of Johann's breathing. On it, mouth breathing, snoring, and repetitive, brief sleep apnea episodes were clearly audible. All-night polysomnography revealed multiple periods of awakening associated with episodes of sleep apnea. During the longest of these, Johann's oxygen saturation level dropped as low as 68%.

A careful examination revealed enlarged adenoids, which had not been visible during the earlier examination. Tonsillectomy and adenoidectomy were performed; within 2 weeks, there were marked improvements in Johann's apnea–hypopnea ratio and oxygen desaturation. His sleep-related breathing became less labored. Six months after the surgery, his weight and height had increased to the 35th percentile. One year later, Johann's growth and development had returned to normal.

Evaluation of Johann

In the vignette, note the lack of apparent sleep disruption as described by Johann's mother. When snoring or excessive mouth breathing is noted in a child, and an audiotape provides suggestive support for episodes of stopped breathing, a polysomnographic laboratory study is mandatory to make the diagnosis and to determine the severity of oxygen desaturation. In young children, as in some adults, awakenings from sleep are not a presenting symptom of this disorder. Often both patients and their families are unaware of the arousals, which may be brief. In a sleep lab, the awakenings/arousals are clearly present—often to the surprise of the patient (or, in this case, Johann's mother). With no other medical condition or substance use to explain his condition, an adenoidectomy was performed that completely relieved his symptoms; this was the proof of the pudding.

Various other disorders can affect sleep, but none of them was a likely suspect in the case of Johann. **Narcolepsy** and **Circadian Rhythm Sleep Disorder** could be ruled out immediately by lack of typical symptoms. Johann had no other mental symptoms (depression, Panic Attacks) that could occasion the diagnosis of **Sleep Disorder Related to Another Mental Disorder**. His pediatrician had ruled out other conditions (such as cystic fibrosis) that could form the basis for **Sleep Disorder Due to a General Medical Condition**; nor, at age 3, did he exhibit any basis for **Substance-Induced Sleep Disorder**. Of course, **Primary Insomnia** is a residual category intended for use when no other more specific diagnosis can be substantiated. Johann's complete diagnosis would be as follows:

Axis I	780.59	Breathing-Related Sleep Disorder
Axis II	V71.09	No diagnosis
Axis III	780.57	Obstructive sleep apnea
	783.4	Failure to thrive
Axis IV		None
Axis V	GAF = 90	(current)

OTHER SLEEP DISORDERS

780.5x Sleep Disorder Due to a General Medical Condition

Many general medical conditions can result in sleep problems (mostly insomnia, but occasionally hypersomnia, parasomnia, or mixed types). Table 13.1 in Chapter 13 presents criteria for Sleep Disorder Due to a General Medical Condition and instructions for coding this by subtype.

Substance-Induced Sleep Disorder

Many psychoactive substances can also produce sleep disturbances. Table 14.5 in Chapter 14 gives the criteria for Substance-Induced Sleep Disorder and specifiers for its subtypes; Table 14.6 provides guidance in coding by type of substance ingested.

Assessing Sleep Disorders

General Suggestions

For conditions such as Sleep Terror Disorder and Sleepwalking Disorder, the diagnosis can almost invariably be made on the basis of history. Because these disorders occur sporadically, expensive studies of a child or adolescent in the sleep lab are unnecessary. In any case where confirmation by observation seems warranted, home videos should prove adequate. Sleep lab studies may be necessary for disorders with greater risk of harm, such as Breathing-Related Sleep Disorder caused by OSAS.

Developmental Factors

Sleep terrors first appear after 18 months of age, whereas sleepwalking first occurs slightly later, during the preschool and school-age years. By adolescence, arousal parasomnias usually either diminish significantly in frequency or disappear altogether.

CHAPTER 24

Impulse-Control Disorders Not Elsewhere Classified

Quick Guide to Impulsive Behavior

Impulse-Control Disorders

DSM-IV places five disorders plus the usual Not Otherwise Specified diagnosis in its section on impulse-control disorders not elsewhere classified. These disorders include Intermittent Explosive Disorder (in which aggressive episodes of physical harm to others or property destruction occur in the absence of other demonstrable psychological or general medical pathology); Kleptomania (in which people act out a pattern of "tension and release" by stealing items they don't need); Pyromania (in which people act out a "tension-and-release" pattern by setting fires); and Pathological Gambling (in which patients repeatedly gamble, often until they lose money, jobs, and friends). However, for reasons described in the chapter introduction, we focus on only one of the impulse-control disorders in this chapter:

Trichotillomania. Pulling hair from various parts of the body is accompanied by feelings of "tension and release" (p. 422).

Other Causes of Impulsive Behavior

Although the phenomenon of "tension and release" can characterize impulsive behaviors connected with substance misuse, it does not do so in other diagnoses, such as Bipolar I Disorder (stealing, gambling, or violent acting out may occur during a Manic Episode—Table 16.1); Schizophrenia (in response to hallucinations or delusions, schizophenic patients may impulsively engage in a variety of illegal or otherwise ill-advised behaviors—p. 296); and Conduct Disorder (fire setting, other property destruction, shoplifting, and various forms of harm to others are all among the criteria—p. 219).

INTRODUCTION

This section of DSM-IV includes several disorders that have as their common ground the failure to control impulses. Otherwise, the group is a mixed bag. The criteria for Pathological Gambling are so similar to those for Substance Dependence that it could be classified as an addiction; indeed, many victims refer to themselves as "addictive" gamblers. Intermittent Explosive Disorder is an evidently rare disorder of adulthood (or late adolescence) that would be difficult to differentiate from normal behavior in young children. The remaining three disorders (Kleptomania, Pyromania, and Trichotillomania) have criteria that are strongly similar:

- The patient's tension level rises until it reaches an unbearable peak.
- Performing the act relieves the tension.
- The patient repeatedly experiences this cycle.
- No other diagnosis or motive better explains the behavior.

Of these disorders, only Trichotillomania commonly begins in early life, and so it is the only one described in detail in this chapter. Although fire setting and shoplifting occur far more often in children and adolescents than clinicians, parents, and society at large might wish, they are much more likely to be seen as part of Conduct Disorder or a Manic Episode—both of which are specifically excluded in the criteria for Pyromania and Kleptomania. Finally, because the use of Impulse-Control Disorder Not Otherwise Specified is even more restricted than that of other Not Otherwise Specified diagnoses (it should be reserved for problems of impulse control that do not meet the cri-

Although Pathological Gambling is not described in detail here for the reason given in the text, it is a disorder that can have its roots in childhood or adolescence. In one study, boys who had been assessed for impulsiveness at age 13 were reassessed in late adolescence for gambling status. The higher the score on impulsiveness, the more likely a boy was to become a problem gambler.

teria either for the other impulse-control disorders *or* for any other disorders in DSM-IV involving impulsiveness), it too is not discussed here.

312.39 TRICHOTILLOMANIA

A "passion for hair pulling" (the literal translation of Trichotillomania) was first described over 100 years ago. Today it is found in at least 1 in 200 persons in the adult population (and actual rates may be several times greater), though it usually begins in childhood. Despite their discomfort, patients seldom complain about or even mention their symptoms, so relatively few mental health professionals—fewer still who specialize in children and adolescents—have ever encountered a case.

Trichotillomania (see Table 24.1 for the full criteria) is defined by a rising sense of tension that is relieved when the patient pulls out a strand of hair. Some recent work suggests a strong connection between it and Obsessive–Compulsive Disorder. However, a substantial number of patients describe the behavior as occurring "automatically" at times when they are thinking about other matters. In some individuals, both forms of hair pulling occur.

The head is most often involved, though the affected hair can be growing on any part of the body—face, brows, lashes, extremities, and (in adolescents and adults) underarms and pubic area. Chewing or mouthing of the hair often occurs; about 10% of patients swallow it. Hair pulling is much more common in children than in adults, suggesting that the usual outcome is spontaneous resolution.

Eve

When Eve was 13, she developed severe abdominal pain that worsened over 4 weeks. At first her family doctor could make no diagnosis, but one evening the

---

TABLE 24.1. Criteria for Trichotillomania

- Repeated extraction of the patient's own hair causes noticeable hair loss.
- The patient feels increased tension just before hair pulling or when trying to resist it.
- The patient feels gratification, pleasure, or relief during the hair pulling.
- These symptoms cause clinically important distress or impair school, work, social, or other functioning.
- The behavior is not better explained by another mental disorder and is not caused by a general medical condition.

---

cramping became so severe that her parents rushed her to the urgent care department of their community hospital. An X-ray revealed something blocking her small intestine. It required surgery to remove the object—a bezoar, or hairball, nearly 2 inches in diameter. That discovery prompted the doctor to look closely at Eve's scalp. "In several patches of scalp the size of a half-dollar, I saw a pattern of thinning of hair, with the characteristic intermingling of long and short hairs growing back in a pattern typical of chronic hair pulling," read the report sent with Eve to the mental health counselor. "This conclusion was subsequently confirmed by a dermatologist."

When questioned about her habit, Eve readily admitted that she had been pulling out her hair, a strand or two at a time, for many months. Though she did not seem to know why it happened, she acknowledged that many times a day she would feel increasingly "wired." After several minutes of rising tension, she would twirl a single hair around her ring finger, then gently tug until the strand came away at the root. As long as no one was watching, she would then roll the strand over and over in her mouth until it was as compact as her tongue could make it. As she swallowed, the sense of tension would evaporate. Although the hair pulling produced no sense of pain, she noted that her scalp seemed to itch where her hair was growing back.

Eve was a slender girl whose figure had barely begun to develop. She wore her blond hair tucked under a knit cap, which she resisted removing. Once the cap was off, it was easy to see why she preferred to wear it. Patches of hair were either missing or thinned; downy, new, short hairs sprouted in some of the patches.

The initial interview revealed no information to suggest another Axis I diagnosis. Eve denied having any other mental or physical problems (among other issues, her mother had reported no evidence of hallucinations, delusions, depression, obsessions, or compulsions). As she slouched in her chair, she grumbled, "I just wish I could stop—I hate wearing that hat, and the kids all call me 'Baldy.' But if I don't do it, I just feel grody."

Evaluation of Eve

Children often do not report the tension-and-release phenomenon; thus many child clinicians complain that the DSM-IV criteria for Trichotillomania do not serve their patients well. Eve, however, spontaneously noted that her sensation of feeling "wired" (or "grody") abated once she had completed her ritual. DSM-IV, noting that many children twist or tug at their hair without sustaining real damage or experiencing distress, advises that the diagnosis should not be made in children unless the behavior has lasted for several months, which was certainly the case with Eve.

In an evaluation of patchy hair loss, **general medical conditions** (especially **dermatological disorders**) must be considered. Eve had no evidence of such a problem, or of another Axis I disorder (such as a **psychosis**, **Obsessive–Compulsive Disorder**, or **Factitious Disorder**) that could explain her symptoms. Her entire diagnosis would be as follows:

Axis I	312.39	Trichotillomania
Axis II	V71.09	No diagnosis
Axis III		None
Axis IV		None
Axis V	GAF = 70	

Assessing Impulsive Behaviors

General Suggestions

Whether they meet the criteria for one of the impulse-control disorders or constitute aspects of another disorder, impulsive behaviors can be difficult to assess accurately because they are perceived as shameful or illegal. Children and adolescents can be expected to hide the facts from clinicians, just as they do from school or legal authorities. For reliable data, clinicians may have to rely on other informants—especially parents and teachers—who can report on behaviors such as jumping to another activity without finishing the first one, shouting in class, or acting rashly without considering the likely consequences. Of course, each of these behaviors must be evaluated in the context of what is usual for a young patient's age, sex, and developmental stage.

Developmental Factors

Several of these behaviors produce important social and economic damage. In that sense, although data are sparse, it stands to reason that younger children who shoplift will steal smaller, less expensive items, and that those with explosively aggressive tendencies will present less of a problem at 6 years than at 16. Because a fire, once set, can quickly get out of hand, fire setting may present as much of a problem in young children as in teenagers.

CHAPTER 25 | Adjustment Disorder

Adjustment Disorder is a popular diagnosis—too popular, according to some writers who believe that clinicians often use it because it lacks the pejorative baggage of, say, Conduct Disorder or even a bipolar disorder. A conservative estimate is that 4% of children develop mental symptoms as the result of some commonplace environmental stressor. The diagnosis is made about as often in boys as in girls, and seems to occur more often among children whose parents are experiencing marital problems.

Agreement between raters (reliability) has often been reported as very low for Adjustment Disorder, partly because clinicians often disagree about the severity of stressors, partly due to the vagueness and paucity of symptoms required (see Table 25.1 for the criteria). A single mental, emotional, or behavioral symptom could qualify, but for inclusion in recent studies, researchers have required criteria more stringent than DSM-IV's—at least three to four symptoms, with five to six the norm. Stressors commonly associated with Adjustment Disorder include divorce, illness of a parent, beginning or changing schools, rejection by peers, and severe personal illness (such as diabetes). When a child or adolescent has been exposed to more unusual stressors (physical or sexual abuse, natural disasters), look first for symptoms of Posttraumatic Stress Disorder. Whereas some writers have included Bereavement as a stressor, DSM-IV specifically excludes it as a precipitant. Adjustment Disorder With Depressed Mood is by far the most common subtype diagnosis made in adults, but for adolescents, With Disturbance of Conduct may be more common yet.

More than half the patients with Adjustment Disorder also have comorbid disorders, such as Conduct Disorder and ADHD. The presence of a comorbid

TABLE 25.1. Criteria for Adjustment Disorder

- Within 3 months of a stressor and in response to it, the patient develops emotional or behavioral symptoms.
- Either of the following demonstrates the clinical importance of these symptoms:
  ✓ Distress that markedly exceeds what you would normally expect from such a stressor
  ✓ Materially impaired school, job, or social functioning
- These symptoms neither fulfill criteria for an Axis I disorder nor represent merely the worsening of a preexisting Axis I or Axis II disorder.
- The symptoms are not caused by Bereavement.
- They don't last longer than 6 months after the end of the stressor (or its consequences).

Depending on the predominant symptoms, code:
  309.0   With Depressed Mood. The patient is tearful, sad, hopeless.
  309.24   With Anxiety. The patient is nervous, fearful, worried.
  309.28   With Mixed Anxiety and Depressed Mood. Combination of the two above.
  309.3   With Disturbance of Conduct. The patient violates rules or rights of others.
  309.4   With Mixed Disturbance of Emotions and Conduct. Combinations.
  309.9   Unspecified. Examples include job problems, physical complaints,
           social withdrawal.

Specify whether:
  Acute: Symptoms have lasted less than 6 months.
  Chronic: Symptoms have lasted 6 months or more (use when stressor is chronic or
    has lasting effects).

Coding Note: Code the specific stressor on Axis IV (for choices, see text).

diagnosis does not appear to affect the rate of recovery from the Adjustment Disorder, which is nearly universal (by definition, it *has* to be). Subsequently, many children with Adjustment Disorder will be found to have another, better-defined illness. Although critics point out that the criteria for Adjustment Disorder are among the flimsiest in DSM-IV, the requirement that symptoms last no longer than 6 months after the stressor resolves may be too restrictive. Some studies report that symptoms last an average of 7 months.

Kerrilynn

Just 1 week after her 12th birthday, Kerrilynn learned that she had leukemia. For several weeks her parents had ignored her complaints that she felt tired and warm, but when her joints began to ache, they finally took her to the pediatrician. After a routine blood test, her doctor consulted with a hematologist, who did a bone marrow smear that left her with a painful right hip. The two doctors spoke with her parents, and then all four of them told Kerrilynn that she had acute lymphocytic leukemia. "What's that?" she asked.

She later admitted to an interviewer that it had frightened her. "I didn't think I'd die," she said, "but I knew it had to be something pretty bad, everyone was so kind." She spent several weeks receiving transfusions and starting chemotherapy, which made her sick. She cried when her hair fell out.

Adjustment Disorder is probably best regarded as a diagnosis of "almost last resort," to be made only after all other possible, more specific DSM-IV categories have been eliminated. The *absolute* last resort would be some form (see Introduction, p. 10) of the powerful statement, "mentally ill, but undiagnosed," which has several advantages:

- It recognizes that a child or adolescent is ill, without forcing a diagnosis before all the data are in.
- Therefore, it decreases the likelihood of an inaccurate diagnosis, especially one that might be pejorative.
- By preventing closure, it encourages ongoing thought about complicated or confusing patients.

According to her father, she "kept it together pretty well" until she returned to school, some 6 weeks after she was diagnosed. Some of her classmates taunted her and called her "Baldy." On the playground, one boy pulled off her wig and for several minutes played keep-away with it. A teacher overheard the class bully explain to her that within a few weeks, she'd be "pushing up daisies."

Although Kerrilynn physically responded well to treatment, she became moody and sullen. She stopped attending her Girl Scout meetings and refused even to talk to friends on the telephone. On several evenings, her mother found her crying in her room, but she refused to talk about her feelings. She repeatedly picked fights with her older sister, whom she said she hated. After 6 weeks, her plummeting grades led to a conference with her school counselor, who reported to her parents that she had two wishes—to be dead and to go to Disneyland. The following day she ran away from home for nearly 6 hours. A policeman found her in the back seat of an abandoned Buick, attempting to have intercourse with a badly frightened 13-year-old boy. "I'm going to die anyway, so I wanted to see what it was like," she told the nurse that evening when she was admitted to the psychiatric ward of a children's hospital.

Kerrilynn and her sister were both wanted children born to middle-class parents. Her developmental milestones had occurred at the expected times. Other than her current illness, there had been no previous operations or major illnesses. She'd experienced menarche at the age of 11, but her periods had stopped shortly before she was diagnosed with leukemia. She had no environmental or drug allergies and no known history of substance misuse. The family history was completely negative for any mental health disorder.

Kerrilynn denied having problems with sleep or appetite, or any somatic symptoms such as heart palpitations or chest pain. She had had no phobias, obsessional ideas, sense of impending doom, or flashbacks or other evidence of reliving incidents from her recent past. She was very interested in learning what delusions and hallucinations were, and finally laughed and said that she was not *that* sick.

For the first several days of her 2-week psychiatric hospitalization, Kerrilynn spent most of her time reading stories about horses. The hospital's classroom teacher noted that she was bright, focused her attention well, and quickly caught up in classes where she had fallen behind during the previous 3 months.

Evaluation of Kerrilynn

As in most evaluations, the first step in evaluating Kerrilynn would be to determine whether she had the symptoms necessary for the diagnosis. In the case of Adjustment Disorder, this might seem almost unnecessary, inasmuch as hardly any symptoms are actually required. However, Kerrilynn's presenting symptoms were important for two reasons: to determine subtype diagnosis, and—far more pressing—to rule out better-defined DSM-IV conditions.

Several symptoms initially suggested a mood disorder: low mood, crying, irritability, and expressing a wish to die (since the alternative was Disneyland, that wish did not seem firmly held, however). By themselves, these would be insufficient to diagnose a Major Depressive Episode, and Kerrilynn did not have vegetative or other symptoms to flesh out the diagnosis of **Major Depressive Disorder**. Of course, the duration had been far too brief for **Dysthymic Disorder**.

She had no symptoms that would suggest **Panic Disorder**, and she denied anything resembling **Obsessive–Compulsive Disorder** or either type of **phobic disorder**. Could her disturbance be a form of **Posttraumatic Stress Disorder**? Being told that she had a life-threatening illness was certainly an awful experience, but she neither relived the experience nor expressed intense fear or horror. She had had no **psychotic symptoms** and denied the **use of substances** such as alcohol. Once she was admitted to the psychiatric ward, it was clear that she had no evidence of a **cognitive disorder**.

However, could Kerrilynn's one or two rather alarming behavioral problems indicate **Conduct Disorder**? For one thing, the time course was wrong: At most, she had been having problems with fighting for only a month or two, not a full year. Her sexual acting out might qualify if she had *forced* the boy, but his participation appeared to have been voluntary, if futile. The running away was brief and occurred only once. Her symptoms of defiance were too brief and too few for **Oppositional Defiant Disorder**. Although a developing **personality disorder** could not be completely excluded, symptoms would have to be present for at least 1 year before any such diagnosis could be made, and **Antisocial Personality Disorder** cannot be diagnosed at all prior to the age of 18. Although the vignette includes no mention of recent deaths in her family, Kerrilynn's clinician would have to establish their absence to rule out **Bereavement**.

Therefore, it seems probable that no other Axis I or Axis II diagnosis could reasonably explain Kerrilynn's symptoms. They *did* occur within 3 months of two serious stressors: first, being told that she had a life-threatening illness, and then the rejection by peers. Indeed, the diagnosis of Adjustment Disorder would seem to fit like a glove, though the passage of time would be needed to be sure that the symptoms really disappeared once the stressors had abated.

Kerrilynn presented with a combination of depressive and behavioral symptoms that would dictate the code number assigned on Axis I. The subtype With Mixed Disturbance of Emotions and Conduct is uncommonly used, but of the six possibilities, it best fit her symptoms. A duration less than 6 months justified the specifier Acute. Although the DSM-IV criteria do not specifically require using the term Provisional for an Adjustment Disorder that has not yet resolved, they should have; her clinician did. Her clinician also decided that there was insufficient evidence even to suspect an Axis II disorder. Her leukemia was mentioned on Axis III. The only sort of health problem that would be listed on Axis IV, even if it appeared to contribute to the development of an Adjustment Disorder, would be problems gaining *access* to health care (such as lack of transportation, insurance, or nearby medical care providers); there were no such problems in this case. Kerrilynn's five-axis diagnosis would therefore be as follows:

Axis I	309.4	Adjustment Disorder, Acute, With Mixed Disturbance of Emotions and Conduct, Acute (Provisional)
Axis II	V71.09	No diagnosis
Axis III	204.01	Acute lymphocytic leukemia, in remission
Axis IV		Rejection by peers
Axis V	GAF = 55	(on admission to psychiatric ward)
	GAF = 81	(on discharge)

Assessing Adjustment Disorder

General Suggestions

The first task is to rule out all other DSM-IV diagnoses. This usually translates into a careful search for the symptoms of Major Depressive Disorder, Generalized Anxiety Disorder, or Conduct Disorder. The second task is to search for stressors, which tend to be everyday problems of nearly any type or severity. If you don't already know, ask the patient about problems in school (grades, peer relations) or at home (parents divorced, illness, one parent imprisoned or away for an extended period on military duty). Younger children may poorly verbalize answers, which can be sought in play.

Finally, as long as symptoms persist, the diagnosis demands frequent reevaluation to be sure that another, potentially more serious diagnosis has not supervened. Many if not most Adjustment Disorder patients also have other Axis I diagnoses, such as Enuresis and ADHD.

Developmental Factors

Depressive symptoms by themselves are much less likely in young children, who well over half the time will have behavioral symptoms. Instead of complaining of feeling tired, sleepy, or not having sufficient energy, children may withdraw or, in contrast, become fidgety, inattentive, and irritable.

| Personality Disorders

INTRODUCTION

DSM-IV lists 10 specific personality disorders, divided into three clusters. Because none of the 10 are often diagnosed in children or adolescents, we do not discuss them individually in this chapter, and thus we have provided no Quick Guide for them. However, we describe them here very briefly for the sake of differential diagnosis.

- *Cluster A.* Generally withdrawn, cold, suspicious, or irrational, these patients are considered by many to have the most severe personality disturbances. Cluster A includes Paranoid, Schizoid, and Schizotypal Personality Disorders.
- *Cluster B.* Some clinicians consider these patients to be intermediate between those in Clusters A and C, and therefore less seriously disordered than those just mentioned. (However, the family of a patient with severe Antisocial Personality Disorder might disagree with this point of view.) They are characterized by behavior that is dramatic, emotional, and attention-seeking; by labile, shallow moods; and by intense interpersonal conflicts. Cluster B includes Antisocial, Borderline, Histrionic, and Narcissistic Personality Disorders.
- *Cluster C.* Anxious, tense, and often overcontrolled, patients with these personality disorders may be thought of as less severely affected than those in the first two clusters. Cluster C includes Avoidant, Dependent, and Obsessive–Compulsive Personality Disorders.

Other causes of long-standing character disturbance include Personality Change Due to a General Medical Condition, in which a medical condition affects a patient's personality but does not qualify as a personality disorder because it originates in physical disease and may not be pervasive (see Table 13.1). A number of Axis I conditions can distort the way a person behaves and relates to others. Such effects are especially likely in the mood disorders (see Chapter 16), the psychotic disorders (see Chapter 15), and cognitive disorders such as dementias (see Chapter 12).

PROBLEMS WITH DIAGNOSING PERSONALITY DISORDERS IN YOUNG PATIENTS

Although some authorities believe that personality disorders can be reliably diagnosed in adolescents, few make that claim for children. With the relationships among child disorders, adult disorders, and adult personality disorders still not well worked out, the study of childhood personality disorders is yet in its infancy. Several features of personality disorders limit their application to juveniles, especially young children:

- The DSM-IV criteria for personality disorders require a lifelong pattern of experiences and features. Children (especially younger children) simply haven't lived long enough to attain this standard.
- When personality disorder diagnoses are made in adolescents, they tend not to be stable.
- Changing diagnostic criteria promote uncertainty in the diagnostic process.
- In fact, as personality disorder diagnoses fall out of favor (consider the case of passive–aggressive personality disorder), even less stability in this diagnostic process can be assumed.
- Many teenagers and adults qualify for several personality disorders.
- According to DSM-IV criteria, the best-validated personality disorder, Antisocial Personality Disorder, cannot be diagnosed before the age of 18.

Consider the behavioral symptoms that constitute the attention-deficit and disruptive behavior disorders (see Chapter 11). Over the past several decades, it has been well documented that these behaviors often predict pervasive social difficulties in later life. (These difficulties will not necessarily be severe ones, however; nor do they imply that individuals will continue to act out in an antisocial manner. In fact, fewer than half of teenagers who qualify for a diagnosis of Conduct Disorder will eventually be rediagnosed as having Antisocial Personality Disorder.) Nonetheless, it is uncommon for children with conduct problems to become adults who have no Axis I or Axis II pathology at all. It is also unusual to the point of rarity for adult personality disorders to develop from a background of normal childhood or adolescent behavior.

Considering all of these factors, we recommend avoiding specific personality disorder diagnoses for all children and for most adolescents. Rather, we prefer to use the generic criteria for personality disorders (Table 26.1), and to indicate on Axis II a level of uncertainty that avoids labeling young patients with pejorative diagnoses and biasing future clinicians' judgments about such patients.

Apart from the difficulty of making personality disorder diagnoses in young patients, these disorders offer opportunities in any patient for confusion with Axis I disorders. Consider the following:

- Histrionic Personality Disorder is found in up to half of patients with Somatization Disorder; many clinicians consider them to be nearly synonymous.
- Schizotypal Personality Disorder is often a precursor to Schizophrenia, Disorganized Type.
- Asperger's Disorder shares a number of features with Schizoid and Schizotypal Personality Disorders.
- It is often difficult to draw a line between Paranoid Personality Disorder and Delusional Disorder.
- For many patients, the line between Conduct Disorder and Antisocial Personality Disorder is crossed at the 18th birthday.
- Although they are described as different disorders, the similarities between Obsessive–Compulsive Personality Disorder and Obsessive–Compulsive Disorder are obvious.
- Social Phobia patients often have Avoidant Personality Disorder—should they therefore really be considered separately?

As if these issues weren't enough, note also that Cyclothymic Disorder used to be a personality disorder (in DSM-II); that Passive–Aggressive Personality Disorder was included in DSM-III and DSM-III-R, but has been remanded to Appendix B of DSM-IV to await further study; and that Borderline Personality Disorder, introduced in DSM-III, is so popular with some mental health professionals that other clinicians mistrust the diagnosis whenever they encounter it. Finally, many patients qualify for multiple Axis II diagnoses, while some experts in the field believe that there may ultimately turn out to be literally thousands of personality disorders!

Further Evaluation of Jim

The case of Jim (see p. 222) is that of a child who amply met the criteria for Conduct Disorder. Which, if any, Axis II diagnosis might be appropriate? Read-

TABLE 26.1. Generic Criteria for Personality Disorders

- A patient exhibits a lasting pattern of behavior and inner experience that markedly deviates from norms of the patient's culture. The pattern is manifested in at least two of these areas:
  ✓ Affect (appropriateness, intensity, lability, and range of emotions)
  ✓ Cognition (how the patient perceives and interprets self, others, and events)
  ✓ Impulse control
  ✓ Interpersonal functioning
- This pattern is fixed and affects many personal and social situations.
- The pattern causes clinically important distress or impairs school, work, social, or other functioning.
- This stable pattern has lasted a long time, with roots in adolescence or young adulthood.
- The pattern isn't better explained by another mental disorder.
- It isn't directly caused by a general medical condition or by the use of substances, including medications and drugs of abuse.

Coding Notes: If the personality disorder is the only diagnosis or the main reason a patient has come for evaluation, (Principal Diagnosis) should be appended to the Axis II diagnosis. For example:
  Axis I   V71.09   No Diagnosis or Condition
  Axis II   301.83   Borderline Personality Disorder (Principal Diagnosis)
A frequently used defense mechanism can be indicated on the Axis II line:
  Axis II   301.0   Paranoid Personality Disorder; frequent use of projection
If the patient's personality disorder has preceded a psychotic disorder (most often Schizophrenia), the diagnosis may be as follows:
  Axis I   295.10   Schizophrenia, Disorganized Type, Continuous, With Prominent
                          Negative Symptoms
  Axis II   301.20   Schizoid Personality Disorder (Premorbid)

ing through the generic criteria for personality disorder (Table 26.1) suggests the following assessment:

Viewed from the perspective of personality, Jim presented with a lifelong pattern of behavior problems and a way of perceiving the world that was strongly different from the expectations of his environment (his mother and school). At least three life areas were affected: cognitive (he perceived the faults in others, not himself); affective (at a minimum, he showed an inappropriate emotional response when the interviewer mentioned the injury to the other child); and interpersonal (he had a long history of bullying). Any evidence for deviant impulse control would have to be sought by the interviewer. These behaviors were present in a variety of situations (home, school, play) and impaired his personal and social functioning.

Could other diagnoses better account for Jim's symptoms? The vignette provides no evidence in support of a **general medical condition** or **substance-**

related disorder. Of the above-mentioned symptoms, only his interpersonal functioning could be explained solely on the basis of his Conduct Disorder, in the criteria for which affective and cognitive symptoms play no role. Although the effects of an occult **mood disorder** could conceivably be argued, a personality disorder would seem the more parsimonious explanation.

In any event, Jim's vignette provides far too few symptoms to define any of the 10 currently sanctioned DSM-IV personality disorders. The one that would seem most likely, Antisocial Personality Disorder, specifically cannot be diagnosed until the age of 18. For a patient who meets the criteria for this disorder except for age, the appropriate diagnosis would be Personality Disorder Not Otherwise Specified, and even the Not Otherwise Specified cannot be used unless the clinician believes that some personality disorder diagnosis is warranted. Such would not be the case for Jim: Although he might well grow up to have a defined personality disorder, he might turn out to have something else—or, improbably, nothing at all. To indicate uncertainty, his Axis II diagnosis would be stated as Deferred, which would keep the clinician thinking until more information (or the passing of time) settled the problem. Jim's complete current diagnosis would therefore remain as given in Chapter 11:

Axis I	312.8	Conduct Disorder, Childhood-Onset Type, Severe
Axis II	799.9	Diagnosis deferred
Axis III		None
Axis IV		Incarcerated in juvenile hall
Axis V	GAF = 41	(current)

Assessing Personality Disorders

General Suggestions

Of course, the most important information in the quest for personality disorders remains that which comes from other people (and previous evaluations). Some of the material gathered on the history of the present illness may provide information about character—repeated suicide attempts, stealing, chronically making excuses. This acknowledged, what techniques might be useful in evaluating the possibility of a personality disorder in a teenager? Consider observation of affect: Is the patient's mood consonant with the content of the discussion? (Borderline Personality Disorder patients may show inappropriate anger.) Does it seem of approximately normal intensity? (A mood that is too bright and eager may indicate Histrionic Personality Disorder, if there is no substance-related disorder or Manic Episode.) Is the mood stable? (Histrionic and Borderline Personality Disorders are associated with excessive lability.)

Be alert for behaviors that can tip you off to personality characteristics: flirtation, inappropriate dress, arrogance. Sometimes spontaneous statements may provide a guide to attitudes about self, others, and events: "Most people think I'm pretty strange," "I don't have any close friends," "I have trouble staying out of trouble," or "The kids are always making fun of me behind my back."

A good screening question for personality disorders probably doesn't exist, but it is certainly fair to request a self-evaluation: "What sort of a person do you think you are?" or "How would you describe yourself?" A follow-up appropriate for an adolescent might be this: "Have you always been that way? When did you begin to be different?" Children and adolescents alike may not admit to attitudes or behaviors if they perceive them as being socially unacceptable. Note that questions about personal attributes can be softened with a prefatory statement that "some kids are this way."

Developmental Factors

We cannot state too forcefully that personality disorder diagnoses should rarely if ever be made before midadolescence. It is true that all adult personality disorders but one are theoretically permissible; in practice, however, the younger an adolescent, the less willing you should be to make any such definitive diagnosis.

| Other Diagnostic Codes

In the field of child and adolescent mental health, many problems that are not themselves mental illnesses can become the focus of clinical attention. For a number of such problems, such as abuse, neglect, and difficulty in dealing with other people, DSM-IV provides codes to use; we list some of them here. At the end of the chapter are some administrative codes that may be applied to patients for whom no clear diagnosis is immediately apparent.

316 PSYCHOLOGICAL FACTORS AFFECTING MEDICAL CONDITION

DSM-IV suggests six sets of psychological factors that can affect the treatment of a medical disorder: Mental Disorder, Psychological Symptoms, Personality Traits or Coping Style, Maladaptive Health Behaviors, Stress-Related Physiological Response, and Other or Unspecified Psychological Factors. Even though clinicians treating children and adolescents may use these designations only occasionally, they can be indispensable. They are all given the same number and coded on Axis I. For example, a severely depressed child with leukemia may have run away instead of accepting a course of chemotherapy. The diagnosis of Major Depressive Disorder would then be coded on Axis I, along with the psychological factor:

| Axis I | 296.23 | Major Depressive Disorder, Single Episode, Severe Without Psychotic Features, With Melancholic Features |
| | 316 | Mental Disorder Affecting Leukemia |

Note that if the child had run away for reasons not related to a psychological problem, the V-code for Noncompliance With Treatment (see p. 443) might be more appropriate.

RELATIONAL PROBLEMS

Relational problems are situations in which people have difficulty in dealing with one another; these are especially common in a child or adolescent mental health practice. If there is no Axis I or Axis II disorder, the problem and its V-code number should be placed on Axis I. If an Axis I or II diagnosis *is* the focus of current treatment, the relational problem is listed on Axis IV, minus the code number. Note that DSM-IV's intent is to apply these codes not just to the identified patient, but to all family members involved in the relational problem. There are no actual criteria for listing relational problems on Axis I, but if there were, they would probably be something like those given in Table 27.1. These "criteria" are brief and appropriately generic, yet they cover a lot of territory. An example of the process of identifying a relational problem is given shortly in the vignette of Scott.

TABLE 27.1. Hypothetical Criteria for Relational Problems

- Two or more individuals have a problem getting along with one another.
- This behavior is the current focus of clinical attention or treatment.
- These symptoms cause clinically important distress or impair school, work, social, or other functioning.
- No Axis I or Axis II disorder can better explain the behavior.
- The symptoms are not directly caused by a general medical condition or by the use of substances, including medications and drugs of abuse.
- They don't last longer than 6 months after the end of the stressor (or its consequences).

V61.9 Relational Problem Related to a Mental Disorder or General Medical Condition

You can use the V-code for the first relational problem, with its somewhat confusing name, if your patient's main difficulty is due to interaction with a relative who has a mental disorder or physical disease. An example would be an adolescent whose problems stem from living with an alcoholic grandparent.

V61.20 Parent–Child Relational Problem

In some cases, parents seek help for their children when the real problems are with the parents themselves—marital conflicts, personal mental disorder, and the like. The diagnosis of parental and interparental disorders is beyond the scope of this book, but you need to be alert to all possible causes of a young patient's troubles. Use Parent–Child Relational Problem when clinically important symptoms or negative effects on functioning are associated with the way a parent and child interact. The problematic interaction may involve over-protection, faulty communication, or ineffective or inconsistent discipline.

V61.1 Partner Relational Problem

Of course, most adolescents will not have a partner (spouse), but when a teen is married or living with a partner, clinically important symptoms or negative effects on functioning may be caused by the way the patient and partner interact. The problematic interaction pattern may be faulty communication or an absence of communication.

V61.8 Sibling Relational Problem

Use Sibling Relational Problem when clinically important symptoms or negative effects on functioning are associated with the way brothers and sisters interact.

V62.81 Relational Problem Not Otherwise Specified

When the need for evaluation centers around relational problems not covered by the above-mentioned categories, use Relational Problem Not Otherwise Specified. DSM-IV suggests the example of problems with coworkers, but a problem with classmates might qualify.

Identifying Relational Problems

Scott

"Scott, come on! It's our turn to go in. The doctor wants to see both of us." Scott didn't look up at his mother, who stood in the doorway of the interviewer's office. He slouched deeper into his chair and turned a page of the magazine he was holding. "Scott, come on!" He still didn't move. With a palms-up gesture of exasperation, the mother disappeared inside the office alone.

"He's always this way with me," she told the therapist when they were seated. "His teachers seem to like him, and he minds his grandfather just fine. I'm the only one who has trouble with him."

The mother's difficulties with Scott had begun 4 years ago. His father, who had been the family disciplinarian, had been killed in a skydiving accident, and she and Scott had had to move in with her in-laws. Scott's behavior had been acceptable for a year, until she won a product liability suit against the parachute supplier and they moved back to California to be near her parents. She got a boyfriend and a job—and, she admitted, probably hadn't spent as much time with Scott as he needed. "And for the last year, life's been nothing but hell. He hasn't been in trouble, and he isn't violent or anything, but we're always arguing and I never seem to win. I think he's actually brighter than I am."

Scott was very bright. Even without studying, he'd maintained above-average grades, and none of his teachers had complained about his classroom behavior. Whenever his mother would suggest that he do his homework, he would smile and continue watching TV or reading a book. Sent to his room, he would listen to music, draw, or just look out the window—in short, do anything but study.

When his mother emerged from the office, the interviewer invited Scott to enter. Pleasant and cooperative, he responded fully to all questions and volunteered other information about his relationship with both of his parents. He had worshiped his father and deeply resented it when his mother eventually began dating again. "I don't care much what she does," Scott said, leaning forward in his chair. "Why should I? She doesn't really care what I do."

Scott denied feeling either anxious or depressed. In fact, his mood was pretty good most of the time. He acknowledged that his mother thought him irritable and angry, but denied that this was so. "If I feel anything, it's contempt," he said. "I can twist her around my little finger."

Evaluation of Scott

The focus of Scott's evaluation was an important interpersonal problem, thereby meeting the first hypothetical criterion in Table 27.1. Before Parent–Child Relational Problem could be listed on Axis I, however, all other possible mental and physical causes for his behavior would have to be ruled out.

The attention-deficit and disruptive behavior disorders would be important to consider on two counts: They are the disorders most commonly encountered in child and/or adolescent mental health clinics, and they cover at least some of the symptoms of which Scott's mother complained. However, Scott's attention span and activity level were normal, and his problem conduct, directed only toward his mother, did not violate the boundaries of person, property, or truth, as would be true for **Conduct Disorder**. Although several of the interactions with his mother could be construed as consistent with **Oppositional Defiant Disorder**, he did not show the typical anger, spite, or loss of temper. Of course, ample academic evidence ruled out **Mental Retardation** and all of the **learning disorders** and **pervasive developmental disorders**. No speech problems were reported or noted, eliminating **Selective Mutism** and any of the **communication disorders**. Although the history includes no mention of problems involving **eating** or **elimination**, the clinician should include questions about these in a review of systems. There were no motor problems reported or noted, eliminating **Developmental Coordination Disorder**, **tic disorders**, and **Stereotypic Movement Disorder**. Scott certainly did have a problem in relating to his mother, but not to other adults (including his grandfather, teachers, and the interviewer), so **Reactive Attachment Disorder** would likewise be ruled out.

What about all the *other* Axis I disorders? Scott specifically denied any symptoms of anxiety or worry, ruling out an **anxiety disorder** (and **Separation Anxiety Disorder**, the remaining "child" diagnosis, which functionally belongs with other anxiety disorders). There is a similar lack of support for a **mood disorder** or **cognitive disorder**. Of course, almost any behavior imaginable can be encountered in the course of **substance use**, and the clinician would need to ask both Scott and his mother about this possibility. Aberrant behaviors are encountered in the **impulse-control disorders** (such as **Pathological Gambling** and **Intermittent Explosive Disorder**), but Scott's behavior was planned, not impulsive. An **Adjustment Disorder** would have had to occur within 3 months of and in response to a stressor (could his mother's dating be considered a legitimate stressor?). The death of his father had occurred too long ago for **Bereavement** to be applicable. Finally, a **personality disorder** (even if there were sufficient symptoms to diagnose one) would have to affect more than one aspect of Scott's life, not just his relationship with his mother.

Perhaps some might argue for a Not Otherwise Specified diagnosis, but what would it be? **Disruptive Behavior Disorder Not Otherwise Specified** might be a possibility, but any Not Otherwise Specified category should be used only when it seems clear that the diagnosis belongs within the general category, and Scott's presentation was far too atypical to indicate a disruptive behavior disorder. Besides, at what point should any clinician relax and "accept the obvious"? The final requirement listed in Table 27.1 serves as a reminder that, just as for Adjustment Disorder, no one can be sure about causation of symptoms attributed to a relational problem until the problem has resolved and the symptoms abate. That is why the cautious term Provisional would be added to the V-code for Scott (and his mother—the V-code would be applied to all members of the family unit in question):

Axis I	V61.20	Parent–Child Relational Problem (Provisional)
Axis II	V71.09	No diagnosis
Axis III		None
Axis IV		None
Axis V	GAF = 75	(current)

PROBLEMS RELATED TO ABUSE OR NEGLECT

One problem with studies of the effects of childhood abuse is that they often conflate physical and sexual abuse, rather than reporting their effects separately. Perhaps this is because the two types of abuse often go together. In general, more severe abuse and earlier abuse are more likely to produce psychopathology. However, most studies don't carefully assess the cause–effect relationship (does the risk factor of abuse clearly antedate the behavior in question?). Children or adolescents may develop substance use problems (alcohol, marijuana, other drugs), sexual acting out and teen pregnancy, depression and low self-esteem, anxiety symptoms, running away, sleep problems (trouble initiating and maintaining sleep), appetite disorders (Anorexia Nervosa), or Conduct Disorder. Adults may develop dissociation, decreased satisfaction with sexual relationships, Posttraumatic Stress Disorder symptoms, eating disorders (especially Bulimia Nervosa), back pain. Up to 20% of female children may be sexually abused in some way; 5–6% of girls suffer severe abuse involving actual or attempted intercourse. Comparable rates for boys are about one-fourth of those for girls.

Although precise information is difficult to obtain, it is estimated that each year about 1 million children in the United States are abused by their parents or other adults. Children abused as infants tend to become much more avoidant, resistant, and noncompliant than do other children. The three categories DSM-IV provides for problems related to abuse or neglect of a young person—Physical Abuse of Child, Sexual Abuse of Child, and Neglect of Child—all receive the same V-code number, V61.21. In each case, specify 995.5 if clinical attention is focused on the child or adolescent as the victim.

OTHER CONDITIONS THAT MAY BE A FOCUS OF CLINICAL ATTENTION

V15.81 Noncompliance With Treatment

Noncompliance With Treatment identifies a patient who requires attention because the patient has ignored or thwarted attempts at treatment for a mental disorder or a general medical condition. An example would be a teenager with Schizophrenia who requires repeated hospitalization for refusal to take medication.

V65.2 Malingering

Malingering is the intentional production of the signs or symptoms of a physical or mental disorder. The purpose is some sort of gain: obtaining something desirable (money, drugs, insurance settlement) or avoiding something unpleasant (punishment, work, military service, jury duty). Malingering is often confused with Factitious Disorder, in which the motive is not external gain but a wish to occupy the sick role, and with the somatoform disorders, in which the symptoms are not intentionally produced at all.

Malingering should be suspected when a patient has or does any of the following:

- Legal problems or the prospect of financial gain
- Tells a story that does not accord with informants' accounts or with other known facts
- Does not cooperate with the evaluation
- Antisocial Personality Disorder

Malingering is easy to suspect and difficult to prove. In the absence of an observation of overt behavior (someone placing sand in a urine specimen or holding a thermometer over a glowing light bulb), a resolute and clever malingerer can be almost impossible to detect. When Malingering involves symptoms that are strictly mental or emotional, detection may be impossible. Because the consequences of this diagnosis are dire (it can alienate patients from their clinicians), we recommend that you make this diagnosis only in the most obvious and imperative of circumstances. Remember that frank Malingering is rare to the point of nullity in children, and probably extremely uncommon even in late adolescence.

V71.02 Childhood or Adolescent Antisocial Behavior

Childhood or Adolescent Antisocial Behavior is supposedly the juvenile equivalent of an adult V-code, Adult Antisocial Behavior, in which clinical attention focuses on antisocial behavior that does not form a recognizable pattern (such as Conduct Disorder or an impulse-control disorder). The diagnosis might be made in an isolated example of criminal activity in which an adolescent has followed the lead of an older person.

V62.89 Borderline Intellectual Functioning

Use Borderline Intellectual Functioning for a patient whose IQ and level of functioning fall within the range of 71 to 84. In the face of other Axis I diagnoses (e.g., psychotic or cognitive disorders), the differential diagnosis between Borderline Intellectual Functioning and Mild Mental Retardation can be quite difficult. Like Mental Retardation, Borderline Intellectual Functioning should be coded on Axis II.

V62.82 Bereavement

It is natural to grieve when a relative or close friend dies. When the symptoms of the grieving process are a reason for the clinical attention, DSM-IV allows a diagnosis of Bereavement—provided that the symptoms don't last too long and aren't too severe. The problem is that grief can closely resemble the sadness associated with a Major Depressive Episode. DSM-IV mentions certain symptoms that can help discriminate between these two conditions. Suspect a Major Depressive Episode in a grieving child or adolescent who shows any of the following:

- Guilt feelings (other than about actions that might have prevented the death)
- Death wishes (other than the survivor's wishing to have died with the loved one)
- Slowed-down psychomotor activity
- Marked preoccupation with worthlessness
- Severely impaired functioning for an unusually long time
- Hallucinations (other than of seeing or hearing the deceased)

In addition, people who are "only" bereaved typically regard their moods as normal. A diagnosis of depressive illness is usually withheld in these cases until after the symptoms have lasted longer than 2 months.

V62.3 Academic Problem

A child or adolescent whose problem is related to schoolwork, and who does not have a learning disorder or other mental disorder that accounts for the problem, may be given the Academic Problem V-code. Even if another disorder can account for the problem, the Academic Problem itself may be so severe that it independently justifies clinical attention. Then you would list both the V-code and the clinical disorder on Axis I.

V62.2 Occupational Problem

Occupational Problem is the work-related equivalent of Academic Problem; examples include choosing a career and job dissatisfaction. Of course, use of this V-code will be rare until late adolescence.

313.82 Identity Problem

Identity Problem may be applied to patients who are uncertain about identity-related issues, such as career, friendships, goals, morals, or sexual orientation. Adolescents who question who they are or what they believe may qualify for this designation.

V62.89 Religious or Spiritual Problem

Patients who require evaluation or treatment for issues pertaining to religious faith (or its lack) may be coded as having a Religious or Spiritual Problem.

V62.4 Acculturation Problem

Acculturation Problem may be useful for children or adolescents whose problems center on a move from one culture to another (e.g., emigrants and immigrants).

V62.89 Phase of Life Problem

Phase of Life Problem is a V-code you can use for a young patient whose problem is due not to a mental disorder but to a life change (e.g., entering school, parental divorce, leaving parental control).

MEDICATION-INDUCED DISORDERS

Medication-induced movement (and other) disorders are important in mental health settings because (1) they may be mistaken for Axis I conditions (such as tic disorders, Schizophrenia, or anxiety disorders), or (2) they can affect the management of children who are receiving neuroleptic medications. Although these disorders are not often encountered in children or adolescents, the following codes may occasionally be appropriate:

332.1	Neuroleptic-Induced Parkinsonism
333.92	Neuroleptic Malignant Syndrome
333.7	Neuroleptic-Induced Acute Dystonia
333.99	Neuroleptic-Induced Acute Akathisia
333.82	Neuroleptic-Induced Tardive Dyskinesia
333.1	Medication-Induced Postural Tremor
333.90	Medication-Induced Movement Disorder Not Otherwise Specified
995.2	Adverse Effects of Medication Not Otherwise Specified

ADDITIONAL CODES

Several other codes are useful for administrative purposes. Two of these codes state that a patient has no diagnosis on Axis I or Axis II. Others provide ways to indicate that you don't know what's wrong, if anything.

300.9 Unspecified Mental Disorder (Nonpsychotic)

Unspecified Mental Disorder (nonpsychotic) may be appropriate if (1) the diagnosis you want to give is not contained in DSM-IV; or (2) you have too little information to make a definitive diagnosis when a child or adolescent is clearly ill and no Not Otherwise Specified category seems appropriate. Once you have obtained more information, you should be able to substitute a more specific diagnosis.

V71.09 No Diagnosis or Condition on Axis I

No Diagnosis or Condition on Axis I means that no major mental disorder or V-code condition is the focus of clinical attention. However, the patient could still have an Axis II disorder, which would then become the principal diagnosis.

V71.09 No Diagnosis on Axis II

No Diagnosis on Axis II means that a patient has no personality disorder or Mental Retardation.

799.9 Diagnosis or Condition Deferred on Axis I

799.9 Diagnosis Deferred on Axis II

The Deferred codes mean that there is not currently enough information to permit an Axis I or Axis II diagnosis to be made. The diagnosis will be changed once enough further information becomes available.

Structured Interviews and Other Reference Materials

Structured and semistructured interviews have both advantages and disadvantages. Whereas they prompt the clinician to cover all the material required by a given set of diagnostic criteria, they may not reveal material that is unusual, complex, or unexpected in a given context. Structured interviews are at their best in selecting a relatively homogeneous group of patients for mental health research purposes; they can also help establish baseline data for individual patients—an especially valuable point for patients whose care may be shared by a number of clinicians. We hasten to point out that often the best test of all remains an interview by a sensitive, experienced clinician.

This appendix consists of three sections. First, we present the Children's Global Assessment Scale (CGAS) in its entirety. Second, we provide brief descriptions of other interviews, schedules, and tests that may prove useful in assessing children and adolescents, along with addresses and references for the instruments themselves or for further information about them. Third, we present a short, annotated bibliography of relevant books and articles.

CHILDREN'S GLOBAL ASSESSMENT SCALE (CGAS)

Rate the subject's most impaired level of general functioning for the specified time period by selecting the *lowest* level that describes functioning; use intermediate values as needed. Rate actual functioning, regardless of treatment or prognosis. This scale is intended for use with children aged 4–16.

100–91	*Superior functioning* in all areas (at home, at school, and with peers); involved in a wide range of activities and has many interests (e.g., has hobbies or participates in extracurricular activities or belongs to an organized group such as Scouts, etc.); likable, confident; "everyday" worries never get out of hand; doing well in school; no symptoms
90–81	*Good functioning in all areas;* secure in family, school, and with peers; there may be transient difficulties and "everyday" worries that occasionally get out of hand (e.g., mild anxiety associated with an important exam, occasional "blowups" with siblings, parents, or peers)
80–71	*No more than slight impairment in functioning* at home, at school, or with peers; some disturbance of behavior or emotional distress may be present in response to life stresses (e.g., parental separations, deaths, birth of a sib), but these are brief and interference with functioning is transient; such children are only minimally disturbing to others and are not considered deviant by those who know them
70–61	*Some difficulty in a single area, but generally functioning pretty well* (e.g., sporadic or isolated antisocial acts, such as occasionally playing hooky or petty theft; consistent minor difficulties with schoolwork; mood changes of brief duration; fears and anxieties which do not lead to gross avoidance behavior; self-doubts); has some meaningful interpersonal relationships; most people who do not know the child well would not consider him/her deviant but those who do know him/her well might express concern
60–51	*Variable functioning with sporadic difficulties or symptoms in several but not all social areas;* disturbance would be apparent to those who encounter the child in a dysfunctional setting or time but not to those who see the child in other settings
50–41	*Moderate degree of interference in functioning in most social areas or severe impairment of functioning in one area,* such as might result from, for example, suicidal preoccupations and ruminations, school refusal and other forms of anxiety, obsessive rituals, major conversion symptoms, frequent anxiety attacks, poor or inappropriate social skills, frequent episodes of aggressive or other antisocial behavior with some preservation of meaningful social relationships
40–31	*Major impairment in functioning in several areas and unable to function in one of these areas,* i.e., disturbed at home, at school, with peers, or in society at large, e.g., persistent aggression without clear instigation; markedly withdrawn and isolated behavior due to either mood or thought disturbance, suicidal attempts with clear lethal intent; such children are likely to require special schooling and/or hospitalization or withdrawal from school (but this is not a sufficient criterion for inclusion in this category)
30–21	*Unable to function in almost all areas,* e.g., stays at home, in ward, or in bed all day without taking part in social activities or severe impairment in reality testing or serious impairment in communication (e.g., sometimes incoherent or inappropriate)
20–11	*Needs considerable supervision* to prevent hurting others or self (e.g., frequently violent, repeated suicide attempts) or to maintain personal hygiene *or* gross impairment in all forms of communication, e.g., severe abnormalities in verbal and gestural communication, marked social aloofness, stupor, etc.
10–1	*Needs constant supervision* (24-hr care) due to severely aggressive or self-destructive behavior or gross impairment in reality testing, communication, cognition, affect, or personal hygiene

Note. From Shaffer D, Gould MS, Brasic J, Ambrosini P, Fisher P, Bird H, Aluwahlia S. A Children's Global Assessment Scale (CGAS). *Arch Gen Psychiatry* 1983; *40*:1228–1231. Copyright 1983 by the American Medical Association. Reprinted by permission.

OTHER INTERVIEWS, SCHEDULES, AND TESTS

In compiling this section, we have tried to focus on what is easily available in conventionally published form or on the World Wide Web. References marked with an asterisk (*) contain the full test text; otherwise, we give authors' or publishers' addresses and, where available, Web sites or e-mail addresses. For further information about individual tests, consult the Web sites given below or standard texts.

General

The **Schedule for Affective Disorders and Schizophrenia for School-Age Children (K-SADS)** is probably the most widely used semistructured interview for patients aged 6–17. Affectionately termed the "Kiddie-SADS," it uses probe questions and DSM criteria to assess current and past episodes of psychopathology in children and adolescents. The clinician adjusts the interview to the developmental level of the patient and uses the patient's (or parent's) language. The K-SADS covers many of the commonly experienced DSM-IV diagnoses, including Major Depressive Disorder, the bipolar disorders, and Dysthymic and Cyclothymic Disorders; Schizophrenia, Schizoaffective Disorder, Schizophreniform Disorder, and Brief Psychotic Disorder; Panic Disorder, Agoraphobia, Separation Anxiety Disorder, Specific and Social Phobias, Generalized Anxiety Disorder, Obsessive–Compulsive Disorder, and Posttraumatic Stress Disorder; Attention-Deficit/Hyperactivity Disorder, Conduct Disorder, Oppositional Defiant Disorder, Enuresis, Encopresis, Transient Tic Disorder, Tourette's Disorder, and Chronic Motor or Vocal Tic Disorder; Anorexia Nervosa and Bulimia Nervosa; Alcohol and other Substance Abuse; and Adjustment Disorder. [Joan Kaufman, PhD, Yale University, Department of Psychology, P.O. Box 208205, New Haven, CT 06520; the K-SADS-PL (Present and Lifetime version) is available online in its entirety at no charge, at http://www.wpic.pitt.edu/ksads/default.htm]

The **Diagnostic Interview for Children and Adolescents (DICA)** categorizes disorders by ICD-9 or DSM diagnoses. It can best discriminate a psychiatric population from a pediatric population on the basis of the Relationship and Academic Problems scales; however, the research is limited. [MHS Inc., 908 Niagra Falls Blvd., North Tonawanda, NY 14120; http://www.mhs.com/index.htm]

The **Diagnostic Interview Schedule for Children (DISC)** has over 200 items that capture information regarding the onset, duration, severity, and associated impairment of child behaviors and symptoms. The DISC is organized into six diagnostic sections: Anxiety Disorders, Mood Disorders, Disruptive Disorders, Substance-Use Disorders, Schizophrenia, and Miscellaneous Disorders. It can be administered by either clinicians or lay interviewers. There are paper and electronic versions for both the identified patient and a parent. [Prudence Fisher, MS, NIMH-DISC Training Center, Columbia University/New York State Psychiatric Institute, Division of Child and Adolescent Psychiatry, 722 West 168th Street, New York, NY 10032; e-mail: fisherp@child.cpmc.columbia.edu]

The **Child Behavior Checklist (CBCL)** is actually a group of assessments that collect data on general functioning from a variety of respondents. Its subscales assess internalizing and externalizing behaviors, including aggression, anxiety/depression, attention, delinquency, sex, social problems, somatic problems, and withdrawal. Separate forms of the CBCL for parents are available for children aged 2–3, children or adolescents aged 4–18, and young adults aged 18–30. There is a Teacher's Report Form for children or adolescents aged 5–18, and a Caregiver–Teacher Report Form for ages 2–5. Self-report forms are available for youths aged 11–18 and for young adults aged 18–30. [Child Behavior Checklist, 1 South Prospect St., Burlington, VT 05401-3456; http://checklist.uvm.edu]

The **Screen for Adolescent Violence Exposure (SAVE)** assesses the exposure of adolescents to violence in the school, home, and community, with excellent reliability and validity. This 32-question screening instrument correlates significantly with objective data on crime and with constructs that are theoretically relevant, such as anger and posttraumatic stress symptoms. [*Hastings TL, Kelley ML. Development and validation of the Screen for Adolescent Violence Exposure (SAVE). *J Abnorm Child Psychol* 1997; *25*:511–520]

The **Global Assessment of Functioning (GAF)** and the **Children's Global Assessment Scale (CGAS)** both reflect the current overall occupational (academic), psychological, and social functioning of a patient—but not environmental problems or physical limitations. The score on each instrument is recorded as a number on a 100-point scale. Both instruments specify symptoms and behavioral guidelines to help determine the score for an individual patient. The GAF is designed for adults and may be useful with adolescents and older children; the CGAS is couched in terms more appropriate for a child. Both scales are inherently subjective, so that their greatest use may be in tracking changes in a level of functioning across time, as assessed by a single examiner. [The GAF may be found in DSM-IV or in James Morrison's *DSM-IV Made Easy*; the CGAS is reproduced above]

Mental Retardation, Intelligence Quotient, Developmental Quotient

The **Wechsler Intelligence Scale for Children—Revised (WISC-R)**; intended for ages 6–16 years, is a revision of a test that has been in use for almost 50 years. The Full Scale IQ score summarizes functioning on six Verbal subtests (Arithmetic, Comprehension,

Digit Span, Information, Similarities, and Vocabulary) and seven performance subtests (Block Design, Coding, Mazes, Object Assembly, Picture Arrangement, Picture Completion, and Symbol Search). [The Psychological Corporation, P.O. Box 839954, San Antonio, TX 78283-3954; http://www.psychcorp.com]

In about 25 minutes, the **Denver Developmental Scale** provides early identification of children (aged 1 month to 6 years) at risk for developmental problems. The 125 items cover four areas: fine motor–adaptive, gross motor, language, and personal–social. [Denver Developmental Materials, Inc., P.O. Box 6919, Denver, CO 80206; telephone: 800-419-4729]

The **Bayley Scales of Infant Development (2nd ed.)** assess the developmental functioning of children aged 1–42 months. [Psychological Assessment Resources, Inc., P.O. Box 998, Odessa, FL 33556; http://www.parinc.com/proframes.html]

In the **Peabody Picture Vocabulary Test—Third Edition**, the patient chooses a picture that best represents a word spoken by the examiner. The score generated equates to IQ, though the publishers discourage the use of the term "verbal intelligence." [American Guidance Service, 4201 Woodland Road, Circle Pines, MN 55014-1796; http://www.agsnet.com/fast.asp]

The **Beery Developmental Test of Visual Motor Integration** assesses visual–motor skills. The child (aged 3–18) copies geometric figures that are arranged in ascending order of difficulty. The 27 culture-free items require about 15 minutes to complete. The test is used to screen children who may need special assistance or services. [Psychological Assessment Resources, P.O. Box 998, Odessa, FL 33556; http://www.parinc.com/proframes.html]

LEARNING DISORDERS

The **Wide Range Achievement Test—3 (WRAT-3)** is easy to administer and assesses reading, spelling, and math skills from ages 5 to adult. It is normed by age, not grade level. [Psychological Assessment Resources, P.O. Box 998, Odessa, FL 33556; http://www.parinc.com/proframes.html]

Communication Disorders

The **Multilingual Aphasia Examination (MAE)** provides a brief (40-minute) evaluation of articulation, oral expression, oral verbal understanding, reading, spelling, and writing, suitable for ages 6 to adult. [Psychological Assessment Resources, P.O. Box 998, Odessa, FL 33556; http://www.parinc.com/proframes.html]

Pervasive Developmental Disorders

The 15 items of the well-validated **Childhood Autism Rating Scale (CARS)** help to identify autistic children, adolescents, and adults, and to distinguish them from those who are developmentally handicapped but not autistic. It also discriminates severe from mild to moderate autism. Based on direct observation as well as historical information, the CARS is suitable for use by lay or professional observers with any child over the age of 2. [Western Psychological Services, 12031 Wilshire Blvd., Los Angeles, CA 90025; http://www.wpspublish.com]

Attention-Deficit/Hyperactivity Disorder

The **Conners Rating Scales** are relatively brief instruments (93 items for parents, 48 for teachers) that assess ADHD. [MHS Inc., 908 Niagra Falls Blvd., North Tonawanda, NY 14120; http://www.mhs.com/index.htm]

Tic Disorders

For any age, the **Yale Global Tic Severity Scale** provides an overall evaluation of complexity, frequency, intensity, interference, and number of motor and vocal tics, including those found in patients with Tourette's Disorder. [*Leckman JF, Riddle MA, Hardin MT, Ort SI, Swartz KL, Stevenson J, Cohen DJ. The Yale Global Tic Severity Scale: Initial testing of a clinician-rated scale of tic severity. *J Am Acad Child Adolesc Psychiatry* 1989; *28:*566–573]

Cognitive Disorders

For older children and adolescents, the **Mini-Mental State Exam (MMSE)** offers a rapid, reproducible way to conduct and score a brief evaluation of the cognitive state. [*Folstein MF, Folstein SE, McHugh PR. Mini-Mental State: A practical method of grading the cognitive state of patients for the clinician. *J Psychiatric Res* 1975; *12:*189–198. Reproduced in *DSM-IV Made Easy* by James Morrison]

Substance Use

Many tools for assessing substance use, several of which can be downloaded free of charge, are described at [http://silk.nih.gov/silk/niaaa1/publication/instable.htm]

The **CAGE** questionnaire is a simple screening device for alcoholism that is widely used because it is easy to remember and quick to administer. However, it may lack sufficient specificity and sensitivity for use in teen populations. [*Ewing JA. Detecting alcoholism: The CAGE questionnaire. *JAMA* 1984; *252*:1905–1907; http://silk.nih.gov/silk/niaaa1/publication/inscage.htm]

The semistructured **Comprehensive Addiction Severity Index for Adolescents** can be administered on paper or by computer in 45–90 minutes, and is intended to guide treatment planning and assess outcome. It assesses symptoms, known risk factors, and consequences of alcohol or drug use within seven main areas of functioning: education status, alcohol/drug use, family relationships, peer relationships, legal status, mental distress, and use of free time. Sponsored by the National Institute of Drug Abuse, the Index is free, but training is mandatory. [Kathleen Meyers, VAMC Philadelphia (116D), University & Woodland Aves, Bldg. 7, Philadelphia, PA 19104; meyershagan@erols.com]

The 30-item **Drug and Alcohol Problem Quick Screen** is a useful office screening tool for the detection of serious problems in adolescents. [*Schwartz RH, Wirtz PW. Potential substance abuse: Detection among adolescent patients. *Clin Pediatr* 1990; *29*:38–43]

Mood Disorders

Mood disorders can be evaluated with the K-SADS, the DICA, and the DISC (discussed above). Here are some additional instruments:

The **Mania Rating Scale (MRS)** was developed to evaluate manic behavior in prepubertal children; its use may discriminate between manic behavior and hyperactivity due to ADHD. The MRS may also help distinguish severity of mania. [*Fristad MA, Weller EB, Weller RA. The Mania Rating Scale: Can it be used in children? A preliminary report. *J Am Acad Child Adolesc Psychiatry* 1992; *31*(2):252–257]

The **Children's Depression Inventory (CDI)** is a self-report, symptom-oriented scale that requires young patients (aged 7–17) to score the severity of their own symptoms over the past 2 weeks. Its 27 items yield five factors: Negative Mood, Interpersonal Problems, Ineffectiveness, Anhedonia, and Negative Self-Esteem. There is also a 10-item short form. [MHS Inc., 908 Niagra Falls Blvd., North Tonawanda, NY, 14120; http://www.mhs.com/index.htm]

The **Suicide Probability Scale** measures suicidal ideation, hopelessness, and social isolation to predict subsequent suicide attempts, suicide verbalizations, and minor self-destructive behaviors. Although it does yield a high number of false positives, when it is used with effective suicide precautions, this scale may be able to lower the risk of suicide in adolescents. [Western Psychological Services, 12031 Wilshire Blvd., Los Angeles, CA 90025; http://www.wpspublish.com]

Anxiety Disorders

For accurate diagnosis of **Posttraumatic Stress Disorder,** children younger than 4 years may require alternative criteria. [*Scheeringa MS, Zeanah CH, Drell MJ, Larrieu JA. Two approaches to the diagnosis of posttraumatic stress disorder in infancy and early childhood. *J Am Acad Child Adolesc Psychiatry* 1995; *34*:191–200]

The **State–Trait Anxiety Inventory for Children (STAIC)** consists of two scales, each made up of 20 self-administered statements, assessing how children feel at a particular moment and how they generally feel. The STAIC is useful for ages 9–12 years; administration time is about 15 minutes. [Psychological Assessment Resources, P.O. Box 998, Odessa, FL 33556; http://www.parinc.com/proframes.html]

Pain Disorder

The **Varni–Thompson Pediatric Pain Questionnaire** uses a visual analogue scale to assess current and worst pain for the previous week. [James W. Varni, PhD, Center for Child Health Outcomes, Children's Hospital and Health Center, 3020 Children's Way, San Diego, CA 92123; jvarni@chsd.org]

Dissociative Disorders

The **Child Dissociative Checklist (CDC)** is a reliable and valid observer report measure of dissociation in children that can be used in research or in screening individual patients. It discriminated well among four test samples: normal girls, sexually abused girls, boys and girls with dissociative disorders, and children with DSM-III-R Multiple Personality Disorder. [*Putnam FW, Helmers K, Trickett PK. Development, reliability, and validity of a child dissociation scale. *Child Abuse Negl* 1993; *17*(6):731–741]

Eating Disorders

The **Eating Disorder Inventory** is a 64-item self-report instrument useful as a screening tool for specific cognitive and behavioral dimensions of persons with eating disorders, as well as a means of distinguishing them from normal dieters. There are eight subscales: Body Dissatisfaction, Bulimia, Drive for Thinness, Ineffectiveness, Interoceptive Awareness, Interpersonal Distrust, Maturity Fears, and Perfectionism. [Psychological Assessment Resources, P.O. Box 998, Odessa, FL 33556; http://www.parinc.com/percouns/EDI232a.html]

The **Anorectic Behavior Observation Scale** queries parents about specific eating behaviors and attitudes in their children. With a cutoff score of 19, its sensitivity and specificity were 90%. [*Vandereycken W. Validity and reliability of the Anorectic Behavior Observation Scale for parents. *Acta Psychiatrica Scand* 1992; *85*(2):163–166]

The **Contour Drawing Rating Scale**, a body image assessment tool, consists of nine male and nine female contour drawings that can be used to measure ideal and perceived body sizes and the discrepancy between the two. The drawings can be split at the waist to compare perceptions of the upper and lower body. [*Thompson MA, Gray JJ. Development and validation of a new body-image assessment scale. *J Pers Assess* 1995; *64*:258–269]

Personality Disorders

Many children aged 12 or older can complete questionnaires themselves. Similar to the adult version, the adolescent version of the **Minnesota Multiphasic Personality Inventory (MMPI-A)** contains 478 items, some of which directly target adolescent concerns. The resulting clinical profile resembles the psychopathology scales of the MMPI-2. [NCS, 5605 Green Circle Drive, Minnetonka, MN 55343; http://assessments.ncs.com/assessments/tests/mmpia.htm]

The 150 true–false items in the **Millon Adolescent Personality Inventory (MAPI)** yield information about impulse control, rapport, personality style, school functioning, and self-esteem in 13- to 18-year-olds. A great deal of research has been published about this increasingly venerable measure. [NCS, 5605 Green Circle Drive, Minnetonka, MN 55343; http://assessments.ncs.com/assessments/tests/mapi.htm]

Abuse and Parental Stress

The 126 items on the **Parenting Stress Index** yield percentile scores in two domains: Child (Adaptability, Acceptability, Demandingness, Mood, Distractibility/Hyperactivity, Reinforces Parent) and Parent (Depression, Attachment, Restriction of Role, Sense of Competence, Social Isolation, Relationship with Spouse, Parent Health). [American Guidance Service, 4201 Woodland Road, Circle Pines, MN 55014-1796; http://www.agsnet.com/fast.asp]

BOOKS AND ARTICLES

General

Ainsworth M, Blehar M, Waters E, Wall S. *Patterns of attachment: A psychological study of the Strange Situation.* Hillsdale, NJ: Erlbaum, 1978.

American Association on Mental Retardation. *Mental Retardation: Definition, Classification, and Systems of Support,* 9th ed. Washington, DC: Author, 1992. Clinicians who treat mentally retarded children should become familiar with this competing classification system.

American Psychiatric Association. *Diagnostic and Statistical Manual of Mental Disorders* (4th ed.). Washington, DC: Author, 1994. The famous DSM-IV is the standard of current American diagnostic thinking in mental health.

American Psychiatric Association. *DSM-IV Sourcebook,* Vol 3. Washington, DC: Author, 1997. Behind-the-scenes discussions of the work that went into the formulation of the DSM-IV section on disorders usually first diagnosed in infancy, childhood, or adolescence.

Chess S, Thomas A. Issues in the clinical application of temperament. In G Kohstamm, J Bates, M Rothbart (Eds.), *Temperament in childhood,* pp. 377–386. New York: Wiley, 1989.

Lieberman A, Wieder S, Fenichel E (eds). *The DC 0–3 Casebook.* Washington, DC: The National Center for Infants, Toddlers, and Families, 1997. An alternative diagnostic classification system for very young patients; includes plenty of examples.

Morrison J. *DSM-IV Made Easy.* New York: Guilford Press, 1995. A one-volume approach to understanding adult DSM-IV diagnoses.

Ollendick T, Hersen M. *Handbook of Child and Adolescent Assessment.* Boston: Allyn & Bacon, 1993. This valuable, though older, reference covers basic issues underlying assessment strategies, the strategies themselves, and specific child disorders.

Robins E, Guze SB. Establishment of diagnostic validity in psychiatric illness: Its application to schizophrenia. *Am J Psychiat* 1970; *126:*983–987.

Spreen O, Strauss E. *A Compendium of Neuropsychological Tests,* 2nd ed. New York: Oxford University Press, 1998. Recent compendium includes descriptions of tests of cognition, intelligence, achievement, attention, memory, language, motor, and other attributes.

Weintraub MI. Malingering and conversion reactions. *Neurol Clin* 1995; *13:*1–450. Among other things, reviews pseudoneurological symptoms and their detection.

Winnicott DW. *Therapeutic consultations in child psychiatry.* London: Hogarth Press, 1971. Source of the famous Squiggles game.

Zeanah CH Jr. (ed). *Handbook of infant mental health.* New York: Guilford Press, 1993. Edited, interdisciplinary analysis of clinical, developmental, and social aspects of infant mental health.

Interviewing

Anglin TM. Interviewing guidelines for the clinical evaluation of adolescent substance abuse. *Pediat Clin N Am* 1987; *34:*381–398.

Barker P. *Clinical Interviews with Children and Adolescents.* New York: Norton, 1990. This work deals with the interviewing process from a largely theoretical perspective (no examples).

Coupey SM. Interviewing adolescents. *Pediatr Clin N Am* 1997; *44:*1349–1364.

Cox A, Holbrook D, Rutter M. Psychiatric interviewing techniques: A second experimental study. *Br J Psychiatry* 1988; 152:64-72. Provides references to a series of seminal papers.

Greenspan SI, with Greenspan NT. *The Clinical Interview of the Child,* 2nd ed. Washington, DC: American Psychiatric Press, 1991. The authors' own developmental perspective, presented with a number of very detailed (though not verbatim) examples.

Hughes JN, Baker DB. *The Clinical Child Interview.* New York: Guilford Press, 1990. This detailed guide to the interview process focuses on school-age children and young adolescents.

Morrison J. *The First Interview: Revised for DSM-IV.* New York: Guilford Press, 1995. Discusses the interview process in adults.

Peterson C, Biggs M. Interviewing children about trauma. *J Trauma Stress* 1997; *10:*279–290.

Pinegar C. Screening for dissociative disorders in children and adolescents. *J Child Adolesc Psychiatr Nurs* 1995; *8:*5–14.

Saywitz K, Camparo L. Interviewing child witnesses: A developmental perspective. *Child Abuse Negl* 1998; *22:*825–843.

Trad PV. *Conversations with Preschool Children.* New York: Norton, 1990. Focuses on the developmental process.

Reviews

Finally, we recommend these articles on childhood and adolescent diagnoses, each of which is subtitled "A review of the past 10 years" and has appeared in the *Journal of the American Academy of Child and Adolescent Psychiatry.*

Beardslee WR, Versage EM, Gladstone TR. Children of affectively ill parents. 1998; *37:*1134–1141.

Beitchman JH, Young AR. Learning disorders with a special emphasis on reading disorders. 1997; *36:*1020–1032.

Bernstein GA, Borchardt CM, Perwien AR. Anxiety disorders in children and adolescents. 1996; *35:*1110–1119.

Birmaher B, Ryan ND, Williamson DE, Brent DA, Kaufman J. Childhood and adolescent depression. Part II. 1996; *35:*1575–1583.

Birmaher B, Ryan ND, Williamson DE, Brent DA, Kaufman J, Dahl RE, Perel J, Nelson B. Childhood and adolescent depression. Part I. 1996; *35:*1427–1439.

Bradley SJ, Zucker KJ. Gender identity disorder. 1997; *36:*872–880.

Cantwell DP. Attention deficit disorder. 1996; *35:*978–987.

Fritz GK, Fritsch S, Hagino O. Somatoform disorders in children and adolescents. 1997; *36:*1329–1338.

Geller B, Luby J. Child and adolescent bipolar disorder. 1997; *36:*1168–1176.

Halperin JM, McKay KE. Psychological testing for child and adolescent psychiatrists. 1998; *37:*575–584.

King BH, State MW, Shah B, Davanzo P, Dykens E. Mental retardation. Part I. 1997; *36:*1656–1663.

March JS, Leonard HL. Obsessive–compulsive disorder in children and adolescents. 1996; *35:*1265–1273.

Pfefferbaum B. Posttraumatic stress disorder in children. 1997; *36:*1503–1511.

State MW, King BH, Dykens E. Mental retardation. Part II. 1997; *36:*1664–1671.

Steiner H, Lock J. Anorexia nervosa and bulimia nervosa in children and adolescents. 1998; *37:*352–359.

Volkmar FR. Childhood and adolescent psychosis. 1996; *35:*843–851.

Weinberg NZ, Rahdert E, Colliver JD, Glantz MD. Adolescent substance abuse. 1998; *37:*252–261.

Zeanah CH, Boris NW, Larrieu JA. Infant development and developmental risk. 1997; *36:*165–178.

In this overview DSM-IV diagnoses, we have made use of the following typographical conventions. DSM-IV section names (the "chapter titles" of the manual, most of which correspond to our chapter titles in Part II of this book) are given in CAPITALS; names of diagnosis groups within sections are given in *italics*. Names of individual diagnoses for which we provide criteria sets in this book are given in **boldface;** names of other diagnoses are given in roman type. Diagnoses illustrated by case presentations are marked with an asterisk (*). (In a few cases, section or group names are also the names of individual diagnoses; in such cases, when we provide criteria sets for these, the names are given in **BOLD CAPITALS** or ***bold italics.***) For all items in boldface, the numbers of the tables where criteria sets are provided are also given. Relative frequency by gender is given when known.

This appendix also states the prevalence of disorders in various age groups ,according to the code given below. In some cases, it is not known when the diagnosis is most likely to be first encountered; in others, a bimodal distribution has been reported.

    0 = Diagnosis is inappropriate at this age
    + = Diagnosis can apply to age group
    ++ = Diagnosis is likely to be first encountered in this age group

Finally, two acronyms are used throughout:

    GMC = General Medical Condition
    NOS = Not Otherwise Specified

Section, Group, or Disorder	Code Number	Table Number	Male–Female Ratio	Infancy	Toddlerhood	Preschool Age	School Age	Early Adolescence	Late Adolescence	Adulthood
DISORDERS USUALLY FIRST DIAGNOSED IN INFANCY, CHILDHOOD, OR ADOLESCENCE										
Mental Retardation		11.1	M > F							
Mild Mental Retardation*	317	11.1		+	+ +	+	+	+	+	+
Moderate Mental Retardation	318.0	11.1		+	+ +	+	+	+	+	+
Severe Mental Retardation	318.1	11.1		+ +	+	+	+	+	+	+
Profound Mental Retardation	318.2	11.1		+ +	+	+	+	+	+	+
Mental Retardation, Severity Unspecified	319	11.1								
Learning Disorders										
Reading Disorder*	315.00	11.3	M = F	0	0	0	+ +	+	+	+
Mathematics Disorder	315.1	11.3		0	0	0	+ +	+	+	+
Disorder of Written Expression	315.2	11.3		0	0	0	+ +	+	+	+
Learning Disorder NOS	315.9									
Motor Skills Disorder										
Developmental Coordination Disorder*	315.4	11.4	M > F	0	0	+	+ +	+	+	+
Communication Disorders										
Expressive Language Disorder*	315.31	11.5	M > F	0	+	+ +	+	+	+	+
Mixed Receptive–Expressive Language Disorder	315.31	11.5	M > F	0	+	+ +	+	+	+	+
Phonological Disorder*	315.39	11.6	M > F	0	+	+ +	+	+	+	+
Stuttering	307.0	11.7	M > F	0	+	+ +	+	+	+	+
Communication Disorder NOS	307.9									
Pervasive Developmental Disorders										
Autistic Disorder*	299.00	11.9	M > F	+	+ +	+	+	+	+	+
Rett's Disorder*	299.80	11.10	F	+	+ +	+	+	+	+	+
Childhood Disintegrative Disorder*	299.10	11.11	M > F	0	+	+ +	+	+	+	+

Section, Group, or Disorder	Code Number	Table Number	Male–Female Ratio	Infancy	Toddlerhood	Preschool Age	School Age	Early Adolescence	Late Adolescence	Adulthood
Asperger's Disorder*	299.80	11.12	M > F	0	0	+	++	+	+	+
Pervasive Developmental Disorder NOS	299.80									
Attention-Deficit and Disruptive Behavior Disorders										
Attention-Deficit/Hyperactivity Disorder*	314.xx	11.13	M > F	0	+	+	++	+	+	+
Attention-Deficit/Hyperactivity Disorder NOS	314.9									
Conduct Disorder	312.8	11.14	M > F	0	0	+	++	+	+	+
Oppositional Defiant Disorder*	313.81	11.15	M > F	0	0	+	++	+	+	+
Disruptive Behavior Disorder NOS	312.9									
Feeding and Eating Disorders of Infancy or Early Childhood										
Pica*	307.52	11.16		+	+	++	+	+	+	+
Rumination Disorder	307.53	11.17	M > F	++	+	+	+	+	+	+
Feeding Disorder of Infancy or Early Childhood*	307.59	11.18		++	+	0	0	0	0	0
Tic Disorders										
Tourette's Disorder*	307.23	11.19	M > F	0	+	+	++	++	+	+
Chronic Motor or Vocal Tic Disorder*	307.22	11.19	M > F	0	+	+	++	++	+	+
Transient Tic Disorder*	307.21	11.19	M > F	0	+	+	++	++	+	+
Tic Disorder NOS	307.20									
Elimination Disorders										
Encopresis . . .	—.–	11.20	M > F	0	0	+	++	+	+	+
With Constipation and Overflow Incontinence	787.6									
Without Constipation and Overflow Incontinence*	307.7									
Enuresis*	307.6	11.20	M > F	0	0	+	++	+	+	+

Section, Group, or Disorder	Code Number	Table Number	Male–Female Ratio	Infancy	Toddlerhood	Preschool Age	School Age	Early Adolescence	Late Adolescence	Adulthood
Other Disorders of Infancy, Childhood, or Adolescence										
Separation Anxiety Disorder*	309.21	11.21	F > M	0	0	+	++	+	+	+
Selective Mutism*	313.23	11.21	F > M	0	+	+	++	+	+	+
Reactive Attachment Disorder of Infancy or Early Childhood*	313.89	11.23		++	++	+	+	+	+	+
Stereotypic Movement Disorder*	307.3	11.24		0	+	+	+	+	+	+
Disorder of Infancy, Childhood, or Adolescence NOS	313.9									
DELIRIUM, DEMENTIA, AND AMNESTIC AND OTHER COGNITIVE DISORDERS										
Delirium										
Delirium Due to [GMC]	293.0	12.1		+	++	++	+	+	+	+
[Substance] Intoxication Delirium*	—.–	12.1		0	0	0	+	+	+	++
[Substance] Withdrawal Delirium	—.–	12.1		0	0	0	+	+	+	++
Delirium NOS	780.09									
Dementia										
Dementia of the Alzheimer's Type	290.xx		F > M	0	0	0	0	0	0	++
Vascular Dementia	290.xx		M > F	0	0	+	+	+	+	++
Dementia Due to HIV Disease	294.9	12.2		0	0	+	+	+	+	++
Dementia Due to Head Trauma	294.1	12.2		0	0	+	+	+	+	++
Dementia Due to Parkinson's Disease	294.1	12.2		0	0	0	0	0	0	++
Dementia Due to Huntington's Disease	294.1	12.2		0	0	0	0	+	+	++
Dementia Due to Pick's Disease	290.10	12.2		0	0	0	0	0	0	++

Section, Group, or Disorder	Code Number	Table Number	Male–Female Ratio	Infancy	Toddlerhood	Preschool Age	School Age	Early Adolescence	Late Adolescence	Adulthood
Dementia Due to Creutzfeldt–Jakob Disease	290.10	12.2		0	0	+	+	+	+	++
Dementia Due to Other [GMC]	294.1	12.2		0	0	+	+	+	+	++
[Substance]-Induced Persisting Dementia	—.—			0	0	+	+	+	+	++
Dementia NOS	294.8									
Amnestic Disorders										
Amnestic Disorder Due to [GMC]	294.0			0	0	0	+	+	+	++
[Substance]-Induced Persisting Amnestic Disorder	—.—			0	0	0	+	+	+	++
Amnestic Disorder NOS	294.8									
Other Cognitive Disorders										
Cognitive Disorder NOS*	294.9			0	+	+	+	+	+	++
MENTAL DISORDERS DUE TO A GMC NOT ELSEWHERE CLASSIFIED										
Catatonic Disorder Due to [GMC]	293.89	13.1		0	0	0	+	+	+	++
Personality Change Due to [GMC]	310.1	13.1		0	0	0	+	+	+	++
Mental Disorder NOS Due to [GMC]	293.9									
SUBSTANCE-RELATED DISORDERS										
[Substance] Dependence*	—.—	14.1	M > F	0	0	0	+	+	+	++
[Substance] Abuse*	—.—	14.2		0	0	0	+	+	+	++
[Substance] Intoxication*	—.—	14.3	M > F	0	0	0	+	+	+	++
[Substance] Withdrawal*	—.—	14.4	M > F	0	0	0	+	+	+	++
SCHIZOPHRENIA AND OTHER PSYCHOTIC DISORDERS										
Schizophrenia	295.xx	15.1	M > F	0	0	0	+	+	++	++
Paranoid Type	295.30	15.2		0	0	0	+	+	+	++

Section, Group, or Disorder	Code Number	Table Number	Male–Female Ratio	Infancy	Toddlerhood	Preschool Age	School Age	Early Adolescence	Late Adolescence	Adulthood
Disorganized Type	295.10	15.2		0	0	0	+	+	++	+
Catatonic Type	295.20	15.2		0	0	0	+	+	+	++
Undifferentiated Type*	295.90	15.2		0	0	0	+	+	+	++
Residual Type	295.60	15.2		0	0	0	0	+	+	++
Schizophreniform Disorder*	295.40	15.4	M > F	0	0	0	+	+	+	++
Schizoaffective Disorder	295.70		F > M	0	0	0	+	+	+	++
Delusional Disorder	297.1		M = F	0	0	0	+	+	+	++
Brief Psychotic Disorder	298.8			0	0	0	+	+	+	++
Shared Psychotic Disorder	297.3		F > M	0	0	0	+	+	+	++
Psychotic Disorder Due to [GMC]	293.xx	13.1		0	0	+	+	+	+	++
[Substance]-Induced Psychotic Disorder	—.–	14.5		0	0	0	+	+	+	++
Psychotic Disorder NOS	298.9									
MOOD DISORDERS										
Depressive Disorders										
Major Depressive Disorder*	296.xx	16.2	F > M	0	0	+	+	+	+	++
Dysthymic Disorder*	300.4	16.5	F > M	0	0	+	+	+	+	++
Depressive Disorder NOS	311									
Bipolar Disorders										
Bipolar I Disorder*	296.xx	16.2	M = F	0	0	0	0	+	+	++
Bipolar II Disorder	296.89	16.2	F > M	0	0	0	0	+	+	++
Cyclothymic Disorder	301.13	16.5	M = F	0	0	0	0	+	+	++
Bipolar Disorder NOS	296.80									
Other Mood Disorders										
Mood Disorder Due to [GMC]	293.83	13.1		0	0	0	+	+	+	++
[Substance]-Induced Mood Disorder	—.–	14.5		0	0	0	+	+	+	++
Mood Disorder NOS	296.90									

Section, Group, or Disorder	Code Number	Table Number	Male–Female Ratio	Infancy	Toddlerhood	Preschool Age	School Age	Early Adolescence	Late Adolescence	Adulthood
ANXIETY DISORDERS										
Panic Disorder Without Agoraphobia	300.01	17.3	F > M	0	0	+	+	+	+ +	+ +
Panic Disorder With Agoraphobia*	300.21	17.3	F > M	0	0	+	+	+	+ +	+ +
Agoraphobia Without History of Panic Disorder	300.22	17.3	F > M							
Specific Phobia*	300.29	17.4	F > M	0		+ +	+	+	+	+ +
Social Phobia*	300.23	17.4		0	0	+	+	+	+ +	+
Obsessive–Compulsive Disorder*	300.23	17.6	M = F	0	0	+	+ +	+	+	+ +
Posttraumatic Stress Disorder*	309.81	17.7	F > M	0	+	+	+	+	+	+ +
Acute Stress Disorder	308.3	17.7		0	+	+	+	+	+	+ +
Generalized Anxiety Disorder*	300.02	17.5	F > M	0	0	+	+ +	+ +	+	+
Anxiety Disorder Due to [GMC]	293.89	13.1		0	0	+	+	+	+	+ +
[Substance]-Induced Anxiety Disorder	—.–	14.5		0	0	0	+	+	+	+ +
Anxiety Disorder NOS	300.00									
SOMATOFORM DISORDERS										
Somatization Disorder*	300.81	18.3	F > M	0	0	0	0	+	+	+ +
Undifferentiated Somatoform Disorder	300.81									
Conversion Disorder*	300.11	18.1	F > M	0	0	+	+	+	+	+ +
Pain Disorder*	307.xx	18.2	F > M	0	0	+	+	+	+	+ +
Hypochondriasis	300.7		M = F	0	0	0	+	+	+	+ +
Body Dysmorphic Disorder	300.7		M = F	0	0	0	+	+ +	+ +	+
Somatoform Disorder NOS*	300.81									
FACTITIOUS DISORDERS										
Factitious Disorder	300.xx	19.1	M > F	0	0	+	+	+	+	+ +
Factitious Disorder NOS*	300.19	19.2		0	0	+	+ +	+	+	+

Section, Group, or Disorder	Code Number	Table Number	Male-Female Ratio	Infancy	Toddlerhood	Preschool Age	School Age	Early Adolescence	Late Adolescence	Adulthood
DISSOCIATIVE DISORDERS										
Dissociative Amnesia*	300.12	20.1		0	0	0	+	+	+	+ +
Dissociative Fugue	300.13			0	0	0	0	+	+	+ +
Dissociative Identity Disorder	300.14		F > M	0	0	0	+	+	+	+ +
Depersonalization Disorder	300.6			0	0	0	+	+	+	+ +
Dissociative Disorder NOS	300.15									
SEXUAL AND GENDER IDENTITY DISORDERS										
Sexual Dysfunctions										
Hypoactive Sexual Desire Disorder	302.71			0	0	0	0	0	0	+ +
Sexual Aversion Disorder	302.79			0	0	0	0	0	0	+ +
Female Sexual Arousal Disorder	302.72			0	0	0	0	0	0	+ +
Male Erectile Disorder	302.72			0	0	0	0	0	0	+ +
Female Orgasmic Disorder	302.73			0	0	0	0	0	0	+ +
Male Orgasmic Disorder	302.74			0	0	0	0	0	0	+ +
Premature Ejaculation	302.75			0	0	0	0	0	+	+ +
Dyspareunia	302.76			0	0	0	0	0	+	+ +
Vaginismus	306.51			0	0	0	0	0	+	+ +
Sexual Dysfunction Due to [GMC]	—.–			0	0	0	0	0	+	+ +
Female Hypoactive Sexual Desire Disorder Due to [GMC]	625.8			0	0	0	0	0	+	+ +
Male Hypoactive Sexual Desire Disorder Due to [GMC]	608.89			0	0	0	0	0	+	+ +
Male Erectile Disorder Due to [GMC]	607.84			0	0	0	0	0	+	+ +
Female Dyspareunia Due to [GMC]	625.0			0	0	0	0	0	+	+ +
Male Dyspareunia Due to [GMC]	608.89			0	0	0	0	0	+	+ +
Other Female Sexual Dysfunction Due to [GMC]	625.8			0	0	0	0	0	+	+ +

Section, Group, or Disorder	Code Number	Table Number	Male–Female Ratio	Infancy	Toddlerhood	Preschool Age	School Age	Early Adolescence	Late Adolescence	Adulthood
Other Male Sexual Dysfunction Due to [GMC]	608.89			0	0	0	0	0	+	++
[Substance]-Induced Sexual Dysfunction	—.—			0	0	0	0	0	+	++
Sexual Dysfunction NOS	302.70									
Paraphilias			M > F							
Exhibitionism	302.4			0	0	0	0	0	+	++
Fetishism	302.81			0	0	0	0	0	+	++
Frotteurism	302.89			0	0	0	0	0	+	++
Pedophilia	302.2			0	0	0	0	0	+	++
Sexual Masochism	302.83			0	0	0	0	0	+	++
Sexual Sadism	302.84			0	0	0	0	0	+	++
Transvestic Fetishism	302.3			0	0	0	0	0	+	++
Voyeurism	302.82			0	0	0	0	0	+	++
Paraphilia NOS	302.9									
Gender Identity Disorders										
Gender Identity Disorder	302.xx	21.1								
In Children*	302.6	21.1	M > F	0	0	+	+	+	0	0
In Adolescents or Adults	302.85	21.1	M > F	0	0	0	0	+	+	++
Gender Identity Disorder NOS	302.6									
Sexual Disorder NOS	302.9									
EATING DISORDERS										
Anorexia Nervosa*	307.1	22.1	F > M	0	0	0	+	+	++	+
Bulimia Nervosa*	307.51	22.2	F > M	0	0	0	+	+	++	+
Eating Disorder NOS	307.50									
SLEEP DISORDERS										
Dyssomnias										
Primary Insomnia	307.42		F > M	0	0	0	+	+	+	++
Primary Hypersomnia	307.44		M > F	0	0	0	+	+	++	++

Section, Group, or Disorder	Code Number	Table Number	Male-Female Ratio	Infancy	Toddlerhood	Preschool Age	School Age	Early Adolescence	Late Adolescence	Adulthood
Narcolepsy	347		M = F	0	0	0	0	+	+	++
Breathing-Related Sleep Disorder*	780.59	23.5	M > F	0	+	+	++	+	+	++
Circadian Rhythm Sleep Disorder	307.45							+	++	++
Dyssomnia NOS	307.47									
Parasomnias										
Nightmare Disorder	307.47	23.2		0	+	+	+	+	+	+
Sleep Terror Disorder*	307.46	23.3	M > F	0	0	++	+	+	+	+
Sleepwalking Disorder*	307.46	23.4	M = F	0	0	+	++	+	+	+
Parasomnia NOS	307.47									
Sleep Disorders Related to Another Mental Disorder										
Insomnia Related to [Axis I or Axis II Disorder]	307.42			0	0	0	0	+	+	++
Hypersomnia Related to [Axis I or Axis II Disorder]	307.44			0	0	0	0	+	++	+
Other Sleep Disorders										
Sleep Disorder Due to [GMC]	780.xx	13.1		0	+	+	+	+	+	++
[Substance]-Induced Sleep Disorder	—.–	14.5		0	0	0	+	+	+	++
IMPULSE-CONTROL DISORDERS NOT ELSEWHERE CLASSIFIED										
Intermittent Explosive Disorder	312.34		M > F	0	0	0	0	0	+	++
Kleptomania	312.32		F > M	0	0	0	0	0	+	++
Pyromania	312.33		M > F	0	0	0	0	0	+	++
Pathological Gambling	312.31		M > F	0	0	0	0	+	++	++
Trichotillomania*	312.39	24.1	F > M	0	0	0	+	+	+	++
Impulse-Control Disorder NOS	312.30									
ADJUSTMENT DISORDER*	309.xx	25.1	M = F	0	0	+	+	+	+	++
PERSONALITY DISORDERS*		26.1								

Section, Group, or Disorder	Code Number	Table Number	Male–Female Ratio	Infancy	Toddlerhood	Preschool Age	School Age	Early Adolescence	Late Adolescence	Adulthood
Paranoid Personality Disorder	301.0		M > F	0	0	0	0	+	+	+ +
Schizoid Personality Disorder	301.20		M > F	0	0	0	0	+	+	+ +
Schizotypal Personality Disorder	301.22			0	0	0	0	+	+	+ +
Antisocial Personality Disorder	301.7		M > F	0	0	0	0	0	+	+ +
Borderline Personality Disorder	301.83		F > M	0	0	0	0	+	+	+ +
Histrionic Personality Disorder	301.50		F > M	0	0	0	0	+	+	+ +
Narcissistic Personality Disorder	301.81		M > F	0	0	0	0	+	+	+ +
Avoidant Personality Disorder	301.82		M = F	0	0	0	0	+	+	+ +
Dependent Personality Disorder	301.6		M = F	0	0	0	0	+	+	+ +
Obsessive–Compulsive Personality Disorder	301.4		M > F	0	0	0	0	+	+	+ +
Personality Disorder NOS	301.9									
OTHER CONDITIONS THAT MAY BE A FOCUS OF CLINICAL ATTENTION										
Psychological Factors Affecting Medical Condition										
[Mental Disorder] [Psychological Symptoms] [Personality Traits or Coping Style] [Maladaptive Health Behaviors] [Stress-Related Physiological Response] [Other or Unspecified Psychological Factors] Affecting [GMC]	316			0	0	0	+	+	+	+ +
Relational Problems										
Relational Problem Related to [Mental Disorder] or [GMC]	V61.9									
Parent–Child Relational Problem*	V61.20			0	+	+	+	+	+	+
Partner Relational Problem	V61.1			0	0	0	0	0	+	+ +
Sibling Relational Problem	V61.8			0	+	+ +	+	+	+	+
Relational Problem NOS	V62.81									
Problems Related to Abuse or Neglect										

Section, Group, or Disorder	Code Number	Table Number	Male–Female Ratio	Infancy	Toddlerhood	Preschool Age	School Age	Early Adolescence	Late Adolescence	Adulthood
Physical Abuse of Child	V61.21			+	+	+	+	+	+	0
Sexual Abuse of Child	V61.21			+	+	+	+	+	+	0
Neglect of Child	V61.21			+	+	+	+	+	+	0
Additional Conditions That May Be a Focus of Clinical Attention										
Noncompliance With Treatment	V15.81			0	0	0	+	+	+	+ +
Malingering	V65.2									
Adult Antisocial Behavior	V71.01			0	0	0	0	0	0	+ +
Child or Adolescent Antisocial Behavior	V71.02			0	0	0	+	+	+	0
Borderline Intellectual Functioning	V62.89			0	0	+	+	+	+	+
Age-Related Cognitive Decline	780.9			0	0	0	0	0	0	+
Bereavement	V62.82			0	+	+	+	+	+	+ +
Academic Problem	V62.3			0	0	0	+	+	+	+
Occupational Problem	V62.2			0	0	0	0	0	+	+ +
Identity Problem	313.82			0	0	0	+	+	+	+
Religious or Spiritual Problem	V62.89			0	0	0	+	+	+	+
Acculturation Problem	V62.4			0	0	+	+	+	+	+ +
Phase of Life Problem	V62.89			0	0	0	+	+	+	+
ADDITIONAL CODES										
Unspecified Mental Disorder (nonpsychotic)	300.9			+	+	+	+	+	+	+
No Diagnosis or Condition on Axis I	V71.09			+	+	+	+	+	+	+
Diagnosis or Condition Deferred on Axis I	799.9			+	+	+	+	+	+	
No Diagnosis on Axis II	V71.09			+	+	+	+	+	+	+
Diagnosis Deferred on Axis II	799.9			0	0	+	+	+	+	+

Index

Definitions are given on pages indicated by *italics*. Criteria are indicated by **boldface**.